EAT
SMARTER

ALSO BY SHAWN STEVENSON:

Sleep Smarter:
21 Essential Strategies to Sleep Your Way to a Better Body,
Better Health, and Bigger Success

EAT
SMARTER

USE THE POWER OF FOOD
TO REBOOT YOUR METABOLISM, UPGRADE
YOUR BRAIN, AND TRANSFORM YOUR LIFE

SHAWN STEVENSON

Little, Brown Spark
New York Boston London

Copyright © 2020 by Shawn Stevenson

Hachette Book Group supports the right to free expression and the value of copyright. The purpose of copyright is to encourage writers and artists to produce the creative works that enrich our culture.

The scanning, uploading, and distribution of this book without permission is a theft of the author's intellectual property. If you would like permission to use material from the book (other than for review purposes), please contact permissions@hbgusa.com. Thank you for your support of the author's rights.

Little, Brown Spark
Hachette Book Group
1290 Avenue of the Americas, New York, NY 10104
littlebrownspark.com

First Edition: June 2020

Little, Brown Spark is an imprint of Little, Brown and Company, a division of Hachette Book Group, Inc. The Little, Brown Spark name and logo are trademarks of Hachette Book Group, Inc.

The publisher is not responsible for websites (or their content) that are not owned by the publisher.

The Hachette Speakers Bureau provides a wide range of authors for speaking events. To find out more, go to hachettespeakersbureau.com or call (866) 376-6591.

ISBN 978-0-316-53791-9
Library of Congress Control Number: 2020944459

Printing 3, 2021

LSC-C

Printed in the United States of America

To my wife, Anne Stevenson. The impact of this book would not be possible without you. Thank you for your endless gift of inspiration. Life with you is food for my soul!

Contents

RECIPES

Author's Preface

If you look up the definition of picky eater in the dictionary, you'll probably see a picture of four-year-old me there holding a fish stick. I remember many days parked in front of the television watching *Cartoon Express* while dipping my fish sticks into copious amounts of ketchup. To me, food was just a delivery system to get as much ketchup into my body as possible. I loved that I always got to eat my favorite foods. And I had the perfect conditions to get away with it.

My earliest memories are from living (and eating) at my grandmother's house in St. Louis, Missouri. It was a magical, happy, peaceful place. Each day my grandmother would pack up my metal lunchbox (which I'm pretty sure is a class II deadly weapon now) embellished with my favorite cartoon character on the outside. The usual lunchbox trappings were a sandwich (white bread, meat, and cheese only, please), potato chips, a fruit roll-up, and a thermos full of that sweet, sweet nectar called fruit punch. I fondly remember taking my lunch to school and often saving half of it to stop and have a picnic with my little cousin, Candi, on our way home. There was a little area where we ducked behind some bushes to sit together, eat, and talk about life. Ya know, kid stuff.

At home with my grandparents, my daily meals generally consisted of some type of "meat," which was usually in nugget form, French fries (which were an important part of my vegetable group), sandwiches, potato chips, canned corn, canned green beans, and the occasional fresh broccoli florets that snuck their way in. Various cereals, orange juice, eggs, and/or sausage for breakfast. Mix in several meals from fast food restaurants and that was my weekly rotation. Nothing more. Nothing less.

Many people may have eaten fast food growing up, but I was *really* about that life. I even had my birthday party at McDonald's and, for me, it was a dream come true. I loved that place. The food (that always tasted the same), the toys in the Happy Meals, and the play area! The only thing that creeped me out a little was the cast of sketchy characters on the McDonald's team. The clown boss himself (think "IT" but with a worse makeup artist), Hamburglar (who was literally a criminal), Grimace (who was severely overweight and apparently in chronic pain, thus the name), and Officer Big Mac (who literally had a huge hamburger for a head). Even though they were weird, they were basically family. Our relationship had me hooked at a very young age and only grew stronger as the years rolled on.

Now, you might think, "How on earth would a good parent/caretaker let you eat that way?" And that's just the thing... my grandparents *were* good caretakers. In fact, I'd argue that they were the best. They taught me the importance of education, spent quality time with me, made holidays and special moments truly enchanting, and they always held me close and were proud of me, even though I was different.

I say that I was different because I was a little biracial kid living in a household with my two older, white grandparents. And this was during a time that it was definitely rare to see a situation like ours. But even though I probably stuck out like a caramel thumb with my curly afro when I was out with them, they never let me feel like I didn't belong. It was much later, outside of their care, that I learned I was different. But we'll get to that in a moment.

My grandmother, like many parents and grandparents, wanted me to feel like I was special. And one of the ways she did that was through food. In many ways, food *is* an expression of love. It's not just stuff we eat. Food can be an act of service, a gift, a means of quality time, a channel for words of affirmation, and, more than anything, food can touch our mind and body like few things can. If you've ever read the book *The 5 Love Languages,* this might sound familiar to you. As humans, we all communicate and receive love through five basic methods: Acts of Service, Giving/Receiving Gifts, Quality Time, Words of Affirmation, and Physical Touch. Food deliciously fits into all of those categories, and that's why food is one of the most powerful things in our universe.

Since my grandmother communicated her love to me through food and she wanted me to be happy, she always bought the foods she knew I'd like. Whether it was homemade, fresh from the microwave, or straight out of a paper bag from a fast food joint, good vibes were attached to those meals. Plus, like many parents and caretakers, she just wanted to make sure the kid ate, period! I was already a skinny child, so getting those calories in me by any means necessary was only the right thing to do. You don't want a kid wasting away on your watch!

Add on top of that the brilliant marketing by food manufacturers. Their messaging led parents to believe that these foods were the right choice for your growing kids. It's fortified with vitamins and minerals and gives your little ones everything they need. Plus, if you wanted some extra insurance, just have the kiddos pop a couple of Flintstones vitamins. And even though it was just glorified candy, at least it might prevent a few kids from getting scurvy.

Now, what's truly strange about this is that my grandmother and grandfather lived their lives differently from many of the people in our neighborhood. My grandmother tended her own vegetable garden (although I never touched any of her bounty), had a lush cellar where she kept jarred foods she prepared, and she even made ice cream from snow, one time. I know the wise saying is to never eat yellow snow, but that vanilla ice cream she made was pretty tasty. What I'm trying to say is that she took a healthier approach to things, as did my grandfather, who hunted and foraged for many years as well. But the pace of life and convenience of heavily processed food eventually got its grips into them too.

Moving Around

While I was sitting at my kiddie table nibbling on fried fish and watching cartoons, I know my grandfather was giving me occasional dirty looks from the kitchen. He was probably wondering why I got to eat what I wanted and my grandma was making him eat something different.

You see, since he had his first heart attack, the doctors recommended that he make some changes to his diet. One of the first things to be nixed was butter. Butter was now to be replaced with a vegetable oil spread. It must be healthier. It says *vegetable* in the name! Plus, the commercials say it's better for you. On the commercials there were two pairs of hands (no faces) and the voices of a man and a woman. The hands were flirting with each other as they spread partially hydrogenated vegetable oil onto bread. I'd never seen hands flirt before. I knew that when I grew up I definitely wanted a relationship with flirty hands too.

With more health problems, including a second heart attack and open heart surgery, the pace of living in a major city had become too much for the old country boy inside my grandfather, so they decided to move back near his hometown, hours away, of Piedmont, Missouri. And that meant after second grade was over, I'd be moving back in full-time with my mom and dad in a different part of St. Louis.

My parents wanted to give me better opportunity, so that's why I spent a few years living with my grandparents. At that time, it was really tough on my parents financially to get by, plus my little brother and sister had come along. Having me there was one extra mouth to feed, but we all made the adjustments and figured it out.

Third grade in a new school was a complete culture shock for me. In the blink of an eye I went from walking to school in a suburban neighborhood to busing to school within the inner city. I have to tell you, I loved riding the school bus. It was more time with friends and more time to goof around. But what I really loved about the new school was the food.

Instead of my grandmother packing me lunch, I now got to pick my own lunch with these magical red tickets. I was on the "free lunch program" designated for low-income households, but it felt like I was rich with that little ticket in my hands! I could pick pizza or chicken nuggets, juice or milk, an average apple or a jazzed up fruit cup, and no one was watching over me to see what I ate.

I adjusted to the new school pretty quickly overall, but one thing I refused to change was the way I ate at home. I remember my mom telling me that I wasn't going to leave the kitchen table until I ate those beans. "Well, guess what, Mom? I'm willing to sit here all night. Are you?"

I eventually just wore my parents down to pure exhaustion and they relented to let me continue eating what I wanted. But now the pickings were a whole lot slimmer. My parents worked long hours to pay the bills, and we also received food stamps to help bridge the gap. When the food stamps would come in it was like Christmas. We would stock up the house with some of my favorites like canned ravioli, ramen noodles, and off-brand cereal. Instead of Froot Loops, we'd have Fruit Rings, instead of Rice Krispies it was Crispy Rice, instead of Cheerios I ate Toasty O's. But it didn't matter one bit to me because I would add so much sugar that by the end it looked like wet, white sand had settled at the bottom of my bowl.

The only problem was there was usually too much month left at the end of the money. Food Stamp Christmas would come and go and we'd be forced to do the best we could afterwards. But this also led to some of my most special food moments in my childhood.

You know how you open the refrigerator and stare into it for a while, like something you actually want to eat will magically appear? Well, it was one of those days. But it was also one of the rare moments that my father was there to make food for us for lunch. He was actually a professional chef and a phenomenal cook. But he worked such long hours and was constantly cooking for other people so he understandably didn't cook that often at home. But, on this day, with nothing but some Texas Toast, some deer sausage that my grandfather made that was tucked away in the freezer, some government cheese, and a cheap jar of pasta sauce... this man made pizzas out of it!

Government cheese sure didn't melt like Kraft cheese slices. Yet, this day, it seemed to melt just right. It definitely didn't taste like a typical slice of pizza. But that wasn't the point. It was the *experience* we all had. Having a food we enjoyed, eating it together, and watching him make something out of nothing really stuck with me for many years to come.

How the Cookie Crumbles

My comfortable eating habits continued into high school and everything seemed to be going as planned. I was getting good grades, on the student advisory committee, a scholar athlete award recipient, and I was even hand-picked as one of the first students eligible to take crossover college credits while still attending my high school classes. Although I was easily handling things academically, my heart was definitely focused on running.

I came in as the fastest freshman athlete by a long shot. But by my sophomore year things started to go sideways. The best description that I have is that it seemed like my body was fighting against me. I started to slow down and I didn't feel like I had the freedom of movement I once had. It all came to a head at track practice one day while doing a 200-meter time trial.

I was at the starting blocks, my coach at the finish line with his stopwatch in hand. Bang! The gun goes off, and I sprint around the curve of the track. Heart racing, blood pumping, eyes focused on what's in front of me. I'm leaning in slightly to my left side as I come off the curve into the straightaway, and as I'm about to straighten out to finish the final 100 meters, I hear another BANG! But this time it was coming from the inside of my body. I had just broken my hip.

Up until that point, I had never really been injured before, so I had no idea what had just happened. It was painful, but it was way more confusing than anything else. My leg wouldn't move like I wanted to, I couldn't stop limping, and my coach told me that I needed to go in for an X-ray and ultrasound.

The physician I saw said it appeared I had pulled a muscle and part of the iliac crest from my hip broke off along with it. "Ah, no big deal! Take some anti-inflammatories, use these crutches, and come in for an occasional treatment and you'll be as good as new in no time." That's the attitude he seemed to have about it, and so I did too. But no one stopped to ask, how did a 15-year-old kid break his hip from simply running? And it wasn't until five years later that I found out the answer.

After about a half a dozen more injuries and my dreams of playing collegiate sports vanquished, I was finally diagnosed with a degenerative bone disease and degenerative disc disease at the age of 20.

I was having leg pain (again) and my doctor sent me in for an MRI of my spine. He put the scan up for me to see and he showed me that I had two herniated discs (L4 and L5–S1) and that was the reason I was having so much leg pain. The sciatic nerves that ran through that area near the discs and down into my leg were being compressed. I was pretty psyched to finally know what the problem was, and so I immediately asked him, "How do we fix this?"

He took a step back from the MRI scans and looked at me. He told me that the discs were herniated because of severe degeneration. He said that he'd actually never seen this happen in someone so young. And he also told me that this was incurable.

My first reaction is that this guy's head mirror must be on too tight. My second thought was, "Why does he even have a head mirror on in the first place? This is the year 2000 and this guy looks like he just stepped out of a *Bugs Bunny* cartoon. I mean, come on, Doc? This can't be that bad. I feel pretty good other than some leg pain, I can't have an incurable condition, can I?"

I asked him again, "Is there anything at all that I can do to fix this?" And, to this day, the next question I asked still baffles me. I had no grounds for asking this question. I had no grounds for understanding why this may have even mattered. But I asked him, "Does this have anything to do with what I am eating? Should I make some changes to my diet?"

To this, he cocked his head to the side and gave me a look of half irritation and half pity. Then he said these exact words: "This has nothing to do with what you're eating." He asserted, "This is something that just happens. And I'm sorry it happened to you. I know you're just 20, but you have the spine of an 80-year-old person. We're going to get you some medication to help you manage the pain. But, I'm sorry, son, this is just something you're going to have to live with."

I left there with my head down, feeling completely deflated. I was trying to process what had just happened and make some sense of it. Little did I know the biggest test was to come. And I was totally unprepared for it.

Starting from the Bottom

Over the course of the next two years, I went from having pain that was sort of a nuisance to chronic, debilitating pain. Even though I was on a slew of different medications, nothing seemed to help. And the sciatic pain was absolutely terrifying. Every time I'd stand up after sitting or lying down, it felt as if I was being electrocuted. A powerful, sharp pain would shoot down my leg so strongly that it would make me physically jerk back. It was painful and it was embarrassing. And since it only happened when I stood up, I subconsciously relented to stay sitting as much as possible.

Sitting or lying down for 95 percent of my days and eating what I affectionately call the T.U.F. Diet (Typical University Food) was definitely not a power combo for maintaining a sexy physique. We'll just say I got fluffy, *real* fluffy. I ended up gaining about 40 pounds in those two years. And even though I had always been the skinny kid in my family, my fat genes kicked in with a vengeance.

Overweight, in chronic pain, and really lost, I was hanging on with my university classes by a thread. I went from a full credit load to barely scraping by with one class. Mustering up the energy to get there, plus the embarrassment of being seen, was just too much mentally. So, most of my days were spent sitting on my couch in my tiny college apartment playing video games and watching TV. The pros: I became awesome at video games. The cons: My condition just became worse and worse.

I continued to seek out help from different doctors. Unfortunately, they all told me the same thing. This condition is incurable. I'm sorry it happened to you so young. Here's some medication to help you deal with the pain.

I felt so incredibly lost. My biggest struggle was sleeping at night because the pain would wake me up, so I was put on other medications for that, too. But it was really just pseudo-sleep because I never actually felt recovered. It was a battle to pull myself out of bed and I spent most of my days in a brain fog that I couldn't snap out of. I needed help and I needed it fast because I was falling apart. And that light at the end of the tunnel would come in the most unexpected way, which brings me all the way back to the beginning of my story.

The Call

During the entire duration of this battle with my health, my grandmother would call to check in on me from time to time. I'd usually just brush her off and tell her that everything was fine. But it was not fine. And in her heart, she knew it.

She hadn't given up on me, and her persistence led to an experience I'll never forget. I was sitting on the edge of my bed one night, pill bottle in my hand, ready to knock a few back to hopefully help me sleep. I stared at the bottle for a while, and my grandmother came rushing into my mind. Even though my well-meaning physicians had given up on me getting better, she never did. From an early age she made me feel like I was going to do something special with my life. Now, here I was ready to throw in the towel just because things had gotten too hard.

I realized that it wasn't just my hopes and dreams on the line, but it was the hopes and dreams of my grandmother and the rest of my family that I was sacrificing by not standing up for myself. Their hopes and dreams lived in me, too. And for the first time I realized that I had been giving my power away.

Even though my doctors had my best interests at heart, they did not walk in my shoes. And they did not have the final say about what was possible for me. What I had not done all of this time was get *educated*. I had no idea what was going on in my body, and I lived with my body all the time! It hit me like a ton of bricks how crazy that was. I had been passing the responsibility of my health off onto other people. Yes, they can be a valuable, supportive force, but the way I lived my life and how I took care of myself was up to me. And in that moment, everything changed.

I decided that I was going to learn everything I could about human health and wellness. In my university classes we learned a lot about disease, but there was very little discussion about what creates a vibrant, healthy human being. We had the typical items tossed at us in a very general way: Eat healthy food and exercise. But the details were dryer than wearing sandpaper nipple pasties in the Sahara Desert.

The legendary UCLA basketball coach John Wooden said, "It's the details that are vital. Little things make the big things happen." And I was dedicated to uncovering the details. I became obsessed with understanding the intricacies of the cellular communities that make us up. I asked important questions like: If my bones and spine are degenerating (losing cells) what are those cells actually made out of? What is all of this extra weight I'm carrying made out of? And what can I do to positively influence what all of these cells are doing?

What I didn't realize at the time was that questions really *are* the answer. On an anatomical level, there are specific regions of the human brain that are driven by questions. In fact, questions trigger a mental reflex known as *instinctive elaboration*. When your brain is posed a question, it instantly kicks into gear to find an answer to it (whether you realize it consciously or not). Your brain *wants* to find the answers to questions (which you can use to your advantage — and we'll talk more about this later!). But the basis of it is asking the *right* questions which will guide you to where you want to be.

I asked, "What are my bones and spine made of?" and that sent me searching down a familiar tunnel that I had only peeked into before. Looking in, you get a glimpse that your bones are made of the nutrients you take in, but only one is standing close to the doorway because it's being pushed there by marketing. If I were to ask you which nutrient do you need for strong bones, you'd probably say, "Calcium!" with great confidence like I did. But I found out that bone formation requires a constant supply of other key nutrients like magnesium, phosphorus, vitamin D, and potassium. Even omega-3 essential fatty acids have been found to contribute to bone mineral density, specifically in the hips!

I was hardly getting any of those things on my drive-thru window diet. My eating habits that were established as a kid were now taking a serious bite out of my bones. How on earth could my body regenerate those tissues if it doesn't have the raw materials to do so? Our bodies are resilient and will do a patchwork job, but without the right materials, your physical building will fall apart. And that's what was happening to me.

Not only that, emerging research has shown that the overconsumption of sugar is a huge contributing factor to bone degeneration. Ever since I was a child, my one consistent food relationship was with *sugar*. We were together through the good times and the bad, but it had stabbed me in the back like a cellular episode of *Game of Thrones*.

Even though the physician who gave me the initial diagnosis said that changing my diet didn't matter, what I was eating *did* matter. And it mattered more than anything I could've imagined.

Every single cell in our bodies is made out of the food that we eat, and, more astonishingly, what we eat largely controls every action that our cells take. There was an entirely new field of science that was soaring to the forefront called *epigenetics*. I first learned about it through a lecture from renowned cell biologist Dr. Bruce Lipton, and it just about knocked my socks right off my feet. The prefix *epi* means "above," and epigenetics is the study of our cellular function *above* genetic control. I was led to believe that I was simply the victim of some bad genetic cards, and that my health problems were something that "just happens." But, in reality, I had elicited the function of several epigenetic factors that were causing my DNA to "print out" lower quality copies of me.

We all have genes for things associated with health (like optimal blood cell function, the production of healthy myelin in our brains, and adequate bone mineral density), but we all also have genes correlated with what we refer to as disease (including abnormal brain cells, dysregulated blood sugar, and suppressed immune system function). What I learned from my conversations with Dr. Lipton was that our environment, our lifestyle factors, and even our diet are controlling how our genes are being expressed every moment. And, today, there are blossoming fields of nutrigenomics and nutrigenetics that are showing us how every bite of food we eat can impact the function of every cell in our bodies. The power isn't just in our hands, it's also at the end of our forks.

Results Speak Louder

After that moment of decision while sitting on the edge of my bed, my life has never been the same. Eating smarter and making some powerful changes to my lifestyle resulted in losing nearly 20 of those unwanted pounds within just a couple of months, I was sleeping better without medication, my energy levels skyrocketed, and—most important for me at the time—I was able to get out of pain.

Within the year I had some new testing done that revealed my bone density had normalized and my two herniated discs had retracted back into their proper position. Where there was once degeneration that caused my discs to look like two crispy slices of poorly cut bologna (weird, but true), the light from the scan now shined through them beautifully. It illuminated my heart and I left there with my head held high and a new mission in front of me.

The transformation I experienced led to a deep passion to help other people experience the same things that I had. I switched all of my studies in college to health and wellness and set off to work with thousands of people over the following decade. To respectfully paraphrase the words of Dr. Martin Luther King Jr., *I didn't see the whole staircase, but I took the first step.* And each successive step led to new things and greater impact. From clinical and corporate work, to writing bestselling books, to speaking on some of the biggest stages, to launching a #1 health podcast. The journey has been out of this world for me, but it all started out of my greatest challenges all of those years ago, sitting alone in the dark. Little did I know that those challenges were there to bring out the best in me. And thankfully I had someone there to remind me of that.

So, today, I want to remind *you* of that. No matter what you've been through, no matter how things might have gone in the past, today marks a new moment in your history. You are powerful beyond measure to affect change in your life, and the power of food is one of the greatest tools to help you do it. Here in these pages you will discover how food impacts your life in a myriad of ways that will change your life forever. You will learn how food affects your body composition, your relationships, your cognitive health, and more. But, most important, you'll learn how it all works in a way you never have before. This is a new way, a smarter way, to become the best version of yourself. The journey awaits, and all you have to do is take the first step.

Shawn Stevenson

EAT
SMARTER

First we eat, then we do everything else.

~*M.F.K. Fisher*

Food is complicated.

It's one of the most valuable, multifaceted things in our universe. It's a key controller of our state of health or disease. It's a social centerpiece that complements the most important moments of our lives. It's the building blocks that create our brain, enabling us to have thoughts, feelings, and emotions. It's the very stuff that makes up our bodies and what we see looking back at us in the mirror. Food isn't just food. It's the thing that makes us who we are.

But food is also ridiculously simple. You just put it in your mouth, chew, and your body handles the fine print. It's because of food's simple side that we sometimes miss how miraculous it is. Still, even if we don't know the details, food is able to work on us, to change us, and to literally shape our lives.

In fact, food has been the basis of every civilization throughout human history. We go, and stay, where the food is. We've grown with food and, in turn, food has grown us. Most experts will attest that it's been our ability to procure and eat certain foods that has enabled us to develop the most complex and powerful brain on our planet. We are thankful for those that have come before us, but shouldn't we also be more thankful for the food they chose to eat?

Over the centuries folks have tasted and tested countless foods to try and figure out what's best for us. And just to be clear, humans have tried to eat *everything*. From tree fruit to bat poop, from corn stalks to sidewalk chalk. You name it, people have tried to eat it. My little sister ate a marble and I even saw David Blaine eat glass one time. But outside of Mr. Blaine's magic digestive tract, the humans of today have leaned heavily on our ancestors to figure out what's good for us to eat. They found health-giving foods, medicines, poisons, and foods that warranted celebration and ceremony. They uncovered that food has a special language that communicates to us humans. And that language is called *flavor*.

One of the many things you'll discover in *Eat Smarter* is how flavor is actually an indicator of the nutrition found in various foods. You'll also learn how that communication has been hijacked and how to clear the line so that you and food can get on the same delicious page again. And, as you'll discover, delicious really is the name of the game.

The problem is that many of us develop the belief that delicious, tasty foods are, by their very nature, bad for you. I've had the thought before while eating, "This tastes too good…it can't be good for me!" Now, just to be clear, there are instances where that's possibly true. But, what if genuinely healthy food that can help you to be leaner, sharper, more energetic, and even defend your body from disease *did* actually taste that good? What if pleasure was one of the missing ingredients from a diet that really works all this time? That's what I've found to be true in nearly two decades of working in the field of health and wellness. It is pleasure that guides most of us to long-term success. However, we tend to be taught that you must suffer your way to the body and health you want. Yet, if you simply think about it logically, suffering does not equal health; suffering does not equal happiness. They are more like polar opposites. And anyone who tells you otherwise is probably just very hungry.

Another thing we're taught to believe is that food is just fuel. "Eat to live, don't live to eat!" Every time you hear someone say that, it would be in your best interest to politely excuse yourself and then run away. Food isn't just fuel. We're not cars! My name isn't Lightning McQueen. Food does provide fuel, but it's also meant to be enjoyed.

Have you ever wondered why food actually tastes good? Well, to make this simple, it tastes good so that you will eat it. True enough, processed food manufacturers have taken advantage of our innate drive to seek edible pleasure. But the wiring to eat tasty things has been there throughout our evolution. It's actually one of our greatest gifts, and in this book you'll learn how to revamp your palate, reset your cravings, and revolutionize your food experiences.

In truth, I'm a nutritionist who no longer believes in food in the conventional sense. Most of the time when people think about healthy food and diet, it's generally in the context of weight loss. People have been programmed to see food from just one angle. And this is a huge mistake. Yes, the right foods at the right time can help someone lose weight. But, to keep it off, and to be happy about it in the process, the meaning of food has to change. People need more reasons to eat healthy food. Their *why* has to be stronger. It's the only way any diet will be sustainable, and it's been overlooked long enough!

What we eat doesn't just affect our weight, it also affects our ability to focus, our ability to communicate with others, and even our ability to make more or less income. Our food choices influence our sleep quality, our body's ability to defend itself from disease, and the quality of our skin and outward appearance; and it can even control how long we're going to live. There isn't a single thing that influences more areas of our lives than our food does. It's time to put some respect on food's name. And learning to *Eat Smarter* is going to transform every area of your life in the most amazing way.

Eat Smarter is broken into three powerhouse sections. Each section will be exploring an area where food is affecting your life, plus the most effective, clinically proven strategies to help you get the most out of what you learn.

In Section One we're going to dive deep into the science of food and fat loss. Most programs take a very calorie-centric approach to try and help people lose fat. But they are utterly missing the point. *There are several game-changing factors that determine what your body actually does with the calories you eat.* This is why two people, at the same weight, can be on the same calorie-restricted diet, and one person can struggle to lose fat while the other person does it with ease. The person who doesn't lose fat isn't broken. It's just that they were never given the full story.

In my university classes I was taught a very shortsighted narrative about body fat. You eat an excess of calories and you gain fat, that's it. But that story is more one-sided than an elephant sitting on a seesaw across from a Chihuahua. Again, *several* factors control how your body handles the calories you consume. We'll be covering each of these factors in depth, but one of the most important is the health of the bacteria that make up your gut, aka your microbiome.

A recent study published in the journal *Cell* found that the presence of a specific type of gut bacteria in mice (A. muciniphila to be exact) actually *blocked* their intestines from absorbing as many calories from the food they ate. This was a groundbreaking and important study, but now human studies are revealing the same thing. Research conducted at the Weizmann Institute of Science has confirmed that there are specific gut bacteria that are more prevalent in folks who are overweight and/or insulin resistant. And lifestyle changes (like smart upgrades to your diet that you'll be learning about) can normalize gut bacteria that are associated with a healthy body weight. In fact, transplanting these human "fat bacteria" into mice caused the mice to gain weight, have increased blood sugar, and higher levels of body fat, while bacteria shared from normal human samples did not. The calorie picture is about to get a whole lot clearer for you with this new research.

In this part of the book we'll also uncover the major factors controlling your metabolism in a way you've never seen before. There are specific fat-burning and fat-storing hormones that simply aren't given enough attention in conventional weight loss programs. We're going to target each of them, in depth, and reveal how certain foods and nutrients affect their performance.

Plus, we'll also break down the three consistent (but overlooked) qualities that guarantee long-term fat loss, no matter what diet you choose. This section will help you to become an absolute master of fat loss, but the story is just going to skyrocket to another level from there. This is the heftiest part of the book because it's laying the groundwork for all of the other incredible things you're going to discover!

In Section Two you'll get to learn how our diets are connected to productivity, creativity, and even our memory. A big part of eating smarter is focused on maximizing brain power. Even though our brain only accounts for about 2 percent of our body's overall weight, it actually consumes 20 to 25 percent of our caloric intake! What we eat automatically affects our brain's performance.

For example, when you ask the question "What are my brain cells actually made of?" a very important (and misunderstood) nutrient comes up: omega-3 fatty acids. The omega-3s you consume from your diet are one of the very few nutrients that actually get to go directly into your brain. As far as your body's concerned, your brain is the most exclusive club in town. And the bouncer at the velvet rope is the equivalent of Dwayne (The Rock) Johnson, kicking uninvited nutrients' asses and taking names later. Omega-3s are welcomed past, and even hugged by the big fella on their way across the blood-brain barrier. This is because omega-3s are a major constituent of what actually holds all of your brain cells together. Without omega-3s, your brain cells can't communicate. And that's just about the worst thing ever.

It's well known that fatty fish are a great source of omega-3s, but can these fish (like mackerel, sardines, and salmon) really make you smarter? A recent study published in the journal *Neurology* found that adults who eat at least one seafood meal per week do, in fact, perform better on cognitive skills tests. Eating and feeling smarter definitely means incorporating some high quality sources of omega-3s. We'll go through exactly what those are, plus how to properly ensure you're achieving your omega-3 needs if you're vegan, vegetarian, or hate fish so much that you can't even watch *Aquaman* without dry-heaving.

This part of the book digs into captivating research on the brain-diet connection, including peer-reviewed evidence on which foods and nutrients can actually increase things like working memory and focus, boost our ability to problem solve, and literally create or kill your brain cells. If you like the idea of having a brain that actually works, then this section is going to blow your mind.

Also in this section, you're going to learn how the food you eat has a direct impact on the health and happiness of your relationships. Not only that, we'll explore the social nature of eating, and how eating with others can have profound benefits on our overall health—from stress relief, to improved digestion, to even making healthier food choices.

One of the biggest revelations you'll uncover is how our food decisions also affect our emotional stability. Being "hangry" (a combination of hungry and angry) is a phenomenon that scientists are taking seriously today (as funny as it may seem). With a drop in blood sugar, the human body naturally responds by releasing the stress hormones cortisol and epinephrine to raise it back up. But the kicker is that those hormones can also lead to strong irritability. The average person can go from grumpy, to grouchy, to full-on Shrek without batting an eye. And this makes us all the more likely to lash out at loved ones or even innocent bystanders, and certain foods (or lack thereof) are usually the culprit.

For instance, a study from the Ohio State University on married couples found that the lower the participants' blood sugar level, the angrier and more aggressive they felt toward their partners. The startling truth is that millions of people create unnecessary drama in their lives each day due to irrational, hangry responses at home, at work, and definitely in traffic. This subsection helps readers discover how eating smarter will help tame their inner beast, and bring them more patience, peace, and happiness throughout the day.

If you've read my previous book, *Sleep Smarter,* then you know that your sleep quality has a huge influence on your mental performance, emotional state, and even your body composition. And you're going to be blown away at just how much the food you eat affects your sleep! Unfortunately, it's not a stretch to say that sleep deprivation is an epidemic in our world today. This part of the book highlights how you can dramatically improve your sleep (and thus your health) by making some upgrades in your nutrition. Among the details is startling new data showing that good sleep is determined by good gut health. Researchers at the California Institute of Technology (Caltech) found that certain bacteria in the gut play an important role in the production of sleep-related hormones and neurotransmitters. Improving and protecting our gut health through smart diet and lifestyle choices can radically enhance our sleep quality. Plus, you need to make sure you're getting in plenty of good sleep nutrients each day. This section will show you how.

Eating smarter isn't just about *what* you eat, because *when* you eat can make a huge difference in the way you look, feel, and perform. In Section Three we will look at the latest science on meal-timing, stress-snacking, fasting, and more. We'll be separating the myths from the facts and covering the latest science on all of these topics.

Mountains of fascinating research are conveying how various forms of fasting can be good for our brains, good for our bodies, and good for our health overall. For instance, research published by the *International Association for the Study of Obesity* found that occasional, smart fasting is more effective for retaining muscle mass than daily calorie restriction. Muscle is our body's fat-burning machinery, and it's one of the things we lose a lot of with a conventional calorie-restricted diet. Without our valuable, lean muscle tissue, our metabolism takes a nosedive (which is one of the major reasons people regain the weight they lose!). Instead of haphazardly cutting calories, simply changing *when* you eat might be the breakthrough you've been looking for. In this segment of the book we'll home in on whether this is right for you.

This section will also introduce *the S.M.A.R.T. method,* a process for addressing stress-driven eating patterns and intuitive eating. According to the American Psychological Association, about one-third of adults report making unhealthy food choices due to the stress in their lives. After reading the previous sections you will have discovered that the foods we eat have a *huge* impact on our emotional well-being and mental health. But life is complex, and our emotions are alive and powerful! Food definitely has an influence on our emotional state, but our emotional state also has a tremendous influence on the foods we choose to eat. This section covers two of the most important aspects of eating smarter: healthfully managing our emotions and mindfulness. You will learn simple tools to help you identify emotional eating patterns, reframe emotional cues, and feel empowered in your food choices to continue eating smarter for life.

To close things out, you'll get access to the Eat Smarter 30-Day

Program. This section brings all of the most pertinent information together in an executable plan. The Eat Smarter Program is complete with daily schedules, delicious recipes from myself and celebrity chef contributors, and bonus tips to make the overall process fun and sustainable.

In just 30 days this body and brain makeover can yield some jaw-dropping results. And you'll be able to share your story, take advantage of expert support and accountability, and continue the process of eating smarter through our exclusive Eat Smarter Group at eatsmarter book.com/community. *Eat Smarter* is not just a book; it's a movement! The results extend far beyond the pages and into real life with a proven program, continuous support, and a community of people who are dedicated to creating the health, relationships, and success that they truly want.

Food is much more than the compilation of nutrients that other programs before this have made it out to be. Food is a complex entity that binds people together. It shapes our bodies, it shapes our communities, and it shapes our world. Every bite of food we take sets off a cascade of remarkable events that you're about to discover. So, let's focus in, have fun, and begin to *Eat Smarter!*

EATING FOR FAT LOSS

CHAPTER ONE

Make the Connections

I'm allergic to food. Every time I eat it breaks out into fat.

~*Jennifer Greene Duncan*

Food and fat have an interesting relationship. In fact, you could even say they're besties. Our body fat has evolved over countless millennia to take what we eat and store it away for safekeeping. And it's really, really good at it.

Your body fat's number one concern is *to keep you alive*. So, trying to get rid of it can be the equivalent of trying to jump out of an airplane. Whether you have on a parachute or not, your fat is going to be fighting you to stay where it is. Even though it might be OK to take the leap and let go, why take the risk if it doesn't have to?

To lose fat effectively, sometimes we have to channel our inner Tom Cruise and pull off some crazy stunts. But part of what makes Mr. Cruise so successful is that he studies what he's dealing with, he prepares, and he shows up ready to execute. Learning about your body fat will take you from mission impossible to sending your fat straight to oblivion. So, buckle up, put on your coolest action-star face, and get ready to become a master in the science of fat loss.

THE MISSING LINK

It's a travesty to have so many diets and fat loss programs without teaching people *how* their body actually burns fat for fuel. Telling people to just burn off more calories than you're taking in is as incomplete as having Netflix without the chill. The truth is, your metabolism is like a unique fingerprint that only you have. And your metabolic fingerprint consists of several key elements that determine how your body interacts with the food you eat. It's much bigger than simply managing calories, and you have the right to know this stuff. Granted, what you discover today is probably going to shock you, but once you understand these moving pieces, you'll be empowered to transform your body like never before.

The first thing to understand is that your body fat is an *organ,* much like your heart, your kidneys, your brain, and your pancreas. Your body fat is an organ whose primary goal is to keep you from taking an untimely dirt nap. Your fat really does care about you (which we'll get to more in a moment), but sometimes it can definitely be a bit clingy.

Even though fat is an organ, most folks tend to think of fat just like cells, or tissues, or scattered droplets of unhappiness throughout your body. But fat is actually remarkably complex. It stretches and communicates throughout your system, releasing its own hormones, giving and receiving information from all of your other cells and organs, and acting as a central bank to manage excess nutrition and to provide resources when needed.

Your life depends on your body fat in many different ways. In fact, it is your *fat* that literally holds all of your cells together! Fat is required to make and sustain all of the membranes of your cells. This is what enables your cells to have structure and the ability to communicate with other cells. Without fat, your cells would literally fall apart, and you'd end up like a large can of fat-free soup on the floor.

Your brain cells are especially dependent on fat. Just like the other cells in your body, your brain cells talk, and they talk with *speed.* Myelin is a fatty substance that wraps around the nerve fibers in your brain and enables them to send electrical communication to and from your brain cells at a lightning-fast pace. Myelin is just one of the fat-dependent structures in your brain, and it's about 80 percent fat! It's ironic that we think so badly about fat, because in reality, we literally can't think without it.

Fat enables the absorption and utilization of essential fat-soluble nutrients like vitamin D and vitamin A (which are both linked to longevity). Fat supports the function of our sex hormones, fat is required to protect us from climate changes and regulate our body temperature, and fat even plays a role in managing our immune system.

Hopefully you're beginning to see that fat is not the enemy. Whether it's storing energy on our waistline or helping us transmit messages in our brain, our fat has a job to do. And the crazy thing is, it's largely responding to the communication you give it. Yes, your fat can actually hear. But a lot of times we're just yelling gibberish at it like we're in an Adam Sandler movie. Fat can hear and fat can talk, but we also need to know which fat we're talking to.

DIFFERENT FLAVORS OF FAT

Another issue we have with understanding fat is that we tend to see it in one, very vanilla way. On a macro level, we have many different types of fat cell communities. We already touched briefly on a fat cell community in your brain called myelin, for example. But for our intents and purposes, we're going to focus on the fat cell communities that are directly linked to our body composition.

A key player in our cellular fat communities are the citizens themselves, the fat cells. Fat cells are called fat cells because of their uncanny ability to store, you guessed it, *fat*. In fact, fat cells can expand their volume more than one thousand times their normal size! Fat can push other cell contents off to the side and crowd in tighter than people trying to see Beyoncé at Coachella.

Our fat cells (also referred to as adipocytes or lipids) are mainly composed of tiny packets of stored triglycerides (each of which consists of three fatty-acid molecules attached to a single glycerol molecule). What's really crucial to understand is that our fat cells literally join together in different communities to work together and get certain functions done. When we're targeting fat loss, one of the cellular fat communities we're talking about is subcutaneous fat.

Subcutaneous fat is the team of body fat that sits right under your skin and is spread throughout your body. Fat on the back of the arms: subcutaneous fat. Fat on the chest: subcutaneous fat. Fat on the bootay: subcutaneous fat. This type of fat has several key functions including storing extra caloric energy, padding your muscles and bones from falls and hits, regulating your body temperature, and serving as a passageway for nerves and blood vessels between your skin and your muscles.

Our ability to store subcutaneous fat is an evolutionary advantage that has enabled humans to store energy that can later be used in times of food scarcity. One of the most important things to realize about eating smarter is that we are totally hardwired to store excess energy as fat. Even though we live in a time when food is abundant, your genes are operating from ancient programs that are hyper-focused on when that next famine is coming. Your body is always intent on saving up calories for a rainy day or zombie apocalypse. Your fat cells are your internal doomsday preppers and they are continuously getting ready for the worst that might come (no matter how weird you think they might be).

The big issue for our fat cells is that we are virtually surrounded by food year-round, yet they are waiting for a famine that never comes. We're going to break down exactly how to clear up the communication so that your fat cells know it's OK to let some of their stockpile go. But first, we've got to uncover where the other communities of fat are hanging out, because they'll have a vital role to play in all of this too.

Visceral fat is a fat community that we store deep inside of our torso, around our organs and under our abdominal muscles. Visceral fat (also referred to as omentum fat) is generally what we're talking about when we think of carrying extra weight around the belly. Yes, we have subcutaneous belly fat too (the stuff you can pinch), but visceral fat makes the belly region protrude out, it's difficult to get a grip on, and it can also be pretty firm to the touch. Visceral fat is the WWE wrestler of your internal organs. It's constantly putting your liver in a chokehold, your pancreas in a suplex, and your intestines in a figure-4 leg lock. The research is clear that visceral fat accumulation can be pretty dangerous. It's been found to contribute more to diabetes and insulin resistance than other types of fat, and recent research published in the *Journal of the American Heart Association* affirmed that carrying extra visceral fat substantially increases our risk of heart disease.

Generally, visceral fat is going to be one of the last places that your body shuttles the excess calories you take in. But there are certain factors that make visceral fat grab the wheel of your body and say, "I'm the fat captain now." We'll go through how fat feeds itself soon, but next up is the unsung lipid, intramuscular fat.

Intramuscular fat is very interesting because we tend to think that muscle and fat are dichotomous and, in many ways, not related. Yet, intramuscular fat is actually used as on-site energy by your muscles to utilize for things like basic movements and moderate exercise. It can act as your muscle's right-hand man, but even this seemingly helpful fat can get backup dancer syndrome and want to steal the show. Researchers at the Boston University School of Medicine affirmed that notable *increases* in intramuscular fat lead to measurable *decreases* in insulin sensitivity.

Want to know what intramuscular fat looks like? Think about the marbling of a steak and you'll know exactly how it appears. Intramuscular fat spreads throughout all of our major muscle groups. Too much can create the appearance of "chubby muscles," but when in balance it's a friendly fat that can support your health and body composition. Now, with that said, there's no fat more impressive and helpful than the one you're going to learn about next.

Brown fat is currently the subject of numerous studies because of the profound effects it has on your metabolism. We've already covered how different types of fat have different roles in your body. The three previous fat communities (subcutaneous, visceral, and intramuscular) are all fat communities that *store* energy (they're all in a class called white adipose tissue). Whereas brown fat (or brown adipose tissue) is a fat community that doesn't store fat . . . it actually burns it!

Brown fat—which is primarily found near the neck, collarbones, upper back region, and along the spine—appears to function in the exact opposite way as white adipose tissue. Brown fat burns energy for heat and it accomplishes this partly through a special protein called *thermogenin*. As infants, we have a much more substantial ratio of brown fat to help protect us from hypothermia. Yet, as we grow older that ratio diminishes quite a bit.

Brown fat achieves its distinguishing brown color thanks to its high concentration of mitochondria, which are metabolic power plants that create energy within your cells. Maintaining a healthy amount of brown fat can be a key ingredient in a robust metabolism. Research published by the Garvan Institute of Medical Research found that, once activated, 50 grams of brown fat could burn an additional 300 calories of energy in a day! Several factors influence how much brown fat we have and how well it does its job, and what you eat definitely has an interesting impact. We'll get to that soon, but first, here is a fat that appears to be sitting on the fence.

Beige fat is the answer to the question, "What if my white fat could get a tan?" Beige fat is fascinating in that it appears to have the flexibility to act like either white fat *or* brown fat. According to scientists at Georgia State University, beige fat has potent potential to fight obesity in much the same way as brown fat (by burning fuel rather than storing it). But beige fat is genetically distinct from brown fat. Brown fat cells are born from stem cell precursors that also produce muscle cells. Beige fat, on the other hand, forms within deposits of white fat cells from beige cell precursors.

It appears that certain lifestyle factors can influence the "browning" of cells within the white fat cell communities. And no matter how Jersey Shore this might sound, this is actually one of the cool ways that your body shifts your metabolic fingerprint beyond the cookie-cutter advice of simply managing calories.

HOW WHAT YOU EAT BECOMES THE FAT YOU SEE (THE BIG PICTURE VIEW)

Now that we know the basics on the various communities that fat can live in, let's talk about how fat cells are born and grow in the first place. And one of the very first things you need to know is that **the number of fat cells in your body will remain relatively constant through-**

out your lifetime. You can cut calories, you can exercise, you can try to fight your fat cells into submission. But that doesn't mean they're going anywhere. Genetically, you have a certain number of fat cells in your cards, and "gaining fat" primarily means packing more stuff into those fat cells. It's generally accepted in science that adult humans cannot directly eliminate fat cells or create new ones, but this is definitely not the end of the story.

Although the number of fat cells we have remains relatively constant, we have fat cells that die and fat cells that are born all of the time. They are not being made because you ate too much, or dying off because you dieted. They are simply replacing each other. According to a report from the Department of Cell and Molecular Biology at Karolinska Institute and published in the journal *Nature,* the average turnover for fat cells is about 8.4 percent a year, with half of the fat cells in your body being replaced every 8.3 years. It's a misconception that you can indiscriminately "kill" a fat cell. When fat cells decide to die off, they are simply being counterbalanced…except for one fat-grabbing catch-22.

The exception to this rule is that when we begin to venture into obesity our genes can start playing by different rules. The scientists at Karolinska Institute found that when people become significantly overweight they start to produce about *twice as many new fat cells annually* as lean people. But, again, they also found the counterbalancing act of fat cell deaths happens at twice the rate among obese people as well.

Now here's the kicker: Even if the obese subjects they studied lost a significant amount of weight, their total number of fat cells in the body remained constant, but the *size* of individual fat cells fell substantially. Researchers at Yale University postulated that this might be one of the reasons that fat is so hard to keep off when you lose it. Those hungry, hungry fat cells are still around and they've been accustomed to holding onto a lot of energy. Thankfully, in *Eat Smarter* you'll learn how to retrain those fat cells and even make some of your fat cells retire permanently.

So, to recap, when we talk about "burning fat" in the conventional sense, we are really talking about burning the fat cell contents, not the fat cell itself. But how are they getting filled up in the first place? That's what we'll address next.

HOW TO GET A FAT BANK ACCOUNT

When I spoke with biochemist Sylvia Tara, PhD, she encouraged people to think of our body's use of fuel like money. Just as currency is used for every exchange in our economy, energy is needed for every transaction in our bodies. When we eat some food it's like instant glucose cash on hand. It's in your bloodstream for easy access and you can use it very quickly if you like. Now, an excess of glucose cash is not safe or smart to have around in your bloodstream, so any extra gets deposited in your internal checking account in the form of glycogen in your muscles and liver. If you need it, you can still access it relatively quickly, you just have to take some time and write a check (like that older fella who got in line in front of you at the grocery store). Now that you've got cash on hand and your checking account is full, it's a good idea to store some energy away for safekeeping as a certificate of deposit. This is when your food currency gets stored as fat. It can hold a lot of energy in reserve, and it's there when you really need it, but it's not as easy to get to.

The process of withdrawing the energy from your fat to use as fuel is often referred to as *lipolysis*. While the process of storing energy as fat in your body is referred to as *lipogenesis* (with *lipo* meaning "fat" and *genesis* meaning "creation"). Remember, with excess energy coming in, you are generally not making new fat cells, you are filling up the fat cells you have with more moola that your body can get to if the situation ever calls for it. But this is the essential thing to understand: Your body's use of fuel works on a hierarchy. It will go for glucose first, then glycogen, and only then will it proactively go through the work of breaking down deposited fat to use it for fuel. We'll be covering how to access fat a little quicker (like a preferred savings account) and, even better, how to avoid storing it when you don't really need to. Next up, we'll break down where all of this energy currency comes from.

CAN I BORROW A CALORIE?

The calorie is the currency that we typically use to describe the value of energy in different foods. It's a socially accepted exchange tool we use, but where the heck did it actually come from?

Leonardo da Vinci never said, "Please pass me those low-calorie cookies while I wrap up Mona Lisa's smirk. I'm so hungry...I wish she could do this herself. I can't wait until they invent selfies!" Leonardo didn't talk about calories because they, like the selfie, were not invented yet.

When the calorie first hit the scene in the 1800s, people had gotten along pretty well without it. In fact, no one was even looking for an energy measurement for food. When the calorie was originally invented, it was used as a measurement tool in physics and engineering, and had nothing to do with nutritional science.

There's a little controversy over who actually invented the calorie. Some references show two Frenchmen, P.A. Favre and J.T. Silbermann, invented the calorie in 1852. Other sources credit a German physician, Julius Mayer, effectively inventing the calorie in a study he published in 1848. However, the earliest records of calorie-talk go back to a French chemist named Nicholas Clement, with lecture notes from Clement defining the term as early as 1819.

When the calorie made the pivot to the science of nutrition, it was in large part due to the work of American chemist Wilbur Atwater around 1887. From there, making its way into popular lexicon, physician Lulu Hunt Peters published an early nutrition bestseller, *Diet and Health, with the Key to the Calories,* in 1918. This book was a smash hit, selling over 2 million copies and triggering a huge change in society's beliefs about food. In it, Dr. Peters encouraged people to start thinking about food in terms of calories. She asserted, "Hereafter you are going to eat calories of food. Instead of saying one slice of bread, or a piece of pie, you will say 100 calories of bread, (or) 350 calories of pie." The shift to food as numbers had begun, and even back then there was no real distinction made between the quality of different foods. Under her system, a person of the same height as her could eat whatever she wanted, as long as she maintained a strict diet of 1,200 calories a day.

It's important to note that during this time, Dr. Peters also began the widespread indoctrination of associating morality with food. In her work, she equated not being able to maintain one's weight with a character defect that needed to be fixed. The words *punishment* and *sin* were now being used around food. This was also the time around World War I, so food rationing was a commonality of the day. It was insinuated that aggressively restricting calories was an act of patriotism. She stated, "That for every pang of hunger we feel we can have a double joy, that of knowing we are saving worse pangs in some little children, and that of knowing that for every pang we feel we lose a pound." Her diet could help you show love for your country, help feed hungry children, and improve yourself at the same time. That's a helluva Groupon deal if I've ever heard one. For better or for worse, Dr. Peters was truly a pioneer, and her own battles with weight problems were the inspiration for her work.

BURNING STUFF FOR ENERGY

So, now we have this commonly accepted unit for measuring the energy in food. But have you ever stopped to think how accurate it really is?

In scientific terms, a calorie is a unit of energy, just like a meter is a unit of distance. One calorie is the amount of energy you need to heat up 1 gram of water by 1 degree Celsius. To measure the amount of calories in food, manufacturers used something called a *bomb calorimeter*. This process involves placing the food source in a sealed container and placing it into another container filled with water. They would then burn the food with electrical energy until it completely incinerates, and afterward they'd measure the water temperature to see how many degrees it was raised (and thus how many calories were supplied to do it).

Now, even though you might be the bomb, you are definitely not a bomb calorimeter. And the way that food energy burns in your body is radically different from burning it up in a container to heat some water. One of the major issues with this method is that the bomb calorimeter measures *all* of the available calories in the product. But most typical foods also contain indigestible components (like fiber) that are generally not burned in the human digestive tract. This, in itself, can lead to inaccurate estimations of the calories in foods. And this is just one tiny factor of several more to come.

With the tedious nature of using a calorimeter, and growing requirements to have caloric nutrient labeling on foods (thanks to the 1990 Nutrition Labeling and Education Act), companies have largely switched to an easier method called the Atwater System to measure their calories. Food manufacturers were now able to simply do some math and come up with the calorie amounts to place on their labels. Noting that each gram of protein contains 4 calories, each gram of carbohydrate contains 4 calories, and each gram of fat contains 9 calories (apparently nothing else matters), the calories listed on your food labels are calculated something like this:

Say you have a bottled smoothie that contains 10 grams of protein, 25 grams of carbohydrates, and 7 grams of fat. Take the protein (10 x 4 calories = 40 calories), the carbs (25 x 4 calories = 100 calories), and the fat (7 x 9 calories = 63 calories), for a grand total of 203 calories going on your calorie label. The calorie label on your food is based on that and that alone, and putting our faith into these gross estimates has haunted so many dieters—until now.

CALORIES: MORE THAN MEETS THE EYE

When it comes to worshipping calories as the chosen leader of nutrition management, if you look hard enough, you'll find some gaps big enough to drive a truck through.

Right off the bat, most calorie counts are inaccurate because they're based on a system of averages that completely ignores the complexity of digestion. As mentioned earlier in this section, you have a metabolic fingerprint that is totally unique to you, and how foods interact with your body is not like anyone else's on the planet. It's pretty cool, but it can also be pretty confusing. So let's put some of these factors of caloric individuality on display so that you're more empowered in your relationship with calories from this day forward.

Basic Energy Exchange

It's an agreed-upon reality that when you eat food you are bringing in new calories. But what's overlooked is the fact that you actually *burn* a significant amount of calories trying to extract new calories from the food you just ate.

Digesting food costs energy. It costs your body calories to chew, to swallow, to produce stomach acid and digestive enzymes, to churn the food and move it through your digestive tract, to mobilize the cells in your small intestine to kick into gear and snatch up nutrients from the food, to move the nutrients to their required places throughout your body, and to ship out all of the metabolic wastes. These are all semi-obvious things that require caloric energy to be used, but the *type* of food you're eating, itself, will determine the net gain in calories you end up with, more than just about anything.

It's generally accepted that protein takes the most energy to digest, with approximately 20 to 30 percent of total calories in the protein going into digesting it. Approximately 5 to 10 percent of the calories in carbohydrates are used just to digest it, and the caloric energy used to digest fats is usually in the range of 0 to 3 percent. Again, it's vital to understand that it costs calories to absorb calories. This is called the *thermic effect of food*.

As a quick example, say you eat 100 calories of protein. Your body will require 20 to 30 of those calories (right off the bat) just to digest and absorb it. In actuality, you're only receiving 70 to 80 calories from the 100 calories you consumed. Proteins may require as much as ten to twenty times more energy to digest than fats because our enzymes must unravel the tightly wound strings of amino acids from which proteins are built. Yet food labels do not account for this expenditure.

Combinations of different foods, macronutrients, and fiber (which costs calories to process, too) will influence how much energy is required to digest the meal and what your net caloric profit actually is.

Digestive Strength and Efficiency

Digestive enzymes in the mouth, stomach, and intestines are required to break down complex food molecules into simpler structures (like amino acids and fatty acids) that travel through the bloodstream to all of our tissues. If your enzyme production is inefficient, whether you're making too many or too few, this will inherently influence how many nutrients and calories you're able to absorb from your food. For example, if you take two people, one who produces lactase (the enzyme needed to break down milk sugars) and one person who doesn't, and give them each a bowl of ice cream, one of them will be able to extract more energy from it, while the other one is probably already in the bathroom unsure if they had to fart or something more (#bettersafethansorry).

Just because you're not digesting more of the nutrients and calories in your food doesn't necessarily mean it's a good thing. Weak digestive firepower can disturb your health, as well as the noses of people around you. We want to encourage strong, robust digestion, and another factor in this is our stomach acid production. Your stomach acid is critical in breaking your food down into more digestible components. Plus, it also aids in the absorption of things like vitamin B12 and magnesium (both essential for supporting your metabolism). Though your stomach acid doesn't get respect in conventional calorie discussions, it's a big player nonetheless, just like the type of food you eat.

The Type of Food Itself

Some foods are simply more digestible than others. And some foods are more giving of their calories than others. Take a recent study published in the journal *Food & Nutrition Research* that set out to find the difference in calories absorbed from a meal of "whole foods" versus a meal of processed foods that each contain the same amount of calories. The researchers gave healthy test subjects sandwiches of either multi-grain bread and cheddar cheese (deemed whole food) or white bread and processed cheese product (considered processed food). The results they saw were shocking.

At the end of the study, they found that eating the processed food sandwich led to a 50 percent reduction in calorie burn after the meal compared to eating the whole food sandwich! The meals were practically the same in terms of proteins, carbs, fats, and calories, but the fact that the food was heavily processed or not led to a huge difference in the number of calories that were stored or burned.

Another thing to consider in this domain is that some foods are actually fighting *not* to be digested. Let's use the plight of some blueberries, for example. Every living thing on the planet is driven, primarily, to extend the life of their species. It's literally in the genes of every life form. That's a human's primary driving force, a zebra's primary driving force, and even a blueberry's primary driving force. And how blueberries sprinkle their seeds around for future generations is by animals (like you) eating them and the seeds playing a little game of ride-the-roller-coaster inside your body to try and make it out the other end intact (and hopefully land in some soil). Biologist Rob Dunn states that it's "a kind of tug-of-war with the food we eat." Sometimes calories from the foods you consume are simply not digested. And, yet again, this doesn't show up in the calorie equation.

Another food that tends to not abide by conventional calorie metrics are nuts, which is highlighted in a peer-reviewed study titled, in short, "Discrepancy Between the Atwater Factor Predicted." This study, conducted by Janet A. Novotny and her colleagues at the U.S. Department of Agriculture, found that when the average person eats almonds, they receive just 129 calories per serving rather than the 170 calories reported on the label.

Calories may seem like a hard nut to crack, but every piece of data that you learn, you'll be able to use in your favor.

How the Food Is Prepared

Now, understanding that certain foods are already more digestible than others, the way that the foods are prepared can also make a substantial difference in how many calories can be absorbed from them. In the introduction to this book, I noted how most experts will assert that it's been our ability to procure and eat certain foods that has enabled us to develop the most complex and powerful brain on our planet. And, by far, it's been our ability to cook those foods that has given us the caloric might to evolve into the people we are today.

Even within a single plant category, the durability of the cell walls can differ depending on how old the plant is, where it is grown, and whether or not you cook it. Let's take spinach for instance. Older spinach leaves tend to have sturdier cell walls than younger leaves and, generally speaking, the weaker the cell walls in the plants we eat, the more calories we can actually extract from them.

Now, if you cook the spinach, the cell walls (that lock away the calories) are easily broken into. The cooked spinach will inherently deliver your body far more calories than uncooked spinach, gram-for-gram. Plus, in the real world, whenever you cook spinach, it seems like an entire jumbo box magically turns into one tiny baby spoonful on your plate. Obviously, cooking can be an easy way to increase the sheer volume you eat.

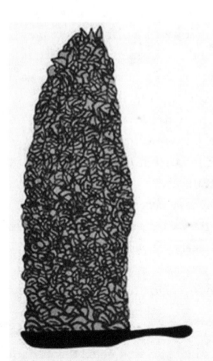

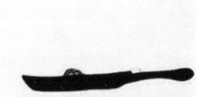

Spinach you start with   Spinach you end with

Researchers at the Department of Human Evolutionary Biology at Harvard University affirmed that the process of cooking starch-rich foods, and even meat, substantially increases the caloric density gained from the foods. So, now you know, whether it's baking, boiling, microwaving, flame grilling, or even flambéing, when you cook your food it brings about a change to its structure, chemistry, and caloric availability. This is not a bad thing at all in most regards (compliments to that big, beautiful brain of yours getting the benefits). But it's just another aspect of calorie conflict that's left out of the equation. And we have one more major area to look at.

The Makeup of Your Microbiome

In the introduction to *Eat Smarter,* I noted a fascinating study published in the journal *Cell* revealing that the presence of a specific type of gut bacteria in mice that actually *blocked* their intestines from absorbing as many calories from the food they ate. Coupling that with recent human studies, data from the Weizmann Institute of Science has confirmed that there are specific gut bacteria that are more prevalent in people who are overweight. And the big kicker is that by transplanting these human "fat bacteria" into mice caused the mice to gain weight, have increased blood sugar, and higher levels of body fat!

Your microbiome is really the final frontier when it comes to understanding your metabolism. The latest information is already eyebrow raising, but there will be a lot more coming down the pike in upcoming years that you will be well ahead of.

A recent study published in the *International Journal of Obesity* revealed that a higher diversity of gut bacteria is directly correlated with less weight gain and improved energy metabolism *independent of calorie intake and other factors.* This is yet another example of how two people can consume the same amount of calories, but one person gains fat, while the other person does not.

Your microbiome diversity plays a major role in how many calories you're extracting from your food. And it's also well noted that certain bacteria are much more apt to absorb more from the carbohydrate/ sugar calories in your food than other macronutrients. It's estimated that every human has one to two pounds of microbes living in their belly. No need to be freaked out—we truly wouldn't be able to survive without them. It's a symbiotic relationship when things are in balance, but when things get out of balance is when all bets are off.

Another study published in *BMC Microbiology* found that individuals who are obese have a significantly higher level of the bacteria *firmicutes* and a lower level of *bacteroidetes* compared to normal-weight and lean adults. It's proposed that a higher ratio of firmicutes to bacteroidetes in their intestines make them more efficient at absorbing calories from food—so instead of being lost as waste, more nutrients make their way into their circulation and eventually get stored as fat. The researchers saw a direct correlation that as body weight goes up, the ratio of *firmicutes* goes up along with it. Once we complete this smarter metabolic picture we've been mapping out, you're going to learn how to optimize your microbiome to optimize your body composition.

Other Tidbits and Ending Calorie Confusion

Hopefully, you now understand that focusing on calories to lose fat is more overrated than the entire *Transformers* movie franchise all rolled into one (no disrespect to Mark Wahlberg or Shia LaBeouf). In addition to what we've already covered, your caloric utilization is also influenced by the response of your immune system to different foods (which requires energy to do its job), how much muscle mass you have (because muscle kicks up your calorie burn), and even the length of your digestive tract itself—all are factors that are not accounted for in our conventional calorie assessment.

The bottom line is that digestion is so complex and fluid that we'll likely never be able to perfectly pinpoint how many calories we'll absorb from a particular food we eat versus someone else. Again, don't get the idea that calories don't have significance: It's a system we have that can give us some guidance, but it's far from being the only thing that matters.

What truly matters are a series of metabolic switches that literally determine:

1. What your body does with the calories you consume
2. Whether or not your body is provoked to unlock stored body fat
3. Whether or not you're storing more fat in the first place

It's time to dig into what's really controlling the show when it comes to fat loss. And *this* is where the magic really happens.

CHAPTER TWO

Your Metabolic Switches

I won't be impressed with technology until I can download food.

~*Unknown*

Much like a computer, we have a set of internal programs that are controlling everything about our biology, including our fat. And there are specific pieces of code we write every day (whether we realize it or not) that dictate exactly what our fat cells are doing on a minute-by-minute basis. Now, what if I told you that you could rewrite your body's fat-storing programs? What if I told you that, just like the 1's and 0's of binary code, you could switch your fat-storing programs on and off? Well, this is exactly what you're about to learn how to do…and you don't need to be jacked into *The Matrix* to get there.

You're about to discover the metabolic switches that are controlling the destiny of your fat. For far too long people have been told blanket statements about losing fat without knowing the truth about how fat-burning actually works. You are Neo in this story, and it's time to free your mind (and some body fat too!).

JUST DOING THEIR JOBS

The first thing you need to know is that fat is not leaving your cells without the help of a couple of key motivators called *enzymes*. Enzymes are biochemical catalysts that are required for nearly *all* metabolic processes in the cells that sustain your life. And there are a few key enzymes that you need to know about in regard to chasing out fat.

Fat is able to exit your cells primarily through the actions of three enzymes called *hormone sensitive lipase* (HSL), *monoglyceride lipase* (MGL), and *adipose triglyceride lipase* (ATGL). Each of these enzymes are like little ushers that help move fat out of your cellular theater after the show is over. Again, without them, the fat would just stay seated in the cell taking up space.

Now, the head usher responsible for the mobilization of free fatty acids from adipose tissue (i.e., lipolysis) is considered to be HSL. It's more easily acted upon by hormones we can influence (thus the name hormone-sensitive), so, for our enzymatic fat loss communication, that's where we're going to put our focus.

HSL is an intracellular lipase that has broad substrate specificity (meaning it can break down all kinds of fat). If you watched the cartoon *Scooby-Doo* when you were younger, you probably remember a time or twenty that someone in the crew had a "skeleton key" that was able to unlock any random door they wanted to get into. While other enzymes are like specialized keys that can break down one type of fat, HSL is like a skeleton key that can open the door to break down many types of fat. Side note: I've been waiting for years to get the recipe for those Scooby Snacks. They looked absolutely delicious.

Moving onward, if we have excess fat we want to lose, we want HSL and its buddies clocked in, on the job, and ready to put forth their best efforts. Now, even though HSL is the head usher in charge of getting fat out of its seat, there's another head usher in charge of getting fat *into* its seat. And if you check its name tag it reads first name: *lipoprotein* last name: *lipase*.

Lipoprotein lipase (LPL) is a key factor in partitioning triglycerides among different tissues in your body. Whether it's putting fat in the front row (subcutaneous fat), in the balcony (intramuscular fat), or in the nosebleed section (visceral fat), LPL is on the job storing fat where it needs to be seated.

So, we have two head ushers that are in charge of getting fat in and out of the cell, but there are some bosses who write their checks that are the managers of their departments. And those bosses are the twin brothers *insulin* and *glucagon* (who both come from their loving mother, *Ms. Pancreas*). Even though they are brothers, they have two very different personalities. Insulin is the more careful and calculating of the two. Insulin is always urging them to "keep saving up" because you never really know when you're going to need it. He always wants to keep the attendees (glucose/potential fat) out of the aisles (the bloodstream). And insulin always wants to keep the theater filled.

Glucagon, on the other hand, is more of a free spirit, and believes in minimalism. Glucagon knows that there is more than enough to go around, and there's no need to hoard and be petty. Glucagon wants people in the theater, but he also wants people to be able to leave if they want and use some energy for an after-party.

Insulin and glucagon both take a proactive job to man the doors of the cellular theater to allow fat in or out. Insulin opens the front doors to the theater to allow fat in. Glucagon opens the exit doors to allow fat out. They hold the keys. And nobody is going anywhere without them. And though insulin is always on duty at the doors, glucagon likes to hang out with the cashier a little bit more (which we'll get to in a moment), so glucagon passes the keys off to his assertive close friend, *adrenaline*.

Adrenaline (also called *epinephrine* by his professors at school) loves to get the fat cell theater cleared out so that everyone can go and kick it after the work is complete. HSL and the other ushers are really motivated to get fat out once adrenaline is around. But, the other huge trigger that sets HSL into action is simply when insulin sits his butt down for a break and stops allowing more fat in.

As we discussed earlier in the book, in order to get to the stored fat cells and start breaking them down for energy, generally we first need to burn through our glucose (cash), then our glycogen (checking account), then we'll be able to begin burning fat (certificates of deposit). Glucagon is a minimalist with an abundance mindset, but he's also responsible for paying the bills. So, after the glucose cash is spent paying for quick supplies, glucagon heads over to the huge cashier located outside of the building called the *liver*.

The liver is the ultimate cashier. Excess cash gets deposited in your checking account here in the form of liver glycogen. And if your checking account builds up and goes over the maximum amount allowed, your liver will automatically begin creating certificates of deposit in the form of fat (lipogenesis) to deal with the excess funds.

Once glucagon arrives at the liver, he begins writing checks for bigger bills and the stored glycogen is converted to glucose, which is then put into the mail (your entire system) to be used as payment at various places. Once the glucose and glycogen is spent, he can command the breakdown of some fat certificates of deposit to pay some bills as well. When we're talking about payment, we're talking about paying for *all* the things your body's thriving business does, supplying energy to your brain, building bones and muscles, keeping your heart beating, and literally everything else you can conceive of to keep you alive and functioning, energy currency is being spent to keep the lights on.

There is one additional form of currency exchange that has to take place to pay the bills. And when we're talking about *burning fat,* this is actually what we're talking about (and this is important!). Lipolysis is the process of freeing fat from the cellular theater, but it's actually burned for energy by your *mitochondria* at the cellular snack bar.

It's well-noted that your mitochondria are the energy powerhouses of your cells. The universal currency of your body is called *adenosine triphosphate* (ATP), and your mitochondria take your fat and "burn it" to convert it into usable ATP (a process called beta oxidation) and burn glucose to make ATP as well (a process called cellular respiration). You can have hundreds or even thousands of these tiny powerhouses throughout most of the cells of your body. And supporting the function of these metabolic Biggie Smalls is a huge key in supporting your cellular theater.

Now, the owner of the entire theater usually goes unseen, but she's always pulling some major strings behind the scenes. The owner of your metabolic theater franchise is the *thyroid gland.* She's incredibly powerful and produces hormones that control your total metabolic rate (the rate at which you burn energy). The thyroid gland is also closely connected to the brain and the gut, and she's a total empath. So a lot of what's going on with the brain and gut influences what's going on with her.

Which brings us to your brain, which is like *The Godfather* watching over the whole neighborhood. He's a mighty regulating force that works to keep eyes on everything (and to make sure everyone important doesn't end up swimming with the fishes). In your metabolic business, your gut is like the second in command. He's always monitoring everybody coming in and out of the neighborhood, making executive decisions, and sending information back and forth with the Godfather to help keep the community in good working order.

If any of these key figures are struggling to do their job, it can throw off the entire system. Hopefully you can see that simply trying to manage calorie currency will never work if any of these players gets lazy on the job, calls in sick, or (heaven forbid) gets whacked. There are many other moving parts to your metabolic community, but this foundation will help you to master your metabolism moving forward.

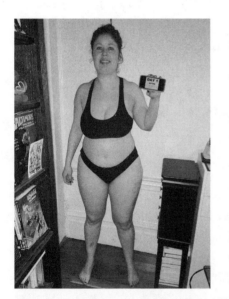 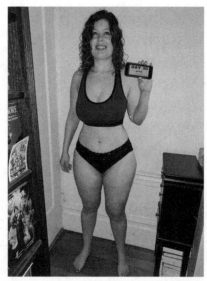

The past month has been a truly incredible, transformative experience for me, and I am so grateful. By the time this new year came along, I was in the worst shape of my adult life—and beyond ready for a change. I said, NO MORE OF THIS!!! I started Shawn's program and then something magical happened—I started feeling soooo good. I wasn't hungry anymore. I started craving nutritious foods. I ate slowly and mindfully and enjoyed each delicious, nourishing morsel. I had so much more energy, and my mood improved immensely.

My whole experience over the past month has felt like coming back to myself. It literally feels like I've become a different person. Taking the "After" photo and making the comparison felt great because I really can see a big visual difference, which matches how I feel. As I write these words, I am filled with so much gratitude for Shawn. This has been a strong start—but I am so excited to take it to the next level, and see what the coming months bring!

Each member of the community leans on each other for success, so now we're ready to jump in on what can lift them up to their very best and what can put a hit out on them.

THE THREE AMIGOS OF BODY FAT GROWTH

There are three major things that can get your metabolic switches jammed and sabotage the jobs of *everyone* in your metabolic community. Any one of these things can make insulin work overtime letting fat in, while another thing might set a fire in your liver cashier's office and start screwing up money management all over the place. So, let's jump in on these *Three Amigos of Body Fat Growth* to see what can cause these problems and how food can fix it.

The first thing to know is that these Three Amigos are just actors trying to play a role and keep the crowds happy. They're not really trying to cause any issues, but when they ride into town and go too far out of their depth, they can really mess some things up. The good news is that you can help turn their acts around and make sure your metabolic movie ends up with a happy ending.

One: Inflammation

Inflammation is a big catchword today, and it can sound like a bit of a sasquatch. It's blamed for a lot of stuff, but hardly anyone ever sees it. And we might even wonder if it's even real. But, unlike a grainy photo of Bigfoot, the latest science has authenticated inflammation in a major way. And understanding the roles of inflammation is absolutely critical to freeing your body of unwanted fat.

This might sound surprising since it's usually framed as the villain, but inflammation is actually essential for your health. Inflammation is a vital part of your immune system's response to injury and infection. It's your body's way of putting out a distress call to your immune system to heal and repair damaged tissue, as well as defend itself against foreign invaders (such as viruses and bacteria). Without inflammation, damaged cells and tissues would never heal, and even small infections could become deadly.

I want to show some serious love to inflammation because it generally gets a bad rap. It does some amazing things for us, but—and it's a big but!—if the inflammatory process goes on for too long or if the inflammatory response occurs in places where it's not needed, it can become dangerously problematic. Chronic inflammation has been linked to conditions such as heart disease, cancer, arthritis, cirrhosis, autoimmune disorders, and, yes, obesity. So, let's dissect how inflammation can gum-up our ability to lose body fat.

Microbiome Mayhem

When it comes to inflammation, your microbiome/gut is truly on the frontlines. Research published in *The Journal of Translational Immunology* affirms that over 70 percent of your entire immune system is located in your gut. And this just makes complete sense. Your gut is a primary point of contact for your body and the external environment. You are literally taking stuff from "out there" and putting it "in you," and your body takes this very seriously because one bite might bring you better health, while another bite might be your very last. Each meal has the potential to overload your gut with sometimes dangerous bacteria, protozoa, fungi, viruses, or toxic substances, so your immune system better be standing at the front gates and ready to handle it.

Since your immune system is predicated on your body's inflammatory response, what you eat can inherently trigger inflammation, and too much inflammation can damage your gut and the entire balance of your microbiome. Inflammation is derived from a Latin word meaning "to set on fire," and eating the wrong things can be like Daenerys Targaryen flying in on her dragon and setting fire to your whole microbiome city. (If you're a *Game of Thrones* fan, I'm sorry if that's still a sore spot!)

We've already covered how your microbiome can literally determine if and how calories are absorbed by your body in Chapter One. Inflammation inherently causes dysfunction in this process, but there's even more to that story. Inflammation in the gut can also lead to abnormal function involving your vagus nerve. Your vagus nerve is a primary pathway in the gut-brain connection. Researchers at the Yale

School of Medicine have found that your vagus nerve communicates information between your gut and your brain about the volume and type of nutrients you have available. And depending on your nutritional status, the function of your vagus nerve can inhibit or stimulate food absorption and intake. Remember, your gut is your brain's second in command, and they're constantly feeding information back and forth. Inflammation can severely mess this whole process up.

Another way inflammation can damage your microbiome and overall metabolism is through overly increased intestinal permeability. Recent data published in the peer-reviewed journal *Cellular and Molecular Life Sciences* reported that the tight junctions of your gut lining act as a selectively permeable barrier that allows in specific nutrients while also limiting the absorption of pathogens, toxins, and larger food molecules. The study goes on to say that disruption to this protective barrier from immune system dysfunction and inflammation can act as a trigger for the development of intestinal *and* systemic diseases.

What's especially important to understand here is that inflammation in the gut can lead to *systemic* diseases (meaning diseases and abnormalities throughout the body). Some of the primary places of concern that this increased intestinal permeability can impact are your thyroid gland, your brain, and your liver (which we'll come back to in a moment). But what's also important to understand is that this inflammation and abnormal permeability doesn't just happen out of nowhere. Research published in the journal *Frontiers in Immunology* cites how diet-induced hyperactive gut permeability is of significant concern right now. Foods commonly eaten today can cause it, and eating the right foods can fix it.

For example, our microbiome influences our health in many ways, but one of the most important is through producing short chain fatty acids (SCFAs—pronounced *ska-fus*). In my conversation with Dr. William Li, Harvard-trained MD and pioneer of over thirty-two FDA-approved treatments for chronic ailments, he shared with me that SCFAs are made by friendly bacteria in our microbiome when we feed them the right stuff.

Eating *prebiotic* plant fibers from foods like asparagus, apples, leeks, and onions have been found to produce substantial gut protection and anti-inflammatory properties. One SCFA called *butyrate* is proven to help reduce inflammation and provide energy for gut cells in the large intestine. Another SCFA, *propionate,* has been found to reduce inflammation and, according to a study published by *BMJ,* it can even help reduce visceral fat!

This is why gut health and eating prebiotics to feed your friendly bacteria is so important. This goes beyond calorie management because it's addressing the things that control your metabolism in the first place. We'll dive in deep on all of the incredible foods to include in your fat loss protocol coming up soon in the next chapters, but we've got one more mighty metabolic force to cover (and it's really going to get you amped—literally!), and before that we've got to check in on how inflammation is picking on your liver.

Liver Shiver

Many people are surprised to find out that liver damage is hovering around the top ten causes of death in our world today. And it's even more shocking once you find out how truly important your liver is. Not only is your liver acting as your internal cashier (storing extra glucose as glycogen and exchanging excess glycogen for fat), but your liver is also responsible for filtering your blood supply (it filters your entire blood supply approximately once every minute!), producing insulin-like growth factor-1 (IGF-1 is another key player in your metabolism), and is also responsible for breaking down insulin (your body's major fat-storing hormone) so it can be eliminated from your system.

Your liver has a lot of other important jobs to do involving your metabolism, but inflammation can definitely sabotage all of it. Recently updated research published in the *World Journal of Hepatology* revealed that inflammation is a huge contributing factor in liver damage. Growing issues like cirrhosis and non-alcoholic fatty liver disease (NAFLD—which is characterized by an excess build-up of fat in the liver) carry a huge inflammatory component, all of which include poor management of fat.

Coupled with data published in the journal *Clinics in Gastroenterology*, physician and *New York Times*–bestselling author Dr. Alan Christianson shared with me that inflammation in the liver can have a huge impact on thyroid function. Your liver is critical in the transport, metabolism, storage, and excretion of thyroid hormones (and many other hormones as well). He stated, "If your liver does not manage the thyroid hormones properly, it can slow your metabolism by hundreds of calories per day."

To make matters more concerning, researchers from Westmead Millennium Institute at the University of Sydney have concluded that *visceral fat is directly associated with liver inflammation and insulin resistance.* Ironically, poor liver function is a causative agent for more belly fat, and more belly fat is a causative agent for poor liver function. This is why reducing overall systemic inflammation is so important. If you're curious what your levels of inflammation may be, a common marker that can be assessed is your blood levels of C-reactive protein (CRP). High levels of CRP are indicative of heart disease, acute infection, or even poor liver function (your liver is actually where CRP is synthesized).

Here are a few notable things that can spark inflammation and depress the function of your liver:

- **Alcohol overload**—This is relatively well-known. Your liver is largely responsible for metabolizing alcohol, and drinking too much liquid courage can send your liver running to cry in a corner somewhere.
- **Carbohydrate bombardment**—Starches and sugar have the fastest ability to drive up blood glucose, liver glycogen, and liver fat storage (compared to their protein and fat macronutrient counterparts). Bringing in too many carbs, too often, can elicit a wildfire of fat accumulation. In fact, one of the most effective treatments for reversing NAFLD is reducing the intake of carbohydrates. A recent study conducted at KTH Royal Institute of Technology and published in the journal *Cell Metabolism* had overweight test subjects with high levels of liver fat reduce their

ratio of carbohydrate intake (without reducing calories!). After a short two-week study period the subjects showed "rapid and dramatic" reductions of liver fat and other cardiometabolic risk factors.

- **Too many medications** — Your liver is the top doc in charge of your body's drug metabolism. When you hear about drug side effects on commercials, they are really a *direct* effect of how your liver is able to handle them. The goal is to work on your lifestyle factors so that you can be on as few medications as possible along with the help of your physician. Your liver will do its best to support you either way, but it will definitely feel happier without the additional burden.

- **Too many supplements** — There are several wonderful supplements that can be helpful for your health, but becoming an overzealous natural pill-popper might not be good for you either. In a program funded by the National Institutes of Health, it was found that liver injuries linked to supplement use jumped from 7 percent to 20 percent of all medication/supplement-induced injuries in just a ten-year time span. Again, this is not to say that the right supplements can't be great for you. This merely points to the fact that your liver is also responsible for metabolism of all of the supplements you take as well. And popping a couple dozen different supplements each day can be a lot for your liver to handle. Plus, the supplement industry is largely unregulated, and the additives, fillers, and other questionable ingredients could add to the burden. Do your homework on where you get your supplements from, avoid taking too many, and focus on food first to meet your nutritional needs.

- **Toxicants** — According to researchers at the University of Louisville, more than 300 environmental chemicals, mostly pesticides, have been linked to fatty liver disease. Your liver is largely responsible for handling the weight of the toxicants (most of them newly invented) that we're exposed to in our world today. Pesticides are inherently meant to be deadly, but just to small organisms (like pests), though it seems to be missed that you are actually made of small organisms, too (bacteria). A study published in *Scientific Reports* found a direct correlation between pesticide consumption, inflammation, and gut damage. Eating organic isn't just a cute, trendy thing to do. It's one of the most important ways to protect your liver, your gut, and your metabolism.

Brain and Thyroid Breakdown

We'll be covering the brain in a major way (and how you can radically improve your memory, focus, and much more) in Section Two. But for our mission with fat loss, it's important to look at the brain's connection with the thyroid, and how inflammation can cause a metabolic meltdown. As we've discussed, your thyroid is largely considered to be the governing force of your metabolism. But your thyroid, like everyone else in your metabolic community, has to check in with the Godfather (your brain). Here is how your thyroid works alongside your brain in a nutshell.

When your body senses low thyroid hormone levels, your hypothalamus (the master gland in your brain) releases *thyrotropin releasing hormone* (TRH). This stimulates the release of *thyroid stimulating hormone* (TSH) from your pituitary gland. (Which, funny enough, looks like a tiny scrotum dangling from the base of your brain—just google "picture of the pituitary gland," but fair warning, you can't unsee it.) TSH then binds to the thyroid gland, and stimulates the release of *thyroxine* (T4; an inactive form of your thyroid hormone). Within the thyroid, a small amount of T4 can be converted to *triiodothyronine* (T3; your active thyroid hormone), however most of it is converted into T3 in other places (mainly by your liver and gut bacteria!). When T4 levels reach their threshold, the release of TRH in your brain is inhibited, and thus the release of T4 slows down. The cycle continues this way when things are in good working order.

Now, this is a lot, and there are many other influences on the process, but hopefully you can see that inflammation in the liver, gut, and even your brain can have devastating effects on your thyroid function.

And, today, we now know that inflammation in the brain and hypo-thalamus itself can be behind severe metabolic damage. A recent study published in the *Annals of the New York Academy of Sciences* reported that hypothalamic inflammation is a double-edge sword to nutritional diseases. The study authors reported that systemic inflammation from things like metabolic dysfunction and excess body fat leads to brain inflammation, and brain inflammation, itself, leads to metabolic dys-function and excess fat.

Now, I'm not sure how many ethical fat-loss programs are sharing with you how important it is to reduce inflammation in your brain to improve your metabolism, but I'll bargain to say it's not many. I want to make sure that you deeply understand this from here on out, and the best way to look at it is that your metabolic rate is like a thermostat. If the thermostat is set a little higher, you will intrinsically be burning more calories automatically. But if your thermostat is set too low, your metabolic rate will be turned down and you will find it difficult to burn fat no matter how many methods of calorie restrictions you try.

Your hypothalamus is sort of like the person who regulates your body's thermostat, and it tells your pituitary and the rest of your organs where it should be set. Think of your hypothalamus as being like the stereotypical dad in your internal household, "You can eat up the food, I'll keep all the bills paid, but no one touches this thermostat but me!" I think all dads have a thing about the thermostat (and the televi-sion remote, if I'm being honest). There's a scene in the movie *Daddy's Home 2* with Will Ferrell and Mark Wahlberg where one of the kids tampered with the thermostat while everyone was asleep, and the dads literally got flaming hot and sweaty, and were shocked that someone else was allowed to try to control the temperature in the house. The dad (the hypothalamus) fought back-and-forth with the kid (the gut, liver, body fat, etc.) to control the temperature and reduce inflamma-tion, but eventually someone has to give up the fight (and this is where we see metabolic dysfunction).

You will automatically be able to support the reduction of brain inflammation by following the Eat Smarter 30-Day Program, avoid-ing the inflammatory foods and influences already noted, and adding the incredible foods we'll be covering in the upcoming chapters. But next up, we've got one more area of inflammation that we need to address.

Your Fat Cells Themselves

Scientists from the Houston Methodist Hospital unveiled concerning new research in the journal *Cell Metabolism*. The report established that when it comes to excessive inflammation and fat storage, the fat cells *themselves* are at least partly to blame. We've established that inflammation is a natural response of your body to injury or infection, and even though your fat cells may be in good working order, when they are overburdened, they appear to issue false distress signals that can send your immune cells into a tizzy. The study found that fat can trigger heightened activity with your immune system, and too many over-filled fat cells can make your body think that you're infected.

This is yet another way that body fat can become a vicious circle of inflammation and more fat storage as a result. The lead investigator, Dr. Willa Hsueh, said that your fat cells are "doing the thing they're supposed to do — storing energy — but reacting negatively to too much of it." This, again, stresses our need to implement methods that reduce body fat *and* reduce inflammation collectively. Managing inflammation is like playing with fire. You need just enough to keep your house warm, cook, and keep everything running. But when it's in excess it can quickly burn your metabolic house down.

Now that we've got the first amigo in the bag, it's time to address amigo number two and continue to crack the code of real, sustainable fat loss.

TWO: Hormone Dysfunction

Current estimates state that you have upwards of 50 trillion human cells that make up your body. Your cells are all like citizens living in a community that are all working together to make you who you are. Now, it can be a wonderful community with a low rate of problems, or it can be a community like the ones seen on *The X-Files* with all kinds of weird stuff going on. A well-run, healthy community thrives on good *communication*. And the entity most responsible for the communication within your cellular community are your hormones.

Hormones are very special chemical messengers that send DMs throughout your entire body. Just like text messages, emails, tweets, and voice memos, hormones can come in many forms and they all play a key role in keeping in touch.

Hormones are produced and sent all throughout your body via your endocrine system (which includes your thyroid, pancreas, adrenals, etc.). Your endocrine system makes hormones that regulate your metabolism, growth rate, sexual function, healing, sleep, mood, and a plethora of other things. Your hormones deliver DMs that literally control *everything* about you. It's an absolutely amazing system when things are working right. But when things are off it can be the equivalent of your hormones drunk texting your cells at 2 o'clock in the morning.

With cellular drunk texting, it might warrant a negative response (i.e., causing an unintended process to be stimulated in your body), it might warrant sympathy (with an overly strong cellular response to try and make things better), or it might even warrant getting blocked by the cell altogether (cellular "resistance" and a downregulation of the receptor site—i.e., the cell is sick of your s%#&).

Right now we're going to hit some points on a few of the major hormonal power players involved in our metabolism. By addressing these hormones we'll be able to create healthy lines of communication in our cellular community.

Insulin

Insulin is one of the most important hormones in human health. It's a hormone that signals our cells to open up to allow in energy. Without insulin, we literally wouldn't be able to supply food to our cells and we'd find ourselves withering away as if Thanos just snapped his fingers.

Insulin is essential for our health, but since it's the major hormone driving energy storage, if it's overactive your metabolism can hit an endgame very fast. Our insulin levels inherently rise when glucose enters our bloodstream. This can be from the food you eat or from the glycogen broken down that was stored in your muscles or liver cashier. Insulin signals your fat cells to open up and absorb all available glucose, fatty acids, and amino acids. But what's important (and often overlooked) is that the presence of insulin also tells your cells to *stop* breaking down stored energy and *stop* using body fat for fuel.

We want insulin to do its job, but we don't want it to be overbearing. Insulin is triggered most aggressively when glucose is in our blood, so we generally have the biggest insulin response when we eat carbohydrates. Now, just to be clear, this is not necessarily a bad thing. Again, insulin is involved in beneficial storage roles when it's in balance, and insulin is even involved in the conversion of your inactive T4 thyroid hormone into the active T3 thyroid hormone to keep your metabolism rolling. However, too much insulin activity (and too much fat being stored in your fat cells) can lead to a downregulation of receptor sites on your cells (meaning that your cells can't properly "hear" insulin's message) and fat, glucose, and other compounds can be left floating in your bloodstream too long, gumming things up and getting unruly.

Not only can this insulin resistance lead to cardiovascular damage but, according to a study published in the *Journal of Gastroenterology and Hepatology,* because your liver is now forced to take on the burden of that excess glucose and fat, this can lead to nonalcoholic fatty liver disease and the rapid accumulation of more visceral fat! Back in Chapter One we covered how dangerous this visceral belly fat is. Now you know one of the fastest ways to make more of it is to overburden your liver and provoke your cells into becoming insulin resistant.

Insulin resistance is caused primarily by the overconsumption of high glycemic (blood sugar spiking) foods *and* inflammation. A study published in the peer-reviewed journal *Circulation* found that systemic inflammation (measured by CRP) was directly linked to insulin resistance. So, is simply avoiding carbohydrates the end-all, be-all solution to getting insulin to stop drunk-dialing everyone? Not exactly. Our other two macronutrients (protein and fat) influence insulin too. Eating protein stimulates insulin release (albeit in a much smaller magnitude) and dietary fats can stimulate insulin indirectly, with the wrong fats even contributing to insulin resistance according to research published in the journal *Clinical Nutrition.*

Yet, when you dig through the evidence you see that, all calories considered, when you shift your percentage of carbs down a bit, and raise your levels of protein and/or fat up a bit, you generally see a favorable response in your metabolism. A big part of that is due to the response of insulin's twin brother, glucagon.

Glucagon

As you'll recall, glucagon's efforts are largely the opposites of insulin. Glucagon's drive is to get stored fat *out* of your fat cells and *out* of your liver to give your body the chance to burn it for energy. Glucagon's favorite line is, "You don't have to go home, but you've got to get the hell out of here!"

One of the other interesting things that glucagon does is decrease fatty acid synthesis (the creation of fatty acids) in fat tissue and in the liver. Simultaneously, it promotes lipolysis in these tissues, which, again, makes them release fatty acids into circulation where they can be broken down for energy. Part of eating smarter is getting glucagon working for you by shifting your protein/carb ratio. An example of this is highlighted in a study published in the journal *Hormone and Metabolic Research.* Scientists at Laval University discovered that, whether you eat a meal of pie or a meal of steak or fish, both immediately elevate insulin and extra glucagon is nowhere to be found. But the incredible thing is that about 30 minutes *after* the higher protein meal of steak or fish, glucagon levels shot up significantly, while baseline levels of glucagon dropped even more after eating the pie. Now, here's the thing, I'm a fan of pie (and other treats too), but there's a way to go about eating these foods that enables your fat-burning hormones to keep doing their jobs and ensuring your fat-storing hormones don't get out of control. Higher quality protein and shifting your protein/carb ratio (*not* a high protein diet) is key to encouraging glucagon.

There's a lot of in-fighting among experts about higher carbs or higher fats, but protein has become the Rodney Dangerfield of the situation, shouting, "Hey, I get no respect!" Another study published in *The Journal of Nutrition* showed that simply increasing protein intake led to enhanced weight loss and reduced blood fat levels in the study participants. Now you know it's because glucagon plays a role, but glucagon can be placed in a brotherly sleeper hold when insulin is acting cattywampus.

Cortisol

One of the things that gets insulin riled up is its good friend cortisol. Cortisol is a lot like Bruce Banner and *The Incredible Hulk*. When it's functioning normally, it's remarkably intelligent, helpful, motivating, and supportive. But when cortisol is elevated and out of balance, all it really likes to do is smash stuff.

Cortisol helps to manage your blood pressure, regulate inflammation, balance your blood sugar, support your thyroid function, and more. But, when cortisol gets angry, each and every one of those systems can get messed up. One of the hardest places hit by an overly aggressive cortisol is your thyroid function. In a conversation I had with physician and *New York Times*–bestselling author Dr. Amy Myers, she shared with me how excess cortisol can depress thyroid activity in many different ways. One is the direct impact the presence of cortisol has by signaling your hypothalamus and pituitary gland to slow down the release of TRH and TSH. Another way is cortisol's ability to convert free T3 (the "gas pedal" of your thyroid metabolism) into *reverse T3* (RT3—the "brakes" of your thyroid metabolism). And yet another way is through cortisol's dirty dancing routine with inflammatory immune cells called *cytokines* that make your thyroid receptors less sensitive to thyroid hormones. And this is just a snapshot of how cortisol can put your metabolism in the corner.

Whether you're eating a low-carb diet or not, stress can send your blood sugar skyrocketing thanks to the action of cortisol. Research conducted at the Washington University School of Medicine in St. Louis demonstrated that cortisol has a muscle-catabolic effect that can rapidly break down your muscle tissue and use it for fuel. This is a process called *gluconeogenesis,* and it's a built-in fight-or-flight mechanism that we developed through evolution. It's super valuable if you're actually in a life-or-death situation with a saber-toothed tiger — wait, lots of people use saber-toothed tiger, so I'm going to use a cuttlefish; those things are super sneaky, and they seem like they have an attitude problem. OK, so if you're in a life-or-death situation with a *cuttlefish,* you want your body to be able to partition extra resources to your bloodstream to fuel your escape (or your fisticuffs situation with the cuttlefish, which I don't recommend). You get away or fight it out, then cortisol and other stress hormones are allowed to return back to normal, and all is well.

Today, most of us don't come face-to-face with a cuttlefish, a saber-toothed tiger, or any real threats to our survival on a regular basis. Yet, scientists have now affirmed that many of us are living with a chronic, low-grade stress that's slowly breaking us down on the inside through many of the hormone-related issues you've been learning about.

We know that today's hyper-stressed combination of work stress, financial stress, family stress, emotional stress, and more can all add to our overall stress load and keep cortisol elevated. But ironically, your diet can stress your body and keep cortisol elevated as well. Eating inflammatory foods, being deficient in key nutrients, and even your emotions around your diet can all add to the same stress that's keeping your cortisol high, thus keeping insulin high, and keeping glucagon in time-out.

Other Hormones Involved in Fat Management

You have approximately 50 hormones circulating and sending messages throughout your body at any given time, and several of them are involved in metabolism. We're just going to touch on a few other key hormones to be aware of.

Testosterone is vital to both men and women because it helps to build and maintain muscle mass. One of the most underutilized ways to help create a healthy metabolism is adding some muscle to your frame.

Muscle is one of the most metabolically active tissues we have. Generally speaking, the more muscle you have, the more calories you burn during activity *and* at rest. And the most incredible thing is that we are endowed with the ability to make more of it if we want! Though we tend to see testosterone as a distinctly male hormone, biochemist Dr. Sylvia Tara shared with me that there is actually more testosterone in a woman's body than estrogen at many times during the month. Men definitely have a higher percentage of testosterone compared to women, and women have a higher percentage of estrogen compared to men. But both are critical to a healthy metabolism and healthy life overall for both sexes.

Testosterone generally decreases fat mass, but can also increase the likelihood of insulin resistance. This is part of the reason that men are more likely to store excess fat on the belly as visceral fat, while women are more likely to store subcutaneous fat on the arms, thighs, butt, and hips.

Estrogen is another important player in our metabolism. Researchers at the University of Houston recently disclosed that excessive or insufficient amounts of estrogen can cause the metabolic network of both men and women to become imbalanced. Abnormal levels of estrogen can directly lead to metabolic diseases and obesity. There are several different forms of estrogen, but the most influential one appears to be *estradiol*. Many people are shocked to find that low levels of this estrogen can cause reduced fat burning, increased appetite, and a redistribution of more fat to the visceral belly fat area. On the other side, too much estrogen is attributed to making an excess of subcutaneous fat. And the ultimate booby trap is that the stored subcutaneous fat can make more estrogen itself! So the more fat you make, the higher the estrogen goes.

And if that weren't concerning enough, these fat cells also have high levels of an enzyme called *aromatase* that can literally steal your testosterone and turn it into more estrogen. And guess what upregulates the activity of aromatase? Big brother, insulin. So, one of the big takeaways is that if we eat to optimize insulin, we'll be able to positively influence estrogen and testosterone as well. But if we let insulin run rampant, we'll see higher levels of fat storage, higher levels of aromatization, and abnormal levels of estrogen. We want estrogen in the Goldilocks position: not too hot, not too cold, but just right.

Human growth hormone (HGH) is a hormone secreted by the pituitary gland at the base of your brain (that gonadal sack of surprises again). Its key role is to promote cellular growth and repair. But, it also plays a role in fat metabolism and body composition. This potent hormone facilitates lipolysis, promotes the utilization of free fatty acids, and stimulates muscle growth. In fact, research highlighted in *The Journal of Clinical Endocrinology & Metabolism* revealed that the amount of body fat you carry is in direct relationship to your body's production of HGH.

Lack of sleep and lack of exercise are well-noted suppressors of HGH. But key nutrient deficiencies and certain styles of eating can make it tank too. Coming up soon you'll learn which foods to eat to support your HGH production and a meal-timing technique that has a profound impact on HGH as well.

Adrenaline is a powerful fat-burning hormone, going back to our example of workers in our cellular theater. Scientists at the University of Missouri School of Medicine found that fat cells have receptors that bind with adrenaline, which signals adipocytes to release stored fat into the system to use for energy. Now, when I think of adrenaline, I think of the movie *Speed* starring Sandra Bullock and Keanu Reeves. Adrenaline can really get your metabolic bus moving! But when it's out of control, a lot of damage can happen along the way. Adrenaline is a major part of our body's fight-or-flight response. It can holler at your fat cells to release energy to fight, flee, or frolic. But yelling too much can make it lose its voice (through damage to your adrenals and other endocrine organs). We want adrenaline to be able to sing confidently, but not to be hoarse for days, months, or even years because of it. Over time it will still be able to speak but it would be the equivalent of mumble rapping. It might have a good beat, but most of your cells won't know what the hell it's talking about.

The fact that adrenaline is a primary fat-burner speaks directly to the power of exercise to stimulate it, but even that has limitations.

What's often overlooked is that there are simple things you can do with your nutrition that can encourage a healthy response of adrenaline as well (and we'll dive into those coming up in Chapter Five).

But now that we've taken a deeper look at some of our major hormonal players, it's time to break down the third amigo that will help bring it all together!

Where Does the Fat Go When You Lose It?

Many diet and exercise programs promise the ultimate reward of losing more body fat. But have you ever stopped to wonder, "Where the heck does my fat actually go when I lose it?" Is there a metabolic lost-and-found? Does it jump to an alternate universe? Or is it actual magic?

The strange reality is that losing fat can seem sort of like magic because we don't really see it leave. The closest approximation we have to seeing fat evicted from our bodies is through the appearance of sweat. Thanks to our conventional calorie-focused health industry, we know that when we're working hard, and breaking a sweat, we are burning away some of those pesky calories. We know that when we see the sweat dripping that's just our fat cells having a good breakup cry as their stored calories are leaving town. But, unfortunately, that's not how our fat's disappearing act actually works.

As we noted earlier, our fat cells are mainly composed of tiny packets of stored energy called triglycerides. When we attempt to "lose fat," what we're really attempting to do is metabolize these triglycerides. Triglycerides are composed of three types of atoms: carbon, hydrogen, and oxygen. And triglycerides can only be broken down by unlocking these atoms through the process of oxidation. Now, here's how fat is able to vanish into thin air.

In a peer-reviewed study published in the *BMJ*, scientists decided to follow the path of these atoms as they are leaving the body. They discovered that when 10 kilograms of fat is oxidized, 8.4 kilograms of that fat is excreted as carbon dioxide (CO_2) via the lungs, while just 1.6 kilograms is released as water (H_2O). In other words, approximately 84 percent of the fat that you lose is eliminated through your breath when you breathe out! And only about 16 percent of the fat you lose is through urine, sweat, and other fluids. Their calculations revealed that the lungs are the primary excretory organ for fat. Plus, if that weren't surprising enough, the researchers estimate that about one-third of weight loss happens as you breathe during a full night of sleep.

Now you know, when fat goes bye-bye it's primarily through your breathing. Cesar Millan may be the Dog Whisperer, but you, my friend, are a fat whisperer.

THREE: Appetite Dysregulation

A big part of fat loss is being able to healthfully regulate our appetite. There are several powerful mechanisms in your metabolic furnace that control your experience of hunger and satisfaction. You're about to discover what they are, but it's also important to understand what you're up against.

Many people are struggling to try and eat less when we're *encouraged* to eat a lot of food in our culture. A great example of this is the all-you-can-eat buffet. "All you can eat" really should mean putting super-weird combinations of food on your plate. As a kid, I would head up to the buffet bright-eyed and bushy-tailed and grab my plate. Then add a slice of pizza with a side of mac and cheese, a piece of fried fish, two pieces of broccoli, and a steak for good measure.

My favorite part was the dessert afterward. You're going to let me, a kid, run this ice cream machine? On many occasions my bowl of ice cream stood taller than my head. And, of course, I added so many toppings that it looked like a volcano just exploded with molten hot diabetes.

Right now we live at a time where we're pretty much surrounded by food everywhere we go. It has its pros and cons, but the reality is that we have largely trained our biology to constantly be eating: big portions, hyperpalatable foods, and easy access all the time. I know I've thought on many occasions about what I'm going to have for dinner while I'm still eating lunch. Our biological rhythms have to be recalibrated, and we also have to optimize our hormones involved in managing our appetite. We'll talk about making some updates to your body's food clock in Section Three, and right now we'll break down what's really controlling your appetite in the first place.

Leptin

Almost poetically, it is our body fat that is controlling our appetite. Being that we are capable of consuming millions upon millions of calories each year, our bodies devised a specific way to inform our cellular community that we are all stocked up on supplies and we can turn our desire to consume more off. Since your fat cells hold the storage supplies, it is your fat cells that release the hormonal email message to the rest of your cells to signal you to stop eating. And the subject line of that email message is one word: *leptin*.

Leptin, derived from the Greek word *leptos,* meaning thin, was just discovered a couple of short decades ago. Prior to that, science widely considered excessive appetite to be a matter of willpower. Fortunately, we've learned that dysfunction of this hormone can be behind many of our challenges with metabolism and food. Leptin is the leader of your body's satiety hormones. It travels from your fat cells into your bloodstream and makes its way to the master controller of your appetite in the Godfather's office, aka your hypothalamus. Leptin literally gives the intel that signals your brain to stop eating. But if leptin is unable to deliver its message, you'll inherently be driven to constantly eat more and more.

Recent research indicates that leptin not only reduces appetite, but is also involved in fat metabolism itself. Learning the essentials on how leptin is expressed or repressed is going to give you a huge advantage in upgrading your metabolism.

Leptin Resistance

Because fat cells produce leptin in proportion to their size, the more body fat we have, the more leptin we produce. According to data published in *The New England Journal of Medicine,* test subjects who are very overweight or obese actually have very high levels of leptin, which you'd *think* would make them full all the time. The underlying issue, however, is a case where there is so much leptin email coming in that it starts to get flagged as spam. After your brain's inbox is constantly bombarded for a while, it will no longer see most of the leptin messages coming in. This downregulation of leptin receptors is known as *leptin resistance,* and it's a major player in difficulty losing body fat. When your brain doesn't properly receive the messages from leptin, it mistakenly thinks you are starving—even though you have more than enough energy stored!

This triggers your brain to change its behavior in order to regain body fat. Your brain will then command you to 1) eat more because it thinks you're starving and 2) dramatically reduce your energy expenditure by slowing down the rate at which you burn calories. So, again, tell me how simply cutting calories is going to help most people when their entire physiology seems to be fighting against them? If we don't address leptin, we are literally pitting people against themselves in a battle of their willpower versus their biology, and our biology will always win out at the end of the fight. By eating smarter you'll be able to purposefully and intentionally improve your leptin sensitivity and get your brain-body connection online again. We'll get leptin whitelisted in your brain's inbox. The first thing we need to do is address the attachments that were causing it to go to spam in the first place.

Put Out the Fire

According to research published in the journal *Endocrinology* and the journal *Gut,* inflammation and abnormalities in your microbiome directly contribute to leptin resistance. As we covered in our earlier discussion on inflammation, damage to your gut can cause metabolic breakdowns in other parts of your body (even your brain!). These studies affirm that by reducing inflammation and improving the health of your microbiome, you'll inherently be able to improve your leptin sensitivity as well.

The Sugarmobile

The sugar we eat ends up driving into our fat cells so fast and furiously, it's as if Vin Diesel is at the wheel. I really don't think most folks realize how quickly your body can convert sugar into fat, and we definitely don't realize how much sugar damages the function of leptin. Our fastest method of delivering sugar to our cells is through the consumption of liquid sugar, which is highlighted in a study published in *The Journal of Nutritional Biochemistry.* The researchers asserted that the consumption of highly concentrated liquid fructose leads to the development of hypothalamic leptin resistance *and* the development of excess visceral fat.

This is what soda and juices do better than anything else to make us gain fat. I remember my mom sending me to the local 7-Eleven just about every day to buy her a Big Gulp fountain soda filled to the brim with Pepsi. Then *Super* Big Gulps came out and she had me bring her those. And eventually the crowning glory of all sodas came out, the *DOUBLE* Big Gulp, and it was now my mission to deliver them to her. No joke, the containers were so big that you simply couldn't grab and go. You had to fold the top of the container together like the triangular top of a milk carton. They wanted to make sure you could squeeze more soda into that pointy top, but I didn't know I was signing up to do arts and crafts at the convenience store. I'm sure if they came out with a *Triple* Big Gulp I would have been sent out for that too. That's the thing about sugar, it makes you want more and more by damaging the function of leptin. Some people might think they have their soda drinking under control, but this could be the #1 thing that's causing your body to be resistant to weight loss.

And if you think that drinking juice is any better, please know from this day forward that your favorite juice is driving a crazy fast car also. In my podcast, *The Model Health Show,* a popular episode took listeners through the entire history of sugar. We looked at sugar's humble beginnings when it was rare for folks to get their hands on it, to today when it's one of the most pervasive things in our culture. One of the things I highlighted was the shocking amount of sugar contained in one bottle of soda. A 20-ounce bottle of Coca-Cola, for instance, supplies 65 grams of sugar (about 16 teaspoons!). While my personal favorite growing up, 20 ounces of 100 percent pure orange juice, is not far behind with 56 grams of sugar (for a whopping 14 teaspoons!). It doesn't matter that it says 100 percent juice. It doesn't matter that it has some vitamins in it. That amount of sugar is going to hyperstimulate insulin, damage leptin, and literally derange the communication between your brain and your body. If you really want some fruit juice, then eat a piece of fruit, otherwise that glass of OJ is going to kick your metabolism in the junk.

Mom, Gluten Won't Stop Hitting Leptin!

A recent study published in the peer-reviewed journal *BMC Biochemistry* revealed some shocking new data. In the study, the researchers found that digested gluten could literally block the ability for leptin to bind to leptin receptors. It was a dose-dependent response, as well. The more gluten present, the more leptin was blocked. In fact, the amount of gluten eaten in a typical meal of bread or pasta was found to reduce leptin binding by up to 50 percent!

Now, gluten has been portrayed in the role of the evil villain in nutrition for many years. Gluten is like the Glenn Close in bread's apparent *Fatal Attraction*. But I don't want you to get your crumbs in a bunch thinking that gluten-containing foods are totally off the menu. Indeed, to play it safe for many folks, it might be a good idea to be careful in flirting with gluten, especially if you're dealing with insulin resistance, leptin resistance, or any inflammation-related problems. This is because data published in the journal *Nutrients* demonstrated that gluten prompts the release of a protein called *zonulin* that increases the permeability of your gut lining (whether you are gluten sensitive or not). As we addressed in our discussion about the microbiome, dysfunction of the tight junctions that make up your gut lining is a key contributor to systemic inflammation. It all goes together like Cruella de Vil chasing after those puppies.

But, as with most things, there are multiple perspectives to consider. Even the researchers in the study noted that the way the gluten was prepared or cooked made a difference in its effects on leptin. Coming up in Chapter Three we'll look at the brighter side of bread most people never see.

However, for the most part, getting into a haphazard affair with gluten can make your metabolic movie end badly.

Ghrelin

If leptin is the captain of the satiety team, the captain of the hunger team would surely be the hormone *ghrelin*. Ghrelin is produced and released mainly by your stomach, with small amounts also released by your small intestine, pancreas, and brain. Ghrelin is dubbed the "hunger hormone" because its release directly stimulates your appetite, encourages increased food intake, and promotes body fat storage. Ghrelin is in a friendly crosstown rivalry with leptin to keep you eating when it senses that food supplies are low.

When your metabolism is running properly, ghrelin just goes on about its business practicing and supporting the metabolic team. But when there are breakdowns with insulin sensitivity, leptin sensitivity, and increased fat storage, ghrelin becomes a team of Monstars that can be really difficult to beat. Research conducted by scientists at King Saud University revealed that after eating a meal, people with normal levels of body fat had a significant drop in ghrelin levels, but test subjects with higher levels of body fat only had a *slight* reduction in ghrelin after a meal. This means that the more body fat someone has, the more they were driven biologically to eat. Because of the higher blood levels of ghrelin, the hypothalamus doesn't get a strong enough signal to turn off the appetite, which easily leads to the overconsumption of calories. Hopefully you can see yet another way that the accumulation of more body fat can become a vicious circle. To address this we have to target the two major areas that coach ghrelin to make the right plays.

I Can't Get No Satisfaction?

When we think about being "full," it generally relates to the physical feeling of newly deposited food in our bellies. We have mechanoreceptors in our gut that respond to being stretched and initiate a feeling of fullness. Certain foods trigger these mechanoreceptors far more than others. Foods that provide more fiber give an assist in this department, as do protein-dense foods. A study published in *The American Journal of Clinical Nutrition* set out to uncover the impact that increasing one's protein ratio would have on levels of ghrelin. The researchers put test subjects on either an "adequate protein diet" (towards the minimum that would prevent degenerative illness) of 10 percent protein, 60 percent carbohydrate, and 30 percent dietary fat, or a higher protein diet of 30 percent protein, 40 percent carbohydrate, and 30 percent dietary fat. The results found that test subjects with a higher protein ratio had higher levels of satiety, a higher resting metabolic rate, and higher levels of fat oxidation. They burned more fat, yet they were more satisfied. And another study found that simply increasing the protein ratio of the first meal of the day led to decreased levels of ghrelin. Again, high-quality protein is often overlooked in the debate about whether dietary fat or carbohydrates are more important, but it has extraordinary effects on regulating our major metabolic hormones.

On the other side, today we have a whole new category of foods that can barely even tickle the mechanoreceptors in our guts. These foods easily enable us to consume hundreds or even thousands of calories without signaling fullness. What foods am I talking about? Well, if you've ever eaten some Cheetos, then you know exactly what I mean. Doritos, Funyuns, Cheez-Its (probably the worst food name ever), Fritos, and, of course, the legendary Lay's Potato Chip itself, whose own marketing bragged that "You can't eat just one."

All of those foods induce a phenomenon known as *vanishing caloric density*. You put it in your mouth, bite down on it for a couple of crunches, and then it seems to just melt into almost nothing. A food scientist from Chapman College, Steven Witherly, states, "If something melts down quickly, your brain thinks that there's no calories in it...you can just keep eating it forever." I don't know about you, but I've personally crushed whole bags of potato chips, and if I was feeling fancy, I'd easily knock down a can of Pringles. (I have no idea why they decided to put them in a tennis ball container, but I guess it's because when I ate them I felt as bougie as if I were sitting courtside at Wimbledon eating each chip with my pinky up.)

Without getting any physical bulk from the food, there's very little reason for the brain to tell you to stop eating. Thankfully, we have a backup system called *sensory-specific satiety* that monitors for big, distinct flavors that can overwhelm your brain. When too much of an intense flavor hits your taste buds, this system responds by shutting down your desire to eat more. Now, this system has evolved to deal with *natural* intense flavors. It was never designed to deal with the cutting-edge, artificial food chemistry we're exposed to today. The most successful snack companies have invested millions of dollars to create complex formulas that entice your taste buds just enough, but don't have a single, overriding flavor note that tells your brain to stop eating. This spawns a situation where ghrelin keeps getting called into the game because you 1) don't have the physical bulk and 2) you have lots of flavor but no real nutrition.

The Science of Flavor

Ghrelin is far more than just a hunger hormone. Today we now understand that ghrelin is also involved in thermogenesis, muscle development, and even bone formation. And what's most important in our mission of maximizing fat loss is ghrelin's role in nutrient detection.

Your brain and other organs are in constant communication making requests for nutrients they need. Omega-3s, chromium, vitamin C, zinc, leucine, niacin, vitamin D... the list goes on and on. There are countless nutrients that humans need to truly thrive, and the way your body signals the request to bring more nutrient supplies in is through *hunger.* If your body is low on magnesium for your muscle function or calcium to help clot your blood, it will heighten your desire to eat to get a chance to bring these nutrients in.

There was a time when our food choices and biological needs matched up. We'd desire different foods, not out of addiction or out of artificial manipulation, but out of cellular intelligence. In the introduction to the book I mentioned that food does, in fact, speak a particular language, and the language food speaks is called *flavor.* Flavor is how food communicates with us and it gives us valuable feedback as to what's actually in the food and what the food can do for us. We've developed this communication with natural foods through a phenomenon we call *post-ingestive feedback.* Essentially, your body learns that certain flavors in foods come along with certain nutrients, and when in need of those nutrients, your hunger will compel you to seek out those foods.

There used to be a time when different foods tasted distinctly like different things. A strawberry tasted like a strawberry, a chicken leg tasted like a chicken leg, roots tasted like, well, roots. The lines were clear. And your taste sensors knew the difference. You weren't going to find something that tasted like something else. But, in recent decades, scientists figured out that flavors are linked to certain chemicals. And many of these flavor chemicals could be isolated. Once isolated, those once unique flavors could be used to artificially flavor things and cause those once clear lines to blur like someone just blew Cheeto dust in your eyes.

Now the flavor of a strawberry is no longer simply found in a strawberry. We can infuse that flavor into sodas, candy, ice cream, cake, and even water. Chicken flavor can now be found in ramen noodles, potato chips, tofu, and more, and actual chicken is no longer required. The flavors need not be exact, but they're close enough to muddy up the waters of your brain trying to see the nutrients that are really in a food.

In talking with award-winning journalist and food researcher Mark Schatzker about his analysis published in his book *The Dorito Effect,* he shared with me that flavors are like nutrition labels built into food. We automatically form flavor preferences once the body links up the ingested flavor of the food we eat to specific nutrients the body receives. I know we can all crave something less than healthy. But haven't you ever really craved something healthy too? Maybe you'd been going on a bit of a pizza bender for a couple of days, and suddenly you have an irresistible desire for broccoli or a fresh salad. As hard as you may have tried to play the role of a Ninja Turtle, your human nutrient needs kicked in and commanded you to get a few nutrients into your system. Your body knew the nutrition label and what it could get. Resetting your flavor palate is critical to turning this cellular intelligence back on and optimizing the function of your hunger and satiety hormones.

Other Hormones Involved in Appetite

As you've seen thus far, there really is an entire symphony of hormonal instruments playing together to regulate your metabolism and appetite. Here are a few other key orchestra members that deserve a little bit more of the spotlight.

Peptide YY (PYY) is another gut hormone that regulates your appetite. It's released by cells in your intestines and colon based on the types and amounts of food coming in. According to data published in *The Journal of Physiology,* PYY is believed to play a major role in reducing appetite and decreasing your risk of excess body fat storage.

Adiponectin has recently gained notoriety as one of the most potent hormones influencing your appetite and fat metabolism. Adiponectin, like leptin, is primarily produced and secreted by fat cells in your adipose tissue (which is how it derives its name). It has been noted to help your body move fat away from the viscera (belly fat) region to the subcutaneous fat region. Low levels of adiponectin have been associated with obesity, insulin resistance, and metabolic syndrome.

Unlike leptin, even though adiponectin is produced by fat tissue, as a person's body fat goes up, its levels paradoxically appear to go down. So, supporting healthy levels of adiponectin is crucial in long-term fat loss. In fact, researchers at the University of Pennsylvania recently discovered that optimal levels of adiponectin can potentially support fat loss *without* increasing appetite. Coming up, we're going to talk about which foods and practices can help you do it!

Glucagon-like peptide-1 (GLP-1) is a hormone produced primarily in your gut when nutrients enter the intestines. GLP-1 has been found to increase the feeling of fullness during and between meals by acting on appetite centers in your brain and by slowing the emptying of the stomach itself. GLP-1 also plays a role in keeping your blood sugar stable.

Neuropeptide Y (NPY) is one the most potent appetite-stimulating compounds found in the brain. It stimulates appetite with a preferential effect on making you want to eat more carbs (yep, this hormone has a diamond studded sweet tooth!). Researchers at the Henri Poincaré University in France uncovered that NPY is also capable of motivating you to eat sooner between meals and delaying your feeling of satiety while eating.

Cholecystokinin (CCK) is a hormone involved in digestion and appetite regulation. When you eat a meal, CCK is called into action to help you secrete bile to assist in digesting dietary fats. It's release also increases satiety to help you feel fuller, faster. Like GLP-1, CCK is produced primarily by cells in your gut and, according to research published in the journal *Physiology & Behavior,* optimizing levels of CCK could play a key role in reducing levels of body fat.

METABOLIC MASTERY

We've successfully broken down many of the key players that regulate your metabolism to truly put the power into your hands. Now that you know *how* your body burns fat for fuel, *how* your appetite is actually controlled, and the Three Amigos that can sabotage the whole thing, you'll finally be sending them on their merry way and tapping into your fat-burning potential.

In the next chapters, you'll learn about some of the most powerful foods and strategies to implement to support your body's metabolic systems and switch your fat-burning hormones and enzymes into the right positions. It's time to take things to another level, so let's do this!

CHAPTER THREE

Fat Loss Essential #1:
Support Your Microbiome

Food is not just eating energy. It's an experience.

~*Guy Fieri*

In the next three chapters, we're going to unveil some of the most powerful foods, nutrients, and eating tips to help you optimize the function of all the metabolic switches that you've learned about. Incorporating a variety of these different foods and strategies will help you stack conditions in your favor to achieve the results that you truly deserve to have.

As you've discovered, real fat loss goes far beyond penny-pinching our calories to try and see some results. We're actually going to target the hormones, organs, and organ systems that determine what your body does with the calories you consume in the first place. This is what eating smarter is all about! And these are all things you have a right to know and utilize to be the best version of yourself.

The food that we eat is *supposed* to be enjoyable and the process of getting healthy is *supposed* to be fun. That's why many of these remarkable foods are put together in delicious recipes incorporated in the Eat Smarter 30-Day Program at the end of the book. Of course, you don't have to wait to start adding in some of these foods to spark an upgrade in your metabolism, but once you put everything together strategically, your results will be absolutely unstoppable. No matter what diet camp you venture into in the upcoming years, I want to make sure you're equipped with the three essentials that actually support long-term fat loss. Whether you go paleo, vegan, keto, pescatarian, vegetarian, or any other approach, these three things are at the heart of real success in any of them. This chapter is dedicated to the relationship between your microbiome and fat loss, and it's a game-changer. The next two chapters will highlight Fat Loss Essentials #2 and #3, and they are equally as powerful. Missing even *one* of these fat loss essentials could spell trouble, and not just for your waistline, but for your health overall. So, intentionally implement these three things and you'll be able to keep your metabolic switches in their proper positions!

SUPPORT YOUR MICROBIOME

Your microbiome is literally the foundation of your metabolism. It's the home for your entire microbial community, and it's the first place that decides what your body will actually do with the calories you consume. We've broken down, in-depth, how this all takes place, but I want to give you one more example of how changes to your microbiome can prevent or encourage more fat loss.

Scientists at Washington University School of Medicine in St. Louis set out to find if changes to the microbiome could affect fat loss in sets of identical twins. Shockingly, they discovered that if one twin had a higher ratio of the bacteria *firmicutes* and a lower ratio of *bacteroidetes* they absorbed more calories than the other twin and were more apt to gain fat while eating the exact same diet!

Building a strong microbiome foundation is critical in maintaining a healthy metabolism. We want to make the most beneficial bacteria feel welcome and comfortable in our gut condominium and keep the less-than-supportive bacteria outside sleeping in a tent. That said, it's important to keep in mind that the firmicutes category of bacteria has important roles to play and are not inherently "bad." But when the ratios of supportive to opportunistic bacteria gets skewed, that's when we put ourselves at a metabolic disadvantage. Let's jump into the ways to remodel our microbiome community.

Diversity in Your Food

The most successful bacterial communities will have diversity as a hallmark. Recent research published in the journal *Nature* revealed that a more diverse microbiome is associated with a greater number of health benefits. And a key driver of your microbiome diversity is diversity in your *food*.

One of the biggest downfalls of typical cookie-cutter fitness diets is the lack of diversity. Chicken, rice, vegetables, repeat. Chicken, rice, vegetables, repeat. This is meal prep gone awry, and we have to start thinking differently about how we eat. It doesn't mean that you have to totally abandon your framework, but simply adding in or swapping out a food each day will make your microbial community thank you. They might even throw a calorie-burning bonfire party in your name.

Rotating in foods like blueberries, almonds, and pistachios can do wonders for supporting more microbiome diversity and a higher expression of one of the most important friendly flora, *bifidobacteria*. Bifido help to make important gut-protecting fatty acids and vitamins in you *for* you. One of the most important vitamins being folate (vitamin B9), which has been found to play an enormous role in methylation (which influences everything from your gene expression to fat metabolism), defending your body from infections, and protecting against fatty liver disease. Plus, bifidobacteria make SCFAs that protect your gut lining and reduce inflammation. Data published in the *Journal of Agriculture and Food Chemistry* affirmed that eating blueberries increases bifidobacteria and positively modulates the diversity of gut bacteria overall, and a study published in the *British Journal of Nutrition* found that eating some pistachios can improve your overall ratio of bifido-bacteria as well.

Eating a diverse array of nuts like walnuts, almonds, pistachios, Brazil nuts, and others will help support microbiome diversity. We tend to go nuts on one type of nut, so mix up your nuts a bit more often. Also, uncooked or dehydrated options are best. Once the nuts are cooked in low-quality oils, you can find yourself bringing in toxic compounds that damage your gut instead of supporting it. The same thing goes for your consumption of an array of berries. How they're prepared matters and you also want a variety. Fresh or frozen are the very best by far, and try to avoid dried fruits (they're hyperpalatable and can easily contain a high amount of sugar). Blueberries are definitely a real power player here in the gut-metabolism community, but occasionally swapping in some raspberries, strawberries, mulberries, blackberries, and others can help round out the diversity team.

One of the most surprising things regarding diversity and the microbiome is that your gut bacteria can actually change dramatically based on what time of year it is! Stanford University researchers revealed that healthy hunter-gatherer tribes have been found to have microbiome shifts that are in sync with seasonal changes made to their diet. The researchers concluded that gut microbes and digestion is cyclical, and in sync with the precise biorhythm of nature in a natural human setting. The problem is, we are no longer in a natural human setting or consistently eating foods that are provided naturally at different times of the year. Many of us have 365-day access to the same foods which, according to data published in *Science Advances,* is having a depressing impact on our microbiome and our metabolism. It's estimated that 75 percent of the world's food is produced from the same 12 plant species and 5 animal species. And the microbiome diversity of families in rural Africa and South America were found to be far greater than that of families in the U.S. and Europe.

Another tip here to support microbiome diversity and your metabolism is to purposefully eat more seasonal foods. This by no means says that you can't eat your favorite foods that might be out of season, this simply means to incorporate more foods that are in season in your area and your microbiome will be grateful for it. You can find resources to help you identify which foods are in season in your local area right now in the Eat Smarter Bonus Resource Guide at eatsmarterbook .com/bonus.

Simply adding a bigger diversity of fruits and vegetables reduces the growth of pathogenic bacteria populations and supports a reduction in waist circumference according to a study published in the journal *Food & Function.* People say, "Eat more fruits and vegetables! Eat more fruits and vegetables!" But why?! Because they're "good for you?" That's just not enough for most folks to make a change. But now you know the deeper story of how adding more (and specifically *diverse*) fruits and vegetables is connected to fat loss. It's the impact it has on your microbiome which, again, is the very foundation for your entire metabolism. And, by the way, if you are someone like me who has lived many years of your life not liking vegetables, it's most definitely because you've never had them cooked deliciously. A basic Brussels sprout is about as appealing as playing basketball in a fresh new pair of Crocs. But actually having them prepared in a tastier, smarter way (see page 372) can make you fall head-over-heels in love with a veggie you may have friend-zoned a long time ago.

Primary Prebiotics

Beneficial bacteria cannot survive without their preferred choices of food. Prebiotics are like appetizers for your friendly bacteria that make them happy enough to stay longer and leave a bigger metabolic tip. When I think of party appetizers, I think of pita and hummus, raw veggies and ranch dressing, and my favorite appetizer as a kid, pigs-in-a-blanket, or as comedian Jim Gaffigan calls them, "the California rolls of the Midwest." Like people, different bacteria like different appetizers, and if you want to make your helpful bacteria happy, then these are some foods to add:

Apples: I never understood the saying, "An apple a day keeps the doctor away." Actually, I don't think anyone did. It just rhymed like an early version of a hip-hop song, so I guess it stuck. The reasons apples (and pears) are lyrically gifted is they are rich in *pectin*. Pectin, as stated by scientists in the journal *BMC Microbiology,* is an excellent prebiotic that enables your gut bacteria to produce the critically important SCFA, butyrate. As mentioned in Chapter Two, butyrate is proven to help reduce inflammation and provide energy for gut cells in the large intestine. While another SCFA, *propionate,* has been found to reduce inflammation and can even help reduce visceral fat! Just to be clear, this is naturally occurring propionate made by your gut flora, not the synthetic propionate that's added to a lot of processed foods that actually increases your risk of visceral adiposity. In addition to apples, great sources of prebiotic foods that help you make propionate are garlic, onions, chicory root, jicama, Jerusalem artichoke, and asparagus.

Asparagus: These green spears are a generally common food that feature a great amount of the prebiotic fiber *inulin*. In a fascinating study published in the journal *Gut,* inulin-derived propionate was found to significantly increase the release of PYY and GLP-1. If you recall from the last chapter, those are two of your body's major hormones regulating satiety and metabolism!

Another form of inulin that's been gaining notoriety in recent years are *Fructooligosaccharides* (FOS), which are also found in asparagus, as well as leeks, onions, and bananas. But note that bananas also contain more total sugar than other commonly eaten fruits like citrus fruits and berries, so definitely be mindful of that. Don't get me wrong, a ripe banana can be better for you than a Pop-Tart, but depending on the health of your hormones and endocrine glands, going ape on bananas might not be the best idea for some people. And keep this little secret in mind: The greener the banana, the higher it is in resistant starch (which we'll get to in a minute!). And adding half of a green banana to a smoothie or incorporating some green banana flour to some of your recipes can add a kick of metabolism support by supporting your friendly neighborhood gut flora.

Cocoa: A randomized, double-blind, controlled study published by *The American Journal of Clinical Nutrition* revealed that polyphenol-rich cocoa has remarkable prebiotic effects in the human body. Study participants consuming a sugar-free cocoa flavanol drink for four weeks significantly increased their ratio of bifidobacteria and lactobacilli populations, while significantly *decreasing* their counts of clostridia (a class of firmicutes associated with fat gain). These microbial changes were paralleled by significant reductions in plasma triglycerides (blood fats) and C-reactive protein concentrations (indicating reduced inflammation). This is yet another reason why chocolate continues to make headlines when it comes to human health. But, let's get this straight. I'm not talking about the Halloween candy version of chocolate. That mutated monster of chocolate will scare your metabolism into submission. What these studies indicate is that the purest forms of chocolate, which come from the seeds where all chocolate originates, *cacao* seeds, is overflowing with potential health benefits. But, the more it's denatured, the closer it goes to the dark side.

In a different way, the dark side is really the light side when it comes to chocolate. Dark chocolate simply means higher levels of cacao and less "other stuff" like milk, sugar, and preservatives. In alignment with the study on chocolate polyphenols, you can go for cacao powder (where the cacao butter is pressed out, leaving a nutrient and fiber-rich powder) or unsweetened cocoa powder, which is cacao powder that's been processed with high heat. There is a loss of nutrients when cacao is exposed to high heat, but, as the study indicates, it's still a wonderful source of polyphenols that can easily be added to shakes, teas, and other cooking recipes.

The polyphenols in cacao and other foods appear to be a prebiotic synergist. Polyphenols are naturally occurring compounds in plants that are generally involved in defense against ultraviolet radiation or aggression by pathogens. According to the latest data, only about 5 to 10 percent of these polyphenols are directly absorbed in the small intestine when eaten, and the rest make their way to the colon to be utilized by supportive bacteria. In addition to dark cocoa, polyphenol-rich green tea and olive oil have been found to support bifidobacteria, bacteroidetes, and other friendly flora too.

The ultimate takeaway is that you can take all of the probiotic supplements you want to attempt to upgrade your microbiome, but those friendly bacteria won't stick around very long without feeding them the stuff they like. Prebiotics are a major key to remodeling your microbiome, and so are the things you're going to learn about next.

Focused Fiber

Many prebiotics fall under the umbrella of a broader, more recognizable term called *fiber*. When thinking of fiber, I used to immediately think of my grandparents. I heard them use the word and I thought it was something you talk about when you get old and your fashion sense starts to go away. I remember my grandmother having my grandfather eat prunes, and I tried one of his prunes one time, and I immediately thought that she must not like him very much.

The truth was, she actually loved him a lot and wanted to ensure that his digestion was robust and healthy. Prunes were the digestive superstar back in the '80s, but our knowledge of fiber and gut health has grown light-years since then.

Fiber facts: Fiber is generally divided into two specific camps: *soluble* and *insoluble*. The solubility of fiber refers to its ability to dissolve in water. So, soluble fiber is a type of fiber that combines easily with water in the gut. When water and soluble fiber meet, it forms a gel-like substance that supports the integrity of your gut lining, supports gut bacteria, and can have profound impacts on your metabolism. A five-year study conducted by researchers at Wake Forest University School of Medicine found that every 10-gram increase in daily soluble fiber intake leads to an additional 3.7 percent reduction in visceral fat accumulation! This study took other lifestyle factors of the 1,114 study participants into consideration, like smoking, sugar consumption, and physical activity. But soluble fiber consumption stood out as one of the most beneficial things for a healthy waistline.

Insoluble fiber does not readily combine with water like soluble fiber does. Instead, it sweeps through the gastrointestinal tract mostly intact while acting as a "bulking agent." When we think of fiber, most of us think of poop. And insoluble fiber gives the poop emoji his photogenic appearance. Plus, according to data published in *The Journal of Nutrition,* insoluble fiber takes on the bulk of the load when it comes to modulating healthy blood glucose levels.

The best fat-burning nutrition approaches are going to contain a healthy combination of both soluble and insoluble fibers. Some of the highest sources of soluble fiber include avocados, sweet potatoes, Brussels sprouts, pears, nectarines, black beans, broccoli, apples, flaxseeds, and carrots. Taking carrots, for example, a study published in the *British*

Journal of Nutrition revealed that a little more than one cup of carrots included with a lunchtime meal led to longer periods of satiety and reduced levels of hunger for study participants. I used to think that carrots were an underground mistake that only cartoon rabbits enjoyed. But, when I had them prepared in the right tasty dishes, I found an extra way to get valuable fiber, vitamin A, and another food that has beneficial effects on leptin.

Some of the best sources of insoluble fiber are berries, beans, lentils, okra, spinach, cocoa, sweet potatoes, whole grains (which we'll talk about momentarily), apples, walnuts, and almonds. Many of these foods also have compounds that feed and support diversity in your microbiome. But another thing to remember about insoluble fiber is that it supports fat loss by influencing the mechanoreceptors in your gut that deactivate hunger hormones and trigger satiety.

Another (often overlooked) way that fiber influences your body composition is by its action to aid in removing metabolic wastes from your body. Not only does fiber help eliminate toxins that can damage your cellular communities, fiber also plays a role in removing excess estrogen from your system. Researchers at the Keck School of Medicine of USC, the University of Hawaii in Honolulu, and the University of Helsinki in Finland uncovered that fiber may play an important role in the metabolism of estrogens and clearing out recirculating estrogens from the body. As you'll recall from Chapter Two, estrogen is absolutely critical to a healthy metabolism for both men and women, but carrying too much estrogen (and not being able to properly clear it) can lead to metabolic diseases and the accumulation of more body fat.

So, now you know, fiber plays a far more important role than simple waste management. But this is definitely not a permission slip to go fiber crazy. Your microbiome adjusts over time to be able to interact with higher levels of fiber. Increasing your fiber intake too quickly can cause gas, bloating, pain, and several uncomfortable conversations with your plumber.

Getting in optimal amounts of fiber is clearly a component in your fat loss equation, but be smart about it. The current RDA of dietary fiber is 25 to 30 grams, yet, many adults in the U.S. only get in about half of that! Research from the *Journal of the Academy of Nutrition and Dietetics* estimate that only about 5 percent of Americans currently meet their daily fiber requirements. With that in mind, any improvement is good improvement, and there's a lot of opportunity to get better in this department. In reality, depending upon your height, weight, digestive wellness, and current state of overall health, anywhere from 20 to even 50 grams of fiber is ideal. It's important to make sure you're meeting your needs, but there's no need to overdo it.

Remember, too much fiber can actually have detrimental effects on your gut health rather than supporting it. But not getting enough will switch off fat loss faster than you can say *Metamucil*. That said, target getting your daily fat loss fiber needs from food first because most fiber supplements tend to lack the food intelligence that ensures your gut is protected and that you're also absorbing all of the nutrients you need from your food. Fiber needs are something that you'll have to gauge a little bit more for yourself. But, as you've learned, most people aren't getting enough, and they're missing out on incredible fat-burning benefits because of it.

Soluble and insoluble are just two attributions that we give to this essential category of dietary fiber. But there are actually several other classifications of various fiber-types, like viscous fibers, fermentable fibers, and one that you really need to know about called *resistant starches*.

Resistant starch: This category of dietary fiber has been garnering a lot of attention the last few years by researchers, and for good reason. A study published in *The American Journal of Clinical Nutrition* found that resistant starch has profound effects on improving insulin sensitivity. While another study published in the journal *Nutrients* revealed that the consumption of resistant starch at breakfast and lunch led to significantly reduced appetite at dinner for overweight and obese test subjects. Again, this kind of information puts the power back into people's hands to help modulate their own metabolism and appetite, rather than haphazardly telling folks to cut calories and just go to war with their hunger. Resistant starches are another underutilized category of nutrition that supports your microbiome and your metabolism, but what the heck are they?

Starches are the main type of carbohydrates consumed in our modern-day diet. Starches ride in a fast car and have a tollbooth speed pass to enter your bloodstream very quickly and increase blood glucose. Resistant starches, on the other hand, are starches that are *resistant* to digestion and pass through your digestive tract without jumping the curb into your bloodstream. Resistant starches function like a soluble, fermentable fiber that feeds and supports your friendly gut flora. Resistant starch can take your friendly flora from battling it out on the playground with unfriendly bacteria, to moving them into safer, sustainable housing like the Fresh Bugs of Bel Air. We've already noted that green banana/green banana flour is a high source of resistant starch, but other rich food sources include cassava/cassava flour, various beans (especially white beans), oats, corn, white yams, potato starch, and cashews.

Did you happen to notice anything interesting about the color of all of these foods high in resistant starch? They all tend to be in the white, beige, and yellow color spectrum. This leads to a reminder that the *color* of natural foods are often a helpful indicator of nutritional content. Yet, again, stressing the need for us to include a variety of different foods in color, flavor, and functionality.

In addition, certain starchy foods can produce a tremendous amount of resistant starch once they are cooked and then allowed to cool all the way down. This includes two foods that are often eschewed by health advocates, which are white rice and white potatoes. If they're cooked, then refrigerated, then warmed when ready to eat, it reduces the impact on blood glucose and increases the amount of microbiome-supportive resistant starch. This goes to show you that it's not just the food, but how it's prepared and utilized that can make all the difference in the world. I'm not saying that white rice and potatoes are superstar health foods, but billions of people have subsisted on them for centuries, so there's got to be more to the story than we realize.

Our food can wear many masks, but there are a couple of go-to fiber foods that are concerning people more than others. Let's slice into them right now.

Bread

Bread has become the Ice Cube of food for many nutrition experts. It's the dough-boy staple that everyone loves to hate. And, true enough, parental advisory is suggested. I have several friends and colleagues who've written entire treatises on the secret, sinister life of modern-day wheat. Today's wheat and all of its soft, doughy offspring are well-documented to contain antinutrients and potentially problematic compounds that can sabotage your health. But is this the full story? Or is bread being toasted for no reason?

One of the big issues with bread (and wheat in general) has to do with a class of plant defense mechanisms called *lectins*. You may be wondering, "Why would a plant need defense mechanisms?" Well, plants, like all other organisms on the planet, have a driving force to live and carry on their species. But, unlike animals, plants can't just get up and run away when they're being threatened. Instead, plants have evolved their own natural defenses that act as small- to large-impact poisons to deter animals from eating or *over*eating them. Some plants have developed a symbiotic relationship with certain animals that eat them and then spread their seeds in other locations when they poop them out (along with a nice bit of organic fertilizer). That said, different animals have different digestive capacities to handle different foods. And humans don't appear to have a very friendly relationship with the lectins found in modern-day wheat.

Data published in the *British Journal of Nutrition* revealed that a lectin in wheat called *wheat germ agglutinin* (WGA) is able to punch its way through your gut lining *intact* and enter systemic circulation in your body. The whole point of digestion is to break food particles down to small, usable parts that are then pulled in through small doors by your intestinal lumen. But WGA steps on the scene with a bazooka and says, "I'll make my own door." The researchers found WGA's intrusive activity can have damaging effects on your immune system, increase inflammation, and more.

But, stick with me, because this story of wheat is going to take a twist you might not expect. Up, first, we're on to the dirtiest "g" word in the world today...*gluten.*

G's Up, Health Down

Gluten appears to be nutritional enemy #1 today. Gluten-free labels are slapped on everything from chips, to body lotions, to flavored water to give people an all-clear that it's safe to use them because gluten isn't around. Like most things, marketers take something with a decent intention and then ride it right into a level of ridiculousness. The other day I saw that a café was offering gluten-free Wi-Fi along with their coffee.

Seriously speaking, cautions surrounding gluten are based on solid science. It's even well documented in countless peer-reviewed studies that gluten can be extremely damaging for people who have an autoimmune condition called celiac disease. For these folks, gluten exposure can result in serious pain, inflammation, osteoporosis (via malnutrition), or worse. It may look like an innocent piece of bread, but for celiac patients, it might as well be a stick of dynamite.

In some rungs outside of celiac disease, gluten still has some major concerns. For instance, *gliadin,* which is one of the proteins that make up wheat gluten, has been found to trigger the intestinal release of the protein zonulin that we touched on in Chapter Two (even in non-celiac patients!). What's so alarming about this is that zonulins not only sound like an alien species on *Star Trek,* but they also have some rather alien effects on our gut lining.

Zonulins are a regulator of intestinal permeability, and when gliadin shows up on the scene, it prompts zonulins to disassemble the tight junctions of the gut lining which then allows gliadin and other wheat proteins to make their way into your bloodstream intact. Physician and *New York Times*–bestselling author Dr. William Davis shared with me that few things have the lockpicking ability to break into places they're not supposed to that gliadin does. So, whether you have celiac disease or not, gluten can disrupt your gut lining and initiate a cascade of problems, ranging from inflammation to autoimmunity.

This leads to the question of, "What in the world is gluten anyway?" Well, to put it simply, gluten is a family of proteins found in grains like wheat, rye, barley, and spelt. As far as functionality in food, gluten is what enables dough to have the flexibility of an experienced yoga instructor. When you see someone beautifully twirling pizza dough over their head, you have gluten to thank for that.

A little fun fact about wheat and gluten: For many centuries wheat flour has been used to make one of the most popular adhesives to do everything from making arts and crafts to hanging up posters for the upcoming jousting match at the royal castle. The sticky potential of wheat is used to make a little product you may have heard of called *paste*.

Other plants can be used to make paste, but gluten gives wheat paste a sticking power that helps it rise above all others. Over time, the gluten in a flour paste cross-links proteins, making it very difficult to release the adhesive. In biology, excessive cross-linking can play a role in conditions such as atherosclerosis through the creation of more *advanced glycation end products* (AGEs). With this holding true, the research indicates that gluten and bread aren't as upstanding as they once appeared to be. But, if anything, gluten is definitely multi-talented. I'll give it that. You can use it to paste pictures in your collage then turn around and use it to make a croissant. Where do you think the name *pastry* came from? Take the base ingredients for paste, then add some sugar, dairy, and other trimmings, and you've got some tasty treats for your sweet tooth. And pasta derives its name the same way. Paste-base, plus a little of this and a little of that. That's *amore*!

And, as weird as it all sounds, people have been enjoying these things for centuries, so it can't be all that bad, can it? The short answer is: It's not.

There's Two Sides to Every Slice

The first thing to note is that the type of wheat proliferating on store shelves today is not the amber waves of grain that our ancestors dined on. Wheat naturally evolved over thousands of years, but only to a modest degree. However, in the last couple of decades the makeup of wheat has been changed *dramatically* under the influence of agricultural scientists. Wheat strains have been hybridized and genetically manipulated to make it resistant to changes in environmental conditions, to make it resistant to pathogens, and (most important for food manufacturers) to increase the speed of growth and yield per acre. This manipulation has essentially resulted in a food that the human microbiome has never seen before. And, in recent years, we're seeing the results of it with growing numbers of celiac disease and gluten-related sensitivities. It's a real thing that's largely related to a less-than-real wheat.

That said, could a higher-quality wheat be better for you? Could it even have some health benefits despite its sketchy attributes? Due to the science surrounding WGA, gliadin, and other issues like phytic acid (that can block the absorption of nutrients like zinc), I avoided wheat like the plague for many years. I seemed to be all the more healthy without it and other controversial foods that are noted to come with gut-punching side effects. Still, seemingly out of the blue, I began developing food sensitivities that started to really concern me.

Foods that I'd been eating for years, from kale to cashews, suddenly started giving me digestive distress in the form of pain, bloating, and occasional nausea. My irritating foods list continued to grow and grow over the course of a couple years, and I just resolved to avoid those foods, because I felt like my normal, healthy, energetic self otherwise. When, suddenly, I realized that I started getting nervous about eating. I would lean on a handful of "safe foods" and I felt like I was rolling the dice when I ate anything outside of those. There was clearly a reason this was happening. And it was time to get to the bottom of it.

As of this writing, I'm inching close to twenty years of working in the field of health and fitness. Over this time, I've prided myself on testing things *first* before I tell another single soul about it. If I don't know what it's like firsthand, then I'm out of integrity to wholeheartedly recommend it to people. So, I spent years at a time experimenting with different diets, foods, and supplements. From plant-based raw food diets, to omnivorous keto diets, to near monthlong juicing diets, and everything in between. I had to know what it did, what it felt like, and what the benefits and pitfalls to each thing were, and it enabled me to reach and help a lot of people. But using my body as the facility for all of these experiments had my personal microbiome ready to put in its two weeks' notice.

Rather than continuing on my game of Russian roulette with different foods to see what would bother me and what wouldn't, I decided to get some advanced microbiome testing done. With the right testing, you can find out which bacteria, yeasts, viruses, or even parasites might be holding up shop in your internal ecosystem. And when my results came back, to my surprise, I had a substantial situation of *gut dysbiosis.* As defined in the peer-reviewed journal *Microbial Ecology in Health and Disease,* gut dysbiosis involves the breakdown of the pivotal mutualistic relationship between gut bacteria, their metabolic products, and the host's immune system. To put it directly, I had an overgrowth of opportunistic bacteria, and was lacking key friendly strains of bacteria that helped keep them in check. I was psyched to know what the issue was, but I was surprised, yet again, by what the solution was going to be.

A physician and friend of mine working on this case with me got me to see, in yet another light, the importance of feeding your friendly flora the right thing. I consumed the right stuff to eliminate the high levels of this pathogenic bacteria strain, I took the probiotics and ate the probiotic foods to bring the levels of friendly flora up, but when I retested a couple months later, the results had barely changed. He looked at the results with me and he and I both knew that I didn't take all his recommendations when we saw the initial results. He said, "Did you add the beans and bread like I suggested?" In my mind I was thinking about all of the negative things attributed to those two foods...the lectins, the antinutrients...no way they could help me *fix* this problem like he suggested. He reiterated, "If you add these sources of resistant starch, in addition to all of the other good things you're doing, you'll be able to turn this around in no time." He wasn't asking me to eat the run-of-the-mill stuff. He implored me to suspend my disbelief and add a slice or two of sprouted grain bread (organic, free from genetic tampering, and free from anything artificial) a few times per week. And on other days add a variety of beans and brown rice (another noted source of anti-nutrients I was avoiding) and just see what the results say.

Reluctantly, I did it. And within a couple of months, all of my digestive distress and food sensitivities went away. My lab results came back with spectacular success and, years later, my digestion is healthy, efficient, and robust. As it turns out, certain grains (even some that contain gluten) can function as an excellent resistant starch that supports friendly bacteria for *some* people.

But what about the potential negative side effects of things like gluten, WGA, and phytic acid? In Chapter Two, I noted a study published in the journal *Nutrients* that demonstrated how gluten prompts the release of zonulin (which increases the permeability of your gut lining). Though I also noted that even the researchers in the study affirmed that the way the gluten was prepared or cooked made a difference in its effects. Many studies are using isolated compounds found in grains, and not the whole foods themselves that are prepared properly and traditionally. Historically, when making bread, it was common to have the grains sprouted and/or fermented, and cooked. All of these things reduce the content of several of these anti-nutrients. Unless your name is Huckleberry Finn, nobody's running around chewing on raw strands of wheat anyway. Just the process of cooking destroys WGA, as demonstrated in a study published in the journal *Food Control*. And another recent study published in the journal *Nutrients* found that levels of WGA are completely undetectable in cooked, whole wheat pasta. Oh, and not to forget phytic acid, a study published in the *Journal of Agriculture and Food Chemistry* found that sprouting grains is an effective way to reduce phytic acid and increase nutrient absorption.

Overall, sprouted and/or fermented grains (especially heirloom grains) are far better than the vast majority of grain-based products on the store shelves. Most grain-based products are heavily refined and contain a tremendous amount of fast-digesting sugars that pathogenic bacteria thrive on, which definitely makes your metabolism suffer as a result. However, data published in *the British Journal of Nutrition* attests that the right type of whole grains can significantly *increase* the ratio of the friendly floras bifidobacteria and lactobacilli for some folks who are not intolerant. And a 16-year meta-analysis published in the journal *Public Health Nutrition* found that study participants who occasionally ate a couple servings of whole grains had a lower body mass index (BMI) and lower levels of visceral fat.

Now, just to be clear, I'm not saying to run out and make a spaghetti sandwich (a real thing I've seen eaten at several family get-togethers). Even a *tiny* exposure to the anti-nutrients contained in grains could be problematic for some people. But we need to work on not being so black-and-white about things that we miss all of the beautiful colors possible. Several health experts insist that "if you simply eliminate bread and other anti-nutrient-containing foods, then boom, all your problems will be solved!" But following any one diet to the detriment of our own health is just silly. We each need to take a smarter approach and allow for the flexibility to do the right things for us, as we are right now, and the person that we will be in the future. Our health is one of the most fluid and changing things in the universe. Everything in our bodies, from our mitochondria to our microbiome, from our heart to our hormones, are constantly varying, evolving, and reshaping themselves. Our food choices need to reflect and support that.

Again, if you are uncertain about your body's response to bread and other grain-based foods, it can likely do your body and metabolism a lot of good to avoid them. I rarely, if ever, eat bread myself today. But I'm also not against folks doing what supports their own health. If you believe that bread is the Darth Vader of the nutritional world, then simply avoid it. But if you feel bread is the handsome antihero like Han Solo, then you have free rein to occasionally add it in if it's prepared more traditionally. I just want to provide you with the facts so that you can make smart decisions on what's best for you and where you are right now.

There are other concerns about carb-dominant, grain-based foods, like their potentially aggressive impact on insulin, for one example. I was taught in my university classes to recommend that people eat seven to eleven servings of whole grains each day. This is just wildly inappropriate for most people, if simply looking at the impact on blood sugar and hormone health alone. Even the sheer amount recommended isn't based on any sound science. Someone just made it up. It could have easily gone something like this:

Government agent 1: Hey, Bill, I'm back from break. Whatcha working on?

Government agent 2 (Bill): Ahh, I'm just trying to come up with some numbers for this new food pyramid. Where'd you go for your break?

Government agent 1: Oh, I just went to 7-Eleven and grabbed a hot dog and Super Big Gulp.

Government agent 2: That's it! You're a genius. Seven to eleven it is!

Government agent 1: Huh? Have you been putting alcohol in your coffee again?

Government agent 2: Yes, but that's beside the point. Seven to eleven servings of whole grains a day has a nice ring to it. That will be the base of the entire food pyramid we'll recommend everyone should eat.

Government agent 1: Sounds good, Bill. Glad I could be of assistance.

Despite the potential digestive problems from conventional grains, and despite the hormone-deranging effects of all those starches, this is what education at the highest levels were teaching just a few short years ago. We've come a long way already, but the beautiful thing is that you no longer have to wait around for the conventional health education system to get their act together. With your knowledge of eating smarter, you'll be far ahead of the curve and equipped with tools, strategies, and insights that will keep you thriving for many years to come. And keep in mind, if you ever feel inspired to get some convenient testing done for the health of your microbiome, I'll always have my recommended resources available for you in the Eat Smarter Bonus Resource guide at eatsmarterbook.com/bonus.

A Quickie on Beans

Beans are another staple for millions of people all over the world. Even though they are still a carb-dominant food, they provide a higher ratio of protein than a lot of other plant-based foods, and they also provide a potentially phenomenal source of resistant starch. But beans can show up with a lot of baggage (and if you open the baggage it's full of lectins). According to the Centers for Disease Control, approximately 20 percent of all food poisoning cases in the United States are the result of lectins in improperly cooked beans. You know the old song, "Beans, beans, good for your heart, but if you cook them wrong you'll end up in the ER."

My friend, and #1 *New York Times*–bestselling author, Dr. Steven Gundry reiterated: "Beans are a great source of resistant starches (that your friendly gut flora can use), as long as you remove those nasty lectins." Dr. Gundry was concerned for his patients who he referred to as "pasta-grain-bean-atarians" who were striving for a healthy plant-based diet, but struggled to pull out these standard sources of protein, even though they were making them sick. He affirmed that most folks would do best to avoid grains altogether, but upon further research into beans, he found that problematic lectins could be effectively eliminated by employing a few different tactics.

He's a big proponent of utilizing a pressure cooker to cook beans, which is one of the most efficient ways to destroy lectins. Various versions of pressure cookers have actually been used for hundreds of years. But, today, the technology (based on a traditional cooking method) is incredible, and a pressure cooker can be one of your best friends in the kitchen. Other methods to reduce and/or eliminate toxins in beans are to 1) soak the beans in water for several hours before cooking and 2) ensure that you thoroughly cook the beans in your conventional pot, slow cooker, etc. until they are tender. Undercooked beans are a sign that there are still lectins lurking.

If beans are a preferred food for you, and now that you are making sure they're properly cooked, here are a couple of ways they can benefit your fat loss mission:

Earlier we covered some fascinating data indicating that a higher ratio of bacteroidetes in your gut, as compared to firmicutes, is directly linked to improved body composition and less weight gain. Beans are among the very best foods to raise your bacteroidetes. In addition to that, a study conducted at UC-Davis and published in *The Journal of Nutrition* revealed that the fiber from beans can significantly increase CCK. As you'll recall, CCK plays an important role in regulating appetite and it could even play a key role in reducing levels of body fat. And this is what appears to be highlighted in a recent study published in *The American Journal of Clinical Nutrition*. Study participants (who weren't even on a calorie-restricted diet!) ended up losing significantly more weight having beans, lentils, and/or chickpeas in their diet versus people who did not. Again, fiber is an essential part of your fat loss protocol, and a variety of different fiber types really is the key. Whether it's green leafy vegetables, starchy tubers, properly prepared beans or grains, nuts and seeds, or low-sugar fruits, now you know why fiber really matters.

So let's head into the next category of foods to supercharge the health of your metabolism by fortifying your microbiome.

Rice Rice Baby

When I was in college, one of the most staunch nutritional rules my professors advocated was to avoid everything "white" and go for the whole grain versions instead. One of the most common foods we were told to nix was white rice. I got it... it was very low in vitamins and minerals, low in (conventional) fiber, and high in blood sugar–spiking starch. But I immediately wondered why cultures from all over the world have been eating white rice for centuries. Did they not get the memo? Was white rice just more sexy to the eyes? Why would they remove what appears to be the most nutritious parts of the rice?

Many generations ago, our ancestors began removing the parts of the rice that make it brown—the bran and the germ—and eating the stripped down white rice instead. Not because white rice was too sexy for its clothes, but because there were pesky gut irritants in the bran and germ. Having the stripped down rice was an easy way to get calories without the digestive distress. My college professors, and the world of popular nutrition at the time, had not taken this into consideration when brown rice was hailed as the fallen king of rice to be recrowned to its hearty throne of fiber.

Well, you've already learned in *Eat Smarter* that white rice has surprising attributes of resistant starch when cooled. Plus, the potential gut irritants have been removed. That's a couple of pros in the battle for rice ruler. But brown rice isn't going to get polished off that easily. Brown rice does, indeed, have a significantly higher amount of nutrients than white rice like selenium, magnesium, zinc and, of course, fiber. The problem is that the potential anti-nutrients can disrupt digestion for some people and even block nutrient absorption.

The winner in the white rice versus brown rice debate? Well, it all depends on your nutritional goals and how you prepare the rice. If you want a source of quick carbs, resistant starch, and to just avoid contact with brown rice's possible anti-nutrients altogether, then white rice is your candidate. But if you want more nutrients, fiber, and enjoy the more earthy flavor, you can place your vote for brown rice. I'd just recommend you purchase sprouted brown rice or soak and sprout the brown rice yourself to drastically reduce the amount of latent gut irritants. Using a pressure cooker to make your brown rice can be an effective way to reduce potential anti-nutrients, too.

Probiotic Foods

While working at a university for many years, I had the opportunity to work with people from all over the world. One of the questions I would always ask people was, "What type of fermented food or beverages did you have in your country?" Whether it was Kenya or China, Brazil or Germany, every culture has some type of traditionally prepared fermented food. It fascinated me to hear about the diversity in types, and it continued to strike me that people have prized cultured foods for thousands of years. And it's even in the name, *culture*!

Civilizations throughout time valued the benefits of fermented foods, and through today's scientific analysis we're finally understanding why. We've already covered how prebiotics and fiber are the substances that make our friendly flora feel supported and welcomed. Now it's time to identify some of the best friendly flora-rich probiotic foods to help support your metabolism and your health overall.

Kimchi

Heavily studied the last few years for its notable anti-obesity benefits, kimchi is gaining massive popularity outside of its original home in Korea. Kimchi is a spicy, fermented vegetable side dish that has a base of cabbage and can include an assortment of other ingredients like ginger, garlic, daikon radishes, carrots, red pepper, fish sauce, scallions, and more. A peer-reviewed study published in the journal *Nutrition Research* found that eating kimchi leads to a significant decrease in body fat, hip-to-waist ratio, and fasting blood sugar for study participants versus those who merely ate the unfermented form of the cabbage dish. Something really cool happens when the bacteria integrate with it, and it has positive effects on our metabolism.

One of the reasons that I really love kimchi is that it's a great source of friendly flora that also comes along with fiber from the vegetables. Kimchi is a dish that many more folks are taking advantage of today. You can make it yourself, you can find it at many authentic restaurants, and you can also find it jarred in many grocery stores. It will be located in the refrigerated section near its close relative, sauerkraut.

Sauerkraut

Growing up, sauerkraut was another food that I saw adults around me eating, and I just didn't understand why. "You mean to tell me you guys are going to eat that stinky, weird-looking stuff when you could be eating mac and cheese instead? No thank you!" The truth is, millions of kids eat sauerkraut every day, I was just indoctrinated into the meal-from-a-box culturescape. And it's actually quite tasty when it's prepared the right way. Plus, equally as important, it has some impressive health benefits that are hard to find anywhere else.

Sauerkraut is one of the most common and oldest forms of preserving cabbage that can be traced all the way back to the 4th century BC. It's a rich source of vitamins and minerals like vitamin C, B vitamins, vitamin K, and iron, and it's also a great source of fiber. These are all players in a healthy metabolism, but sauerkraut has some more specific actions as well. A study published in the journal *PLOS ONE* found that a probiotic strain found in sauerkraut (lactobacillus) can potentially defend against fat gain by modulating genes associated with metabolism and inflammation in the liver and adipose tissue. Bacteria aren't just assistant managers of our metabolism, they also influence our genetic expression!

Earlier in this chapter we discussed the critical importance of having diversity in your microbiome to support your metabolism. Research cited in the journal *Applied and Environmental Microbiology* demonstrated that one serving of sauerkraut can provide around 30 different strains of bacteria. But make sure to avoid purchasing pasteurized, off-the-shelf versions of sauerkraut, because the vast majority of the probiotics will have been destroyed. Typically, probiotic-rich sauerkraut will be found in the refrigerated section, but still check the label to be sure. Also, keep an eye out to avoid unnecessary additives and preservatives. It should be cabbage, water, salt, and that's it. Some brands might spruce it up by adding some other veggies, but real sauerkraut doesn't have anything artificial.

Yogurt

I wonder about the very first time anyone ever tried fermented dairy a few thousand years ago. It was probably a big brother, little brother situation.

Big brother: Hey, the milk is gone bad again. I dare you to still have some.
Little brother: No way, dude. That's gross.
Big brother: Come on...I'll let you wear my new loincloth to school tomorrow if you do.
Little brother: Deal!

However it might have gone down, someone discovered many centuries ago that the beneficial bacteria resulting from cultured milk had some significant health benefits. Yogurt is made from milk that has been fermented by friendly bacteria, mainly lactic acid bacteria and bifidobacteria. A recent study published in the *British Journal of Nutrition* found that yogurt consumption was able to reduce biomarkers of chronic inflammation and endotoxin exposure in many of the test subjects. Keeping in mind that inflammation is one of the *Three Amigos of Body Fat Growth*, the researchers postulated that yogurt is able to reduce inflammation by improving the integrity of the gut lining.

Another study, conducted by researchers at the University of Connecticut, uncovered that yogurt has a strange, unexpected superpower. The researchers gave test subjects some pretty crappy, high-calorie/low-quality food for breakfast. They wanted to "stress their metabolism" and see if there would be any influence if they consumed yogurt beforehand. One group was given a serving of yogurt just prior to their meal, while another group was given a serving of non-dairy pudding. The test subjects were then instructed to eat a total of 900 calories of breakfast food you'd find at a typical fast food restaurant—two sausage biscuits and two hash browns. They had them fast for several hours beforehand so they were hungry enough to get it all down, and then set out to monitor their biomarkers over the next several hours. Here's what they found...

Test subjects who had yogurt prior to their meal had significant reductions in certain endotoxin markers (endotoxins are toxic substances bound to your bacterial cell walls). The researchers also noted that in obese participants, post-meal glucose levels dropped back to baseline faster in the yogurt group. This indicates that this fermented food can improve glucose metabolism in some people.

Now, yogurt is as broad of a term as someone saying they're an artist. We've got everything from sculptors, to musicians, to "sandwich artists" at Subway. Not saying either one is more artistic, but they're definitely not the same thing. In the same vein, there's so many different versions of yogurt, it can be hard to keep up with it all. Fat-free yogurt, low-fat yogurt, or full-fat yogurt. Sweetened yogurt or sugar-free yogurt. Artificially flavored and colored yogurt marketed to kids and Greek yogurt marketed to anyone who had to read *Odyssey* in high school. There's organic yogurt, yogurt with live cultures, grass-fed dairy yogurt, and yogurts made from nondairy sources. Again, yogurt is a very broad term, so here's a few things to look for if you're hankering for some.

A multiyear study that included over 18,000 women found that a greater intake of high-fat dairy products (including yogurt) was associated with less weight gain than study participants consuming low-fat dairy products. Go for full-fat yogurt if it suits your fancy, it's better for your hormones and better for your microbiome. Also, shoot for naturally sweetened, low-sugar or sugar-free yogurt or you could be shooting up your insulin levels. Many conventional yogurts actually contain as much sugar as two glazed donuts. Our inner Homer Simpson knows exactly what a donut is, but many yogurts hide under the guise of being healthy. Don't fall for it the next time you're at your local grocery store or Kwik-E-Mart. Add your own fresh fruit or low-glycemic natural sweetener to give your plain yogurt a glow up without all of the sugar. Additionally, organic and grass-fed varieties contain less potential allergens that disrupt your gut health rather than support it.

What if you're lactose intolerant or dairy is just not your cup-o-cheese? It may seem strange, but yogurt may be suitable for some people with lactose intolerance. This is because the bacteria turn most of the lactose (milk sugar) into lactic acid, which is also why yogurt has a sour bite to it. Plus, today there is a wide array of nondairy yogurt options, from coconut milk to oat milk–based, and more. Though keep in mind that the overwhelming majority of research on the benefits of yogurt has come from dairy yogurt. Nondairy options haven't been studied much as of yet, but that's not to say they're not viable options.

Natto, Miso, and Tempeh

If there were a food that would have paparazzi chasing it around to try and capture some of its controversy, it would definitely be soy. Soy is one of the most widely used foods in our world today. Its historic use hails from several countries in and around Asia dating all the way back to 9000 BC. Traditionally, soy has been utilized by many long-lived cultures as a rich source of protein and as a staple for several different fermented foods. So, with its long history of use, why has it become so controversial?

Well, for starters, cultures that regularly consumed soy did so in small amounts. We're talking a couple of ounces a day, at most. Whereas today, millions of people are consuming massive amounts of highly processed soy in the form of soy burgers, soy hot dogs, soy milk, soy cheese, soy nuggets, soy ice cream, soy cereal, soy bacon, soy sandwich slices, and there's even a big mound of soy "meat" molded together in the shape of a ham for the holidays. Things have gotten soy out of hand that its more noble origins have been lost along the way. Just from a simple place of logic, this much newly invented processed food cannot be that good for you. In addition to that, the sources of soy, and the way that it's prepared, have taken a turn into a sketchy neighborhood.

Many of the concerns over increased soy consumption have to do with anti-nutrients and its potential influence on our hormones. For our intents and purposes, we'll take a brief look at how it can potentially impact our metabolism.

Soy contains problematic lectins like those similar to wheat. They're under a category of *soybean agglutinins* (SBAs) that have been found to cause inflammation and increased intestinal permeability. The phytic acid and protein inhibitors in soy have been revealed to block the absorption of key minerals and amino acids that can depress your metabolism as well. Additionally, soy also contains *goitrogens* that can negatively impact the thyroid by blocking iodine absorption, and research published in the journal *Biochemical Pharmacology* found that phytoestrogens in soy can potentially block the production of thyroid hormones. Now, this sounds like soy has some serious explaining to do. The paparazzi cameras are flashing, and soy has been dressing really weird lately.

Back in the day, nearly all of these potential concerns were eliminated through traditional preparation. Soybeans were consistently fermented to decrease the amount of problematic compounds and increase the action of beneficial bacteria. Today's science affirms the effectiveness of traditional fermentation with a study published in the journal *Food Research International,* noting that the fermentation of soybeans successfully removes up to 95 percent of the lectins present. Even customary preparation of tofu involved the use of fermentation and bacteria. Probiotic-rich foods like natto and tempeh, originating from Japan and Indonesia respectively, have some remarkable health benefits too. Natto is one of the best natural sources of vitamin K2, and a new study published in the *European Journal of Clinical Nutrition* revealed that optimal vitamin K2 levels improved the function of adiponectin (one of the hormones from Chapter Two that influences your appetite and your fat metabolism). The study also found that test subjects experienced greater amounts of weight loss, reduced levels of visceral fat, and reductions in abdominal fat mass overall.

Research conducted at the Institute of Food Technology of Plant Origin at Poznań University of Life Sciences in Poland demonstrated that tempeh is a notable source of prebiotics *and* probiotics, with several of the most beneficial strains of friendly bacteria that support human metabolism. And data published in the peer-reviewed journal *Pharmaceutical Biology* uncovered that fermented tempeh has far greater antioxidant capacity than uncultured soy does alone, with antioxidants acting as another defense against chronic inflammation.

Miso, another staple from Japan, is a traditional seasoning produced by fermenting soybeans with salt and a fungus called *koji.* This fermented paste is used for things ranging from sauces, to pickling vegetables or meats, to mixing with soup stock to create the renowned miso soup. Data published in the *Journal of the Japanese Society for Food Science and Technology* found that study participants who consumed miso with their meal had improved insulin function and a faster normalization of post-meal blood glucose levels.

Natto, Miso, and Tempeh may sound like a more cultured version of the Jonas Brothers, but they've got the music to back it up. They hit a variety of flavor notes and versatility that enables them to be used in a plethora of dishes. Again, it's important to remember that these benefits are seen with a *small* amount of soy in the diet which, according to data from the American Thyroid Association, doesn't appear to have deleterious effects on thyroid function. But once we venture into a battle of the bands that includes regular consumption of the Frankenfood versions of soy, all bets are off.

Kombucha

Kombucha is the hottest thing to hit the streets since the invention of yoga pants and jeggings. There's a ton of anecdotal evidence purporting that kombucha can be supportive of everything from weight loss to enhanced digestion. Though there currently isn't a lot a clinical evidence on the benefits of kombucha, this summation will share with you some of the things that we know.

Kombucha is a fermented black tea (or sometimes green tea) with origins tracing back at least two thousand years. It's made by adding specific strains of bacteria, yeast, and sugar to the tea, then allowing it to ferment for a week or more. The birthplace of this process is often attributed to China or Japan, but today you can regularly find kombucha in grocery stores, restaurants, and I'm pretty sure I saw an ice cream truck selling kombucha on tap before.

Early data, like that published in the *Journal of Microbiology and Biotechnology,* revealed that kombucha has antioxidant effects that could be protective of your liver (which you'll recall is a major player in your metabolic function). Another study featured in the *Journal of Food Biochemistry* found that the bacteria in kombucha can potentially reduce the ratio of pathogenic microbes and support the proliferation of friendly microbes.

What's unique about kombucha is that it also features the metabolism-boosting effects of black and green tea. Research in *The American Journal of Clinical Nutrition* showed that these teas have thermogenic properties that promote fat oxidation beyond that explained by caffeine itself. The combination of nutrients in tea have a synergistic effect on burning fat that you'll be hard-pressed to find anywhere else.

You can definitely utilize teas, but if you choose to utilize their fermented cousin, kombucha, there are a few words of caution. One, be mindful of the sugar content. The bacteria in kombucha are supposed to eliminate the vast majority of sugar, but (depending on how it's made) there can sometimes be a hefty amount left behind. Two, be careful about the alcohol content. Some batches of kombucha have been found to contain up to 3 percent alcohol (close to what's found in beer). You might be showing up to get a dose of friendly flora but end up dancing on top of the conveyor belt at Whole Foods instead. Check the label, but also check in on how this (and any other food or beverage) makes you feel. Your body is the ultimate guidance when pinning down your preferred source of fermented products, and we've got just a couple more options to cover.

Pickles

Pickling is another valuable method of food preservation dating back thousands of years. At a time before the invention of modern refrigeration, pickling was a primary way to preserve various foods for future consumption. With origins spanning across Africa, India, Asia, and Europe, besides being able to keep food edible longer, pickling was found to have some surprising additional benefits.

Pickles (and pickle juice) have been found to provide beneficial flora, improve digestion, support healthy blood glucose levels, and even reduce inflammation. Recently, thanks in part to a study published in *Medicine & Science in Sports & Exercise,* pickle juice has become popular for athletes as it was found to work better than water at reducing muscle cramps. Pickles (and pickle juice) have naturally occurring electrolytes and antioxidants that support performance and metabolism.

When we think of pickles, we generally think of the offspring of cucumbers. But you can "pickle" just about anything. Around the world, people are pickling everything from peaches, plums, and berries to prawns, fish, and eggs. Many of these pickled foods are prized in their various cultures for their taste and their health benefits. Pickled cucumbers are definitely a favorite here in the U.S., and it's something that I enjoyed growing up, especially *hot* pickles. Pickles can be flavored different ways using salt, sugar, hot peppers, and/or a variety of different herbs. Now, just a word to the wise: Fermentation is a way to make pickles, but pickles are not always fermented. Instead of pickling using the traditional method of fermentation, sometimes food manufacturers use vinegar to make the cucumber twerk its way into pickle form. Vinegar, itself, is made by a fermentation process, but, if it's pasteurized, it has lost its potential probiotic powers.

Kefir

This fermented, probiotic-rich drink dates back thousands of years as well. The name *kefir* appears to originate from a Turkish word that means "feeling good." Which immediately makes me wonder if the actor Kiefer Sutherland's parents knew that and secretly named their son "Feeling Good" Sutherland. He's helped to create some absolute classics, by the way. Thanks for helping us to feel good, Kiefer!

The probiotic drink kefir was originally made from milk by adding what came to be known as *kefir grains* (which are not actually grains, but rather, they're cultures of bacteria and yeast) to goat's milk or cow's milk. Today, there are several other kefir beverage options like coconut kefir and even water kefir. They're often developed into a fizzy drink that can be a tasty upgrade from conventional soda that also provides antioxidants, vitamins, minerals, and support for your microbiome.

I recently did a keynote speech for the students and faculty at Dalhousie University in Halifax, Nova Scotia, Canada, and I was intrigued to find out that their biology department was doing research on the probiotics found in kefir. Their data, published in the journal *PLOS ONE* demonstrated that these probiotics could be helpful for both the treatment *and* prevention of several gastrointestinal issues. Additionally, a study cited in the *Journal of Functional Foods* asserts that traditionally made kefir can potentially reduce liver triglycerides and improve fatty acid metabolism. This is pretty impressive stuff to sip on, and yet another viable source of probiotics to include on a regular basis.

METABOLIC FURNACE

When it comes to fat loss, supporting your microbiome is of the utmost importance. Hopefully, what you've learned thus far has shined a bright light on a subject that has remained in the dark for far too long. Eating smarter will enable you to enhance the function of your metabolism by optimizing your microbiome at several different levels. By ensuring the regular intake of prebiotics, resistant starch, and fiber (in general), you'll ensure that you are providing your friendly gut flora the nutrition they need to keep the foundation of your metabolism in good working order.

In the Eat Smarter 30-Day Program (page 355), you'll have access to smarter food lists featuring the foods we've covered and several more that you can utilize from each category. During the program, each day you will target at least one or two prebiotic foods, one to two servings of resistant starch, and 20 to 50 grams of fiber (depending on your individual needs) from a variety of foods and fiber types based on the recommendations from this chapter. As for probiotic foods themselves, strive to include at least three to four servings of fermented foods and/or beverages each week. Again, quality matters a lot, and I have some of my favorite resources in the Eat Smarter Bonus Resource Guide that I'll keep updated for you online as new products and innovations come along.

Your body's metabolic furnace is ignited by your microbiome. But the rest of your Three Fat Loss Essentials will fan the flames of transformation even more. So, it's time to level up with our next one!

CHAPTER FOUR

Fat Loss Essential #2: Mind Your Macros

Real food is the stuff that fuels real life!

~*Kristina Turner*

Macronutrients are a gigantic focus in the world of health and nutrition today. But there are some major holes in many people's game that can leave them falling short of winning their fat loss trophy.

If nutrition was starting a basketball team of macronutrients, its stars would be the Big Three: protein, carbohydrates, and fat. They make most of the headlines and take up the most space on the stat sheet for many folks, but you can't have a full team without some other key players. The underrated "glue" of the macronutrient team would be water. He doesn't get a lot of credit, but you'd never have any dunks, tear drops, or swishes without him. The fifth player in the macronutrient starting lineup is alcohol. Alcohol is like the Dennis Rodman of the team. He can get you a few points and grab you some unexpected rebounds, but he might end up kicking someone or get married to... himself. And no squad would be complete without a sixth man coming off the bench. On the macronutrient team, that would be fiber. He's a great role player, he keeps everything moving, and brings a lot of value to the team. We've already covered fiber in the last chapter, and thanks to that new data, he might win the award for most improved player. But now it's time to cover all of your Starting Five in a way that you've never heard before. What you're about to learn will enable you to put these players in the right position for yourself and bring your fat loss championship home!

POWER-DUNKING PROTEIN

In Chapter Two we talked about how protein is the most underrated player today when people are talking about the Big Three macronutrients. Many people think it's just a one-dimensional player that builds muscle. But protein can do a whole lot more than dunk on you.

Protein is actually an all-around player that can help you manage blood glucose, burn body fat, and even help regulate your appetite. Researchers at the University of Kansas Medical Center used fMRIs and discovered that adding more protein, specifically for your first meal of the day, literally decreases the signals in the brain that stimulate appetite and lead to overeating. A performance like this should be making front page news! But it will take all of us to help spread the word about it.

Remember, part of protein's allure is the fact that it's a building block of your valuable muscle tissue (which helps you burn more calories simply by having more of it on your frame). But another aspect of protein's fat-burning skills is that you actually burn more calories digesting protein than digesting any of the other Big Three. As a refresher, 20 to 30 percent of total calories in the protein you eat goes into digesting it, while approximately 5 to 10 percent of the calories in carbohydrates are used just to digest it, and the caloric energy used to digest fats are generally in the range of 0 to 3 percent. It's the thermic effect of food, and protein lights up the scoreboard like nothing else can.

In order to garner more respect for protein's gameplay, earlier in the book we also noted a study that was published in *The Journal of Nutrition* showing that increasing protein intake led to enhanced weight loss and reduced blood fat levels in the study participants. To take it a Eurostep further, Danish scientists at Copenhagen University Hospital published research featured in *The American Journal of Clinical Nutrition* revealing that, over the course of a five-year study, no macronutrient reduced the amount of belly fat for study participants more than protein had. The scientists noted that the outstanding results were particularly from animal-based protein. Don't worry if you'd rather be an animal on the court than eat one. We'll cover some proven plant-based options in a moment.

This is so important to understand because as our society's recommended ratio of carbohydrates has gone up (see: the old-school food pyramid that jacked a lot of people up), but our collective consumption of *high-quality* protein has actually gone down. Many experts would lead us to believe that we are consuming excessive amounts of protein and running around eating meat and cheese sandwiches that have two pieces of fried chicken for a bun. Yes, this does actually exist thanks to the Voldemort-level scientists at KFC, but most folks are not eating that stuff. Millions of people have been fighting hard going on and off the diet train that proposes they eat sinister amounts of whole grains, magically huge amounts of skimpy salads, and Weasley low-calorie snacks. But encouraging optimal amounts of protein has been overlooked long enough. In fact, research conducted by the U.S. military and cited in the peer-reviewed *Journal of Nutrition* uncovered that, despite the generally accepted belief that protein intake above the RDA increases cardiometabolic risk, higher-protein diets are associated with *lower* BMI, *lower* levels of visceral fat, and an *improved* cholesterol profile compared to protein intakes at RDA levels. Their data took into account an array of other factors including age, sex, carbohydrate intake, and physical activity. And the scientists found, surprisingly, that a higher ratio of protein can actually *lower* your risk of developing cardiometabolic disease.

Now, before you go out and try to score career highs with protein, there are a couple of caveats you need to know about. At no point did any of the data advocate a *high* protein diet, just a *higher* protein diet (meaning a shift in the percentage of protein as compared to the carbohydrates and fat someone is consuming). Especially if it's on the low side, changing that ratio of protein can have some remarkable benefits. But if protein is overused, and you are consistently nibbling on things like that Voldemort sandwich, it can increase your risk of problems to the tune of damage to your microbiome, constipation, excessive stress to your liver, heart, and kidneys, and even something clinically we refer to as *halitosis* (lesser known as stank breath).

You might be thinking, "I thought people in the U.S. were already eating *too much* protein." But if you look at the dietary intake stats from the U.S. government, you see that the number of people not getting enough of the RDA amount of protein is nearly equal to the number of people who are at or surpassing the RDA amount of protein. Keeping in mind that the RDA is considered to be low by some standards (and generally, the recommended amount is just enough to keep you from a protein deficiency–related disease). In fact, brand-new data is affirming that certain populations of U.S. citizens are definitely not getting enough protein.

A study conducted by researchers at the Ohio State University and published in *The Journal of Nutrition, Health and Aging* revealed that as we age our protein requirements are even more important. The research analyzed study participants age 51 and up for nearly ten years and found that approximately 46 percent of the oldest participants did not consume enough protein on a regular basis. This led to higher rates of muscle loss, increased risk of fractures, and higher levels of other nutrient deficiencies. The study reported that people who didn't eat enough protein were also less likely to get in sufficient amounts of key micronutrients (which we'll get to soon). One of the study authors stated that, "Despite the protein craze in America, the data shows there's still a big gap in adults' protein intake." Some folks are overshooting their intake of protein (especially of low-quality, nutrient-deficient sources) while some folks are drastically undershooting their intake of protein.

Part of eating smarter is getting clear about where you reside on this protein spectrum and ensuring that you're getting the right amount of protein for *you* where you are right now in your life. Your protein requirements are a unique part of your metabolic fingerprint. There are generally two camps—Camp 1: Protein doesn't matter that much and Camp 2: Protein is everything. Both camps need to do some team building exercises, because the answer usually exists somewhere in the middle. My goal is for you to be mindful about getting enough of this critical, fat loss–supporting macronutrient, but without going so hard in the paint with excess protein that you end up fouling out (in terms of rebound fat gain and overstressing your internal organs).

So, how do you find out the right amount of protein for you? Referencing back to a study from Chapter Two that was published in *The American Journal of Clinical Nutrition,* researchers put test subjects on either an "adequate protein diet" (toward the minimum that would prevent degenerative illness) with 10 percent of their caloric intake coming from protein, or a higher protein diet where 30 percent of their caloric intake was coming from protein. The results clearly showed that test subjects with a higher protein ratio had a higher resting metabolic rate, higher levels of fat oxidation, and higher levels of satiety. They burned more fat *and* they were more satisfied. That's what I'd call all-star gameplay!

This study echoes many other studies affirming that hitting around 30 percent protein in your macronutrient ratio appears to be the most effective for fat loss. Please note, you, as a unique individual, may require a little more or a little less to put your metabolism in the right position. You have the free rein to test, and the results will be seen in the way that you look, feel, and perform. But going off of our comprehensive target of 30 percent, you can find the number of grams to aim for by multiplying your calorie intake by 0.075. For example, on a 2,000-calorie diet you would calculate 2,000 x 0.075, which is 150 grams of protein. For many folks struggling to lose fat, this number might be a far cry from where they're at. They're battling their metabolism by cutting more calories, when they really just need to shift their macronutrient ratio. The good news is that it's never too late to adjust and test.

Another prominent way of determining your protein needs is by aiming for a particular amount based on your body weight. This is yet another method that has a broad range of recommended amounts. The U.S. RDA is currently 0.4 gram protein for each pound of body weight. So, for a person weighing 170 pounds, this translates to 68 grams of protein per day (170 x 0.4 = 68). According to some experts, this could be enough to maintain basic functioning for the average person, while other experts assert that it's nowhere near enough for optimal function. Your protein needs will depend on several unique factors that contribute to your metabolic fingerprint, like your gender, age, ethnicity, and current level of activity. For example, the more physical work you put in, the higher your protein needs will tend to be. The International Society of Sports Nutrition's daily protein recommendation is 0.9 gram protein per pound of body weight for athletes. So, for a 170-pound person, that's 153 grams of protein each day. That's more than *twice* the baseline RDA. But neither one is right or wrong, there's only identifying what's right for *you*. And eating smarter gives you the insights to do so.

Quality over Quantity

You want to know one of the most overlooked reasons that adequate, high-quality protein is so important? Well, remember all of the remarkable hormones we've covered that actually control your body's ability to burn fat, build muscle, and regulate your appetite? Guess what they're primarily made of? That's right...protein.

Without the core building blocks, your body simply can't efficiently make and regulate your hormones. Fat loss and fat gain will be as random as Justin Timberlake and Andy Sandberg getting together and giving us such musical hits as "Motherlover," "3-Way," and let us not forget about their holiday gift-giving song. Random, but sometimes it works.

But instead of being random, we want to ensure that you're giving your body the raw materials that it needs to really thrive. Most of the studies on protein are not making a distinction between the quality and source of the protein. Many studies are using conventionally raised animal foods that are often eating an abnormal diet, given growth hormones, and regularly fed antibiotics to help nullify the diseases they develop as a result of their abnormal conditions.

Did you know that it's been a regular practice in the conventional dairy and beef industry to feed cows candy? This is in no way a joke. If you want, you can see the cows eating candy (wrappers and all) through the video in the Eat Smarter Bonus Resource Guide at eat smarterbook.com/bonus. Now, I don't mean to be Captain Obvious here, but isn't candy something that's clearly unhealthy for us humans? At least as humans, we've adjusted to eat thousands of different foods and have a very diverse digestive capacity. But cows? Cows haven't learned how to harvest corn, cook soybeans, or make candy. Yet, those are three of the most common things that some of the conventional cattle are fed today. And the results are not just business as usual. These animals are sicker, just like we would be. According to a report from the FDA Department of Health and Human Services, over 80 percent of all antibiotics sold in the U.S. are for use in food-producing animals. Antibiotics are used as treatment, prevention, and (surprisingly to most people) as a tool to increase the weight gain of cattle.

All the way back around the 1940s it was discovered that feeding subtherapeutic levels of antibiotics to cows improved feed efficiency (more output of meat or milk for a given amount of feed) and the animals would gain weight faster which, according to data from Kansas State University, is a result of alterations in the animals' microbiome — decreasing the amount of "lean bacteria" and increasing the amount of "fat bacteria" that shuttles more calories into the animals' tissues. And if you think that this whole process would have an effect on the nutrition that people get from these animals, then you would win this round of factory-farm family feud.

The research isn't clear yet whether or not this rampant antibiotic use has a direct impact on humans consuming conventionally raised beef and dairy products, but here's what we do know:

- According to peer-reviewed research published in the *British Journal of Nutrition,* the beef from animals fed an abnormal diet contains up to five times *less* omega-3 fatty acids than what's found in grass-fed beef. This is a crucial missing factor for our metabolism and overall health, as data cited in the *European Journal of Clinical Nutrition* reports that these omega-3 fatty acids have anti-obesity effects and improve levels of adiponectin (noted to reduce appetite and move fat away from the viscera [belly fat] region to the subcutaneous fat region).

- Research from the College of Agriculture at California State University–Chico that was published in *Nutrition Journal* asserts that grass-based diets elevate precursors for vitamin A and E, as well as increasing disease-fighting antioxidants like glutathione and superoxide dismutase activity compared to grain-fed (primarily corn and soy-based) beef.
- Grass-fed beef contains about twice as much of the valuable fatty acid, *conjugated linoleic acid* (CLA). Scientists at the University of Wisconsin School of Medicine and Public Health found that higher intake of CLA is associated with greater reductions in body fat.

If you're going for beef to fulfill some of your protein requirements, then quality truly does matter. There's a whole spectrum: from grass-fed/grass-finished to grass-fed/grain-finished to grain-fed/grain-finished to screw it, let's just give them candy. Grass-fed is clearly healthier. If not for avoiding the potential problems from rampant antibiotic use, then simply for the fact that you're getting more *nutrition* along with the protein that helps to support healthy hormone function. Improving your quality is one way you can actually eat *less* protein but activate *more* satiety and fat-burning hormones.

The same thing holds true for chicken, pork, fish, bison, lamb, and any other commonly eaten animal-based foods. The vast majority of data shows that when these animals are allowed to eat their natural diet, their food products are more nutritious. If you eat meat, it would be in your best interest to avoid eating animals raised using antibiotics, synthetic hormones, and abnormal diets. When it comes to eating animal foods, it's not, "You are what you eat," it's really, "You are what you eat ate."

Vegetarian and Plant-Based Proteins

There are more versions of vegetarian eating than there are remakes of *Spider-Man*. One of my favorite sentiments is hearing people say, "I don't eat meat, I just eat fish" (common pescatarian lingo). Ah, I'm pretty sure that fish is meat. Maybe you should just say that "I don't eat land meat." That would sound weird, but it would definitely make more sense. Full disclosure: I was pescatarian for a while, too.

There are vegetarians who don't eat meat (including fish, for goodness' sake) but include eggs and dairy in their diet. Some vegetarian approaches exclude meat and eggs, but still include dairy. Some folks go completely free from all animal foods, grabbing the title originally coined in the 1940s called *vegan*. And some folks are vegan but they do have a little honey or other bee products. They'd be called a *beegan* (which I think wins the award for the cutest name). So, as I said, many different versions, and I'm proud to say that I've been all of them.

One of the most common questions I would get, and I know many vegans and vegetarians still face this question daily, is, "Where do you get your protein?" You can do really well on a plant-based diet, and the truth is just about every commonly eaten plant food has a fraction of protein in it, whether it's a bean or a berry. But the even bigger truth is, based on the protein data we've already covered, that we all need some dense, high-quality sources of protein to really assist our hormone function and our metabolism. So, we're going to go through some of the most well-researched sources going from vegetarian to vegan and from more whole food-based to more processed.

Eggs

Some experts cite eggs as the world's healthiest food, while others warn of the questionable amounts of fat and cholesterol. You can check out more on cholesterol in the "Are You Cholesterol-Right?" box on the next page, but for our purposes here just know that cholesterol is a building block for all of your sex hormones (kind of important) and cholesterol plays a key role in the maintenance of your brown adipose tissue (your body fat that burns fat!), according to a large-scale study conducted at ETH Zurich. There are many types of cholesterol, and it's essential to know that the cholesterol in food is not the same thing as the cholesterol that's in your blood. That said, peer-reviewed evidence conducted by scientists from the Department of Nutritional Sciences at the University of Connecticut revealed that eating eggs, specifically, does not translate to increased risk of heart disease and problematic ratios of cholesterol. In fact, eating eggs was found to *decrease* heart disease risk.

There's an extraordinary amount of data stating that eggs are a health-affirming, viable source of whole food protein, based on science and not assumptions. In this regard, for meeting your protein needs, eggs fit the bill at approximately 34 percent protein by weight, 64 percent fat (mostly in the yolk—which is also where you'll get an array of powerful antioxidants like lutein and zeaxanthin), and a negligible amount of carbohydrates. Studies published in both the *International Journal of Obesity* and the journal *Nutrition Research* found that eating eggs for the first meal of the day can improve levels of satiety hormones, reduce levels of the hunger-hormone ghrelin, and enhance overall weight loss.

Are You Cholesterol-Right?

There was a time when cholesterol was more confusing than a Picasso painting, but thankfully the latest science is creating a clearer picture of this valuable nutrient. Many people are surprised to find out that you can't actually survive without cholesterol. It's essential for maintaining the membranes of trillions of cells in your body. Cholesterol supports the permeability and fluidity of cell membranes and enables your cells to remain stable at varying temperatures. Cholesterol is also the building block for your steroid hormones (including your sex hormones and hormones that control your metabolism), it's needed to make bile so that you can digest dietary fats, and it's needed to make essential fat-soluble vitamins like vitamin D.

Cholesterol is so important for the function of your brain that your brain actually makes cholesterol itself. In fact, the human brain has a higher concentration of cholesterol than any other organ in the body. Most of that cholesterol is in the myelin sheaths that surround your nerve cells to enable lightning-fast transmission of electrical impulses that govern thought, movement, spatial awareness, and so much more.

When you hear about cholesterol, you usually hear about *low-density lipoprotein* (LDL) and *high-density lipoprotein* (HDL), which, contrary to popular belief, are not actually cholesterol at all. These are both *carriers* for cholesterol, and other things like triglycerides and phospholipids, for that matter. LDL helps transport cholesterol where it needs to go throughout your body, but it doesn't get any credit for the good things it does. It's just labeled as "bad" cholesterol and depicted as the Grinch Who Caused Heart Disease in the media. The biggest flaw with this theory, right off the bat, is that a study conducted by researchers at UCLA all the way back in 2009 looking at the data of over 130,000 patients revealed that nearly 75 percent of people hospitalized for a heart attack did not have high cholesterol!

Now, this is not to say that the grinch in the media (aka LDL) can't slide into town and cause some trouble. But saying it's "bad" and it's the major causative factor in heart attacks and heart disease is as misleading as saying a pair of pliers can cut your electricity bill by 100 percent.

Today we know that LDL has different particle sizes that allow it to do its job, and the smaller, denser particle size appears to be a little more concerning than the bigger, fluffier LDL carriers. We also know that inflammation radically increases the probability that LDL can cause traffic jams in your arteries, according to a massive meta-analysis published in the peer-reviewed journal *Nutrients*.

HDL helps to scoop up leftover cholesterol and ship it back to the liver to be recycled or excreted (your liver is the prime production spot for cholesterol to be made for bodily use outside of the brain). Again, LDL helps take that precious cholesterol your liver makes and delivers it where it needs to go. It's not inherently a bad guy. The most important markers to consider are your overall cholesterol ratio (having a good balance of HDL to LDL), the LDL particle size, blood glucose levels, and levels of systemic inflammation. All of these things can be tracked by a knowledgeable physician if you ask for them.

Dairy

If you're looking for another controversial category of foods, look no further than the dairy department. Dairy includes milk and foods made from milk—primarily cow's milk in the U.S., but this could include goat's milk, sheep's milk, yak's milk, and you'd be surprised how many folks are humping around sipping on camel's milk these days.

Many cultures have been consuming dairy foods for thousands of years. Though, in the grand scheme of things, dairy has not been a part of the human evolutionary story for very long. But, to that point, neither has a huge percentage of foods we commonly eat today. This includes all grains and, believe it or not, most of the healthiest fruits and vegetables you can name that don't remotely resemble what our ancestors ate thousands of years ago. It may come as a surprise, but even our innocent lettuce has been bred over the years to contain less and less of the compounds that gave it psychoactive properties. That's right, eating a salad back in the day might've gotten you higher than Snoop Dogg baking cookies at Martha Stewart's house. That said, the argument that it's a newer food or that it's strange for humans to drink milk from another animal has not prevented many cultures from surviving and, in some cases, thriving with a diet that includes dairy. But, before someone pours that frosty cup of mammal milk, there's a few things you should know.

Though some populations do very well on dairy, estimates show that upward of 75 percent of the world's population are lactose intolerant. As noted in our review of yogurt as a fermented food, lactose is milk sugar, which is the primary form of carbohydrate found in dairy. Most humans stop producing the lactase enzyme (which is needed to break down lactose) early in childhood. As a result, consuming lactose-laden dairy could cause an array of issues ranging from pain, gas, and bloating to full-blown nausea and flare-ups of irritable bowel syndrome (IBS). If you're lactose intolerant, even a little gas makes you not fun to be around. I literally put my oldest son out of the car one time (in the rain) when he was including more dairy trying to "bulk up" and let one go. I love you, but you're going to have to hit the showers.

Another recent discovery is that of dairy or milk allergies. This is a situation where your immune system becomes hyperactive due to the exposure of certain proteins found in the milk. This can also be linked to digestive issues, as well as immune responses affecting many things ranging from your skin to your lungs.

There's a well-noted connection between asthma and allergies and milk intolerance. Data published in the journal *Frontiers in Pediatrics* found that about 45 percent of children with asthma also have dairy and other food allergies, while a study cited in the *Journal of Asthma and Allergy* showed that children with food allergies (dairy included) are up to four times more likely to have asthma or asthma-related symptoms. This is not saying that dairy is the cause of the issue, but it's a connection you need to be mindful of, especially if you have little ones you're caring for. If you have asthma and/or allergies, consuming dairy could potentially worsen your symptoms.

With all of this said, there are certain populations of people who have the genetic cards to eat dairy without issues, while other folks can enjoy dairy based on the quality or how it's prepared. Remember, many people who are lactose intolerant can eat fermented dairy (like yogurt and kefir) thanks to the action of friendly microbes eating the milk sugar. Also, lots of people with milk allergies find they can utilize butter since all the milk sugar and milk protein has been removed (unless a few sneak by). Other folks can have things like whey protein without issue even though they may be sensitive to lactose or casein (another milk protein). All of this, again, really just depends on you and your unique metabolism. I just want to make sure you have the facts so that you can make the best decision for yourself.

This brings us to why dairy can even be a viable protein source in the first place. A study conducted at Brigham and Women's Hospital at Harvard Medical School found that participants who regularly consumed whole-fat dairy had lower levels of obesity, lower levels of blood fats (triglycerides), lower levels of inflammation, and higher levels of insulin sensitivity. Another study published in the *European Journal of Clinical Nutrition* found that dairy consumption increased circulating levels of PYY, which you'll recall from Chapter Two is a hormone that works to reduce appetite and decrease your risk of excess body fat storage. Put this together and dairy (specifically *full-fat* dairy) can help knock out the Three Amigos of Body Fat Growth for *some* people.

Remember, the fat is where it's at when it comes to dairy—that's where you'll access the metabolism-boosting benefits of CLA we talked about earlier, plus the powerhouse fat-soluble vitamin K2 that activates your satiety hormone adiponectin. And just to be clear, again, grass-fed dairy contains more vitamin K2 and, according to scientists at the University of Wisconsin–Madison, it also contains up to 500 percent more CLA than standard grain-fed dairy!

If you choose to use dairy foods as a protein source, please be mindful that the quality matters a lot. Also, keep in mind that, depending on the dairy food you might choose, the amount of protein you're getting might pale in comparison to the amount of fat and carbs. Take milk, for example. When it's whole milk, it's actually about 48 percent fat, 31 percent carbs, and only 21 percent protein. It's more fat and carb/sugar dominant than the fraction of protein you're getting. For some folks, that may fit into the overall macro ratio you're looking for, but for other people, not so much. There's reduced-fat milk ("2%") that will have about 10 percent less fat and a little bit higher ratio of carbs and protein. And then there's skim milk, or should I say, "No thank you, I prefer to have white water on my cereal, please" milk. But with both, you're missing out on the valuable benefits of fats, and they're still higher in liquid carbs than protein.

There are obviously several factors to consider with dairy, though if it's right for you, you have the freedom to go for it. But if your milkshake doesn't bring all the boys to the yard, and instead only brings gas to people's noses, you might want to let the dairy go and take advantage of something else.

Beans, Peas, and Lentils

We've already covered how this category of food can impressively affect your metabolism by supporting the health of your microbiome. But beans, peas, and lentils are also another go-to food for protein for billions of people around the world.

Take chickpeas, for example. It's a ridiculously popular food today thanks to being the main ingredient in the gloried "dip" called hummus.

I put dip in quotations because I've seen people dig hummus out of a container with pita bread, veggie slices, their fingers, and even a pen cap one time. People who love hummus tend to love it in a social misconduct kind of way. But the chickpeas themselves (also called garbanzo beans), when prepared properly to reduce the potential lectins and anti-nutrients, are a viable source of protein with a slightly higher ratio of fat and less carbs than some other beans.

A study published in the *Journal of the American Dietetic Association* found that test subjects consuming about 3 ounces of chickpeas per day had reduced levels of insulin resistance. In Chapter Two we discussed how carbohydrates are the most instigating of insulin and fat-storage of the Big Three macronutrients. Yet, although beans (including chickpeas) are carb-dominant foods, their rich proportion of fiber and bioavailable protein actually has a normalizing effect on insulin.

If chickpeas and hummus were the popular kids in school, then navy beans would be the one who turned out to be super-hot later on in life (like "Dang...I knew I should have talked to navy beans when I had the chance!"). Seriously though, navy beans are another suitable source of plant protein. Research conducted at the University of Toronto uncovered that incorporating navy beans into the diet led to reductions in waist circumference, reductions in insulin resistance, and reductions in overall calorie consumption.

Soy and all of its tabloid-worthy outfits like tofu, natto, and tempeh are included here in the bean family, as well. As you'll recall from our discussion on fermented soy foods, one of the major concerns about soy is its anti-nutrients. Fermentation is one method, but sprouting soybeans before making foods like tofu can reduce phytates and other anti-nutrients by up to 81 percent, while also increasing protein content by up to 13 percent. This is according to data published in the *Journal of Food Science and Technology.*

Another study cited in *The American Journal of Clinical Nutrition* found that including a small amount of soy-based foods like tofu, natto, and tempeh in the diet led to favorable changes in fasting glucose levels. Unlike soybeans, which are also a notable source of protein, tofu has a higher ratio of protein and a lower ratio of carbohydrates because it's made from condensed soy milk (where much of the carbs have been removed). Tofu is a major go-to for plant-based protein today, but it's important to keep the *quality* of the tofu in mind, and to also remember that the long-lived cultures utilizing soy for thousands of years were not going soy balls to the walls with it. It was part of their overall variety of proteins that also included things like fish, vegetables, and an assortment of other foods.

Black beans are another staple food for cultures all over the world. A recent study published in the journal *Nutrients* found that eating black beans can aid in reducing insulin resistance and reducing systemic inflammation, as well. They're also an excellent source of folate (vitamin B9) which, according to data cited in *Nutrition Research Reviews,* low levels may have a direct correlation with having a higher BMI and risk of obesity. As noted earlier, folate is also essential for methylation that influences everything from your gene expression to fat metabolism.

Speaking of folate, you'd be hard-pressed to find a better source than lentils. At around 30 percent protein, lentils are a little higher in protein than the rest of its legume buddies. Some adventurous scientists, who could've easily been the Super Mario Bros. themselves, put together a study where test participants were given either lentils, chickpeas, navy beans, or yellow peas before giving them access to all-you-can-eat pizza. The results, published in the *British Journal of Nutrition,* found that all of the legumes led to a lower blood glucose response, but lentils reduced caloric intake even more than the rest of the group. Eating lentils appears to increase satiety hormones, decrease hunger hormones, and nourish the friendly flora in your microbiome.

No matter what beans, peas, or lentils you choose from, it's important to know that they are still carb-dominant foods. Just because they're a denser source of protein than most plant foods does not mean that they will keep you in the macronutrient ratio you want to be in. Black beans are about 70 percent *carbs,* 26 percent protein, and 4 percent fat. Kidney beans, another popular bean, are approximately 69 percent carbs, 27 percent protein, and 4 percent fat. And even the small but stout lentils are 68 percent carbs, 30 percent protein, and around 2 percent fat.

If you try to tomahawk dunk too many servings of beans in your body to try and meet your protein needs, you might find that you accidentally slip and land in a bigger pants size. We have to be conscientious about our carbohydrate intake (as you'll learn about in a moment), but this is not to say that beans can't be an excellent add-in. This is even more true for beans because, within that carbohydrate fraction, there is also a hefty dose of dietary fiber. Fiber is that sixth man coming off the bench to "net" those carbs, which drops the overall carbohydrate load. Net carbs are essentially the carbohydrates that are actually absorbed by the body during a meal. To calculate the net carbs, you simply take the total amount of carbs from the food and subtract the total amount of fiber. For example, if you're eating ½ cup of black beans, that would be about 20 grams of carbs and 8 grams of fiber. So, 20 minus 8 would give you 12 grams of net carbs actually hitting your bloodstream. It's less of an impact, but still something to be aware of.

Some folks even include an occasional serving of beans on their keto diet because of the fiber and reduced net carb load, though, obviously, it can't be the major protein source because a bean too many would kick you right out of ketosis. Beans really boil down to how you use them and they're one of many options for you to take advantage of. Beans are not a "complete protein" because they don't contain all of the essential amino acids (the protein building blocks that the human body can't make and must obtain through diet). But mixing and matching with other protein sources and diversifying your foods can ensure that you're getting all of your aminos and also hitting the macronutrient ratios you want.

Nuts and Seeds

This category of foods is another sensible source of protein on a plant-based diet (and any other type of diet, for that matter). Similar to beans, nuts and seeds are not protein-dominant, so you need to be mindful of not going too hard on them to try and achieve your protein needs. Nuts and seeds are fat-dominant, which means they do, in fact, contain more calories per gram than a lot of other foods. Yet, if the nuts and seeds are sourced and prepared properly, their natural dietary fats can provide a huge assist for your metabolism.

Almonds are probably the nut that gets most of the spotlight today, and for good reason. A fascinating new study published in the journal *Nutrition Research and Practice* sought out to find if the *timing* of almond intake during the day would have different effects on the body. One group was assigned to eat about 2 ounces of almonds before eating a meal, while another group was assigned to eat the 2 ounces between meals as a snack. The study also had a control group that didn't include almonds at all. After the results were compiled at 8- and 16-week intervals, here's what they found…

The group of study participants who ate the almonds before their meal lost significantly more body fat and even reduced visceral fat compared to the control group who didn't include the almonds. While the participants who ate the almonds between meals didn't have a significant improvement in body composition compared to the control group, they did have reduced total cholesterol numbers and a significantly improved cholesterol ratio.

Almonds are a fat-fighting food, but they appear to work best when including a handful at the beginning of your meal. And, as I mentioned earlier in this section, uncooked or dehydrated options for nuts and seeds are best. Once the nuts are cooked in low-quality oils, you will reduce the nutrition, increase inflammation, and potentially damage your microbiome. Dehydrated nuts and seeds still have the nice crunch that we're looking for, and you can get them made with a variety of tasty spices and flavors as well.

Within the domain of almonds, there's a ton of other lower-carb, almond-based options out there today, like almond flour, almond butter, and almond milk. You can buy unsweetened ready-made almond milk in just about any grocery store now, and you can even make it yourself using a nut milk bag (literally the worst product name ever). Compared to conventional milk that's 48 percent fat, 31 percent carbs, and 21 percent protein, unsweetened almond milk is about 71 percent fat, 15 percent protein, and 14 percent carbohydrates. It's a little lower in protein but significantly lower in liquid sugar if you're minding that macro ratio.

Peanut Butter and Jealous

Probably the most popular nut in the world is actually a legume in disguise. In reality, peanuts are more like peas than pistachios. But part of the confusion likely lies in the fact that peanuts have "nut" in their name. Archaeological records show that the historic use of peanuts dates back thousands of years in South America. But it wasn't until a few hundred years ago that the distribution and growth of peanuts was spread to places like Asia, Africa, and North America.

Peanuts blend easily into the nut crowd versus other legumes thanks to their taste, culinary uses, and nutritional profile. Like nuts, peanuts are fat-dominant and have a notable ratio of protein. Peanuts are approximately 73 percent dietary fat, 16 percent protein, and 11 percent carbs. And in clinical trials peanuts performance is on par with almonds in helping to improve fasting glucose levels, which was cited in a 12-week study published in the journal *Nutrients*.

Now, let's be honest...peanut butter is a whole mood. The smell, the taste, the endless combinations with things ranging from jelly to chocolate. Peanut butter was a huge part of millions of people's lives growing up. But, today, unfortunately peanuts have shot up on potential food allergen lists. A mycotoxin common to peanuts called *aflatoxin* is sometimes thought to be the issue, but a report cited in the journal *Food and Nutrition Sciences* found that approximately 89 percent of aflatoxins are eliminated through conventional processing of peanut butter. Though not all aflatoxins are eliminated, not all peanuts have aflatoxins to begin with. Still, this could be enough to cause issues. Plus, there are other viable theories as to why there's been an enormous spike in peanut allergies in the past couple of decades. Many of these theories link the increase to immune system dysfunctions and/or abnormalities in the microbiome.

If you feel peanuts and peanut butter contributes to health and happiness for you, go for it. But if you're peanut butter and jealous that you can't join in the peanut fun, there are a plethora of alternatives to take advantages of today, ranging from cashew butter to almond butter or sunflower seed butter to pumpkin seed butter (if your system says to skip nuts—and their camouflaged friend the peanut—altogether).

There are several other nuts with remarkable benefits to take advantage of, from walnuts and hazelnuts to Brazil nuts and pecans. We'll cover more of them in upcoming sections, but we can't talk about nuts without including their little cousins in the seed family.

When it comes to protein, the seed that would win MVP in the category would be hemp seeds. Hemp seeds are actually one of the very few complete protein sources you'll find within a single plant. It's a little low on the lysine side, but it's there with the other eight essential amino acids nonetheless. Hemp seeds are upward of 25 to 30 percent protein by weight and have an excellent ratio of essential fatty acids as well. Three tablespoons of hemp seeds will easily give you 10 grams of highly digestible protein, with only a tiny fraction of carbs and a plethora of vitamins and minerals. You can sprinkle some on salads, or add them to smoothies, desserts, entrées, and more.

Pumpkin seeds are another viable plant protein source to utilize. They're about 20 percent protein by weight and a study cited in the peer-reviewed publication *Journal of Diabetes and Its Complications* found that pumpkin seeds have the potential to help reduce blood glucose levels and provide other anti-obesity effects in addition. Also in the study, the scientists incorporated flaxseeds which provide a notable portion of protein, as well as valuable fiber to help support the health of your microbiome.

There's a wide array of nuts and seeds to take advantage of to meet your protein target. But keep in mind that nuts and seeds are fat-dominant foods that can throw in a lot of extra calories along with the protein if you go overboard. To help balance things out, let's take a look at one of the true, natural sources of protein-dominant plant-based food.

Spirulina, Chlorella, and AFA

When I found out about spirulina many years ago, it nearly blew my mind. First of all, I had no idea that humans were actually out there snacking on algae. Spirulina has been a major protein source for various human civilizations spanning thousands of years. Its use has been traced back to the ancient Aztecs of Mesoamerica and all the way to the nation of Chad in Africa. Its rise back to popularity began in the late 1980s when NASA initiated research proposing that this nutrient-dense protein source could be utilized in space by astronauts. When I watched *The Jetsons* cartoon as a kid, they imagined flying cars and getting a hot three-course meal at the push of a button. In reality, we still haven't gotten our souped-up DeLoreans yet, and the best futuristic food we can come up with is actually something from thousands of years ago.

Spirulina (and its blue-green algae companions) mimic the action of land plants by using photosynthesis to turn sunlight into concentrated chlorophyll. These algae just do it way better. Spirulina is one of the most chlorophyll-rich foods in the world, and it's also the most dense source of protein ever discovered. Spirulina is upward of 71 percent protein by weight! It's a true protein-dominant, plant-based food that's also a complete protein. Just to be clear, it's upward of 71 percent protein by weight, but this doesn't mean that it weighs very much. One tablespoon will give you about 4 grams of protein. So, to equal the amount of protein in a typical 6-ounce chicken breast, you'd need to eat about a half a cup of powdered spirulina. Which, clinically speaking, is a buttload of spirulina.

Just because it has a high protein ratio doesn't mean that it has the actual density to make up the lion's share of your protein needs. However, there's something really noteworthy about the protein in spirulina (and other edible algae) that you won't find anywhere else. The protein is of such a high quality, and it's so packed with additional nutrition, that it does things for your body that other conventional foods can't hold an algae-scented candle to.

Spirulina is so rich in nutrition that the United Nations has been working to utilize it to help stamp out global malnutrition. It has an abundance of antioxidants, vitamins, minerals, and other essential nutrients that we'll talk more about later. But for our immediate focus on metabolism, here's what the data shows:

- In a recent double-blind, placebo-controlled study, participants who received spirulina lost significantly more weight and had a greater reduction in BMI than those taking a placebo.

- A study published in the *Journal of Medicinal Foods* uncovered that having just 2 grams of spirulina a day had outstanding effects on reducing blood glucose levels over the course of a two-month study period.
- A fascinating recent study cited in *Annals of Gastroenterology* demonstrated that patients with nonalcoholic fatty liver disease (NAFLD) having 6 grams of spirulina per day for six months had substantial improvement in metabolic function indicating improved liver performance and overall improvements in reported quality of life.

Spirulina is clearly a potent food to add, but now let's take a look at its sister from another mister, chlorella.

Chlorella appropriately received its name by being one of the most chlorophyll-rich foods on the planet. And when it comes to supporting metabolism, that's what gives this food a superstar edge. A study published in the peer-reviewed journal *Appetite* found that chlorophyll can aid in weight loss and reduce the urge to eat hyper-palatable foods. In an earlier chapter we talked about how food manufacturers have been working furiously to create hyper-palatable foods that compel you to keep eating more. Eating foods rich in chlorophyll is one of the ways to take back control of your appetite.

What's also interesting is that chlorophyll has been found to increase the release of GLP-1 which, according to research published in the *Journal of Endocrinology,* has the potential to trigger body fat redistribution. This literally means that high-chlorophyll foods could spark the *decrease* of visceral fat and the healthy *increase* of subcutaneous fat (which appears to be more protective against metabolic diseases). The interaction between food and our bodies is truly amazing once you realize this stuff. Chlorella is not only a great source of chlorophyll, but it's also approximately 50 percent protein by weight and loaded with incredible micronutrients, as well.

The last of the most popular, historically utilized algae in this category is *aphanizomenon flos-aquae* (AFA) blue-green algae. Researchers from the Department of Nutritional Sciences at the University of Connecticut found that AFA is incredibly effective at supporting metabolism by reducing the production of inflammatory cytokines. Additionally, they uncovered that AFA may be able to prevent fatty liver disease, at least in part by inhibiting lipogenesis (the creation of fat) within liver tissues. AFA is about 60 percent protein by weight, at the top of the list of high-chlorophyll foods, and a powerhouse source of vitamins, minerals, and essential fatty acids.

Grains

We went in pretty deep discussing the pitfalls and potential upsides of incorporating certain grains into your diet earlier in the last chapter. Based on the overwhelming amount of data, it's pretty clear that a grain-heavy diet is not ideal for fat loss and overall metabolic health. However, that's not to say that grains can't be used as a supportive food in the diet, or even as a complementary source of protein. A few of the grains that are at the top of the charts in protein are quinoa, oats, and amaranth.

Amaranth is making a rise in popularity, but it's another food that has origins dating back thousands of years. Even when I first said the word *amaranth* I immediately felt like I was transported back into medieval times — "Hark, who goes there? Art thou trying to swipe my satchel of amaranth?!" Satchels were the fanny packs of their day, and obviously great for carrying amaranth. Though even prior to medieval times, amaranth was cultivated by the ancient Inca, Maya, and Aztec civilizations as a consistent food in their diet.

Amaranth is naturally gluten-free, rich in fiber, and possibly the highest protein grain on the block. As a comparison, amaranth contains about twice the amount of protein that you'd find in brown rice. Keeping in mind that *all* grains are still carbohydrate-dominant foods, amaranth and its other vowel-heavy friends, oats and quinoa, have a higher ratio of protein than most other foods in the category. These three are each around 15 percent protein, 13 percent fat, and 72 percent carbohydrates.

A study published in *Molecular Nutrition & Food Research* found that amaranth is another food that can help fend off inflammation by preventing the activation of inflammatory precursors. Oats appear to have a beneficial impact on levels of PYY (one of our major hormones influencing appetite and body fat storage), according to data cited in the journal *Nutrition Research*. With quinoa, you're getting another one of the very few plant-based foods that are also complete proteins. Researchers from the Department of Food Science and Microbiology at the University of Milan uncovered that quinoa reduced blood sugar and triglyceride levels more than other gluten-free grains that were tested. All three of these grains hit each of the Three Amigos of fat gain in their own way helping to reduce inflammation, balance hormones, and normalize appetite.

Protein Powders

Nothing says "I work out" more than a shaker bottle full of those powdered grains. And everyone who's ever mixed up their protein powder in a shaker bottle has had one of three things happen (if not all of them).

1. You forgot to clean your shaker bottle after using it, and then you open it several days later, only to be hit by a smell that sets your nose hairs on fire with an aroma that could best be described as hot dumpster juice.

2. You add your protein and liquid to your shaker bottle and start giving it the shake of a lifetime, only to discover the lid was not properly closed and now it looks like a wet powdery crime scene around you.

3. You "thoroughly" shake your protein mix in your shaker bottle and take a swig, only to find you're swallowing clumps of what feels like mud-covered sand.

Protein powders are one of the most popular supplements in the world today. And that's the important thing to remember…they are *supplements*. Meaning they are supposed to "supplement" an already-healthy diet that includes plenty of whole food sources of protein. That said, intelligently produced protein powders can definitely be used in support of reaching your protein and metabolic performance needs. Let's take a quick look at some of the most widely used options.

Whey protein may seem relatively new, but it has origins dating back thousands of years. There are even reports that Hippocrates, who's widely considered to be the father of modern medicine, prized whey as a treatment for his patients to restore vitality and boost the immune system. One resource stated that he not only had patients consume whey protein, but he also recommended bathing in it. Hearing that, I wouldn't be surprised if Hippocrates ran a high-end spa and eyebrow-arching place (to relax in a tub of whey and get your eyebrows fixed after your stinky ancient Greek shaker bottle blows them off).

Just to be clear, Hippocrates used fresh whey, which he called *serum.* Conventional whey protein starts off in a similar way coming from milk. It's the liquid that separates from the curds during the cheese-making process. But that liquid is then filtered and dried to attain its familiar powdered form. From there, depending on the manufacturer's practices, flavors, sweeteners, and preservatives are added.

Remember this: *The quality of the whey protein depends upon the diet of the cows that it is produced from.* "You are what you eat ate" applies here, too. Beyond that, there are several different forms of whey protein supplements. For simplicity's sake, let's take a look at the main two. There are whey protein *concentrates,* using heat, acid, and/or enzymes to extract the protein from the whole food, resulting in 60 to 80 percent protein and a combination of 20 to 40 percent carbs and fat. And there are whey protein *isolates,* adding an additional filtering process that removes more of the carbs and fat, resulting in a product that's 90 to 95 percent protein. Because there is less roaming lactose (milk sugar), whey protein isolates tend to be much more digestible for those who are lactose intolerant.

There are several other types of protein supplements available on the market today from both plant and animal sources. But the vast majority of clinical evidence supporting the benefits of using a protein supplement are from studies done on whey. A randomized, double-blind study published in *The Journal of Nutrition* found that overweight test subjects who were instructed to consume whey protein daily for 23 weeks lost more fat mass, had a greater loss in waist circumference, and had a greater reduction of circulating ghrelin levels (our major hunger hormone) compared to test subjects taking daily soy protein or an isogenic carbohydrate drink. What's really interesting about this study is that the test subjects were not instructed to make any other dietary or lifestyle changes. Just adding more protein led to these results.

Now, another study published in the *Journal of the International Society of Sports Nutrition* sought to uncover the influence on body composition and muscle performance of whey protein versus beef protein isolate (another animal-based protein option) versus a carbohydrate-based drink. This experiment, conducted on experienced weight-training men and women, found that the whey protein and beef protein isolate groups both had substantial improvements in their body composition (with an increase in lean body mass and a reduction in fat mass) compared to the carb-sipping group. Plus, their 1-rep max lift in the dead lift and bench press were significantly improved, too.

One other significant thing about whey protein is that it's also a potent source of *branched chain amino acids* (BCAAs). BCAA supplementation has been found to directly increase the creation of new mitochondria in muscle tissue. As we discussed earlier in *Eat Smarter,* it is within your mitochondria that fat is actually "burned" for energy. The creation of more mitochondria (also referred to as mitochondrial biogenesis) is one of the reasons protein supplementation appears to have such a profound impact on our body composition.

There is an overwhelming number of studies validating the effectiveness of whey protein, but there are many other options rising in popularity. The next one (another vegetarian-based, but not fully vegan option) is egg white protein. This protein supplement is an excellent source of the muscle- and mitochondria-supporting BCAA leucine. And one of the most popular plant-based proteins, pea protein, was recently found to promote gains in muscle thickness equal to that of whey protein in strength training study participants (versus a placebo). There are protein supplements based on hemp seed, brown rice, soy, quinoa, and many others (and even combinations of several of them). The most important thing is to mind the quality, and avoid protein supplements that have artificial or high glycemic sweeteners, artificial colors, fillers, or any other unnecessary ingredients that don't have any nutritive value. And most important, make sure that it feels good for *your* body.

When we get into protein powders and other supplementation, it's a largely unregulated industry as of now. Recently, Harvard Health Publishing did an exposé citing research that screened 134 products for 130 types of toxins and found that many protein powders contained heavy metals (lead, arsenic, cadmium, and mercury), bisphenol-A (BPA—a xenoestrogen found in plastics), pesticides, or other contaminants. Many of the toxins were in negligible, trace amounts, while some were present in significant quantities. Now, there will be trace amounts of some heavy metals and pesticides even in whole, organic foods, simply by the nature of things circulating in our giant earth-bubble environment. But, blatant and dangerously high levels of those things is what you want to be cautious of. Be mindful of your supplement sources and choose products from companies that care deeply about their products and are doing things the best way possible.

And even though they can be incredibly helpful, you don't *need* to include a protein powder if you're getting in plenty of whole food sources of protein. This can be properly raised chicken, beef, fish, pork, etc. Or vegetarian and plant-based options like eggs, dairy, beans, nuts, etc. like we've discussed here in this chapter. A study published in *The American Journal of Clinical Nutrition* found that the ingestion of whole eggs immediately after resistance training resulted in greater stimulation of protein synthesis than the ingestion of egg white protein (despite being the same amount of protein). There's something magical about the interaction of nutrient-rich whole foods on our bodies that simply can't be replaced. But smart supplementation, from ethical sources, can give us that extra edge we need in the protein department.

The Protein MVP (Most Valuable Point)

Like we discussed in the previous section, it's important to include a variety of foods when it comes to supporting your microbiome and your metabolism overall. This applies to your sources of protein as well. For most folks, that's going to be a combination of plant and animal sources. But, ultimately, you get to decide the ratios and what feels best for your body.

A lot of times when we're not seeing the results we want on a particular diet, we tend to think that we are the real problem and we just need to work harder to make the diet work. You think you need to "paleo harder" or "vegan harder." No, maybe you just need to adjust some small things that the framework doesn't include. And just to be clear, there are some wonderful frameworks that are absolutely life-changing for people. But many folks end up struggling long-term, while even more people simply don't see the incredible results that others do. This is partly because each framework has a clear set of rules: Do this, don't do that, and you will achieve all of your wildest dreams. And maybe you will for a while. But health is fluid and success is fluid; it's not an end destination you arrive at and maintain with the same, exact approach that got you there. You need to be able to adapt and pivot. Because at some point, that set chain of rules could be the very thing that imprisons you.

When we think of protein, we tend to think of the ultra-dense sources of protein, but essentially all foods have a ratio of protein. We just want to ensure we're including more foods with a higher protein ratio more often (especially if we determine we are lacking in this department). *Eat Smarter* is here to give you the tools and insights you need to progress, adapt, pivot, and create an exceptional level of health and fitness for a lifetime.

Up next, we've got another one of the Big Three on your team to help you grab your big victory.

CROSSOVER CARBOHYDRATE

Carbohydrate is the flashy, durable, all-pro player on your macronutrient basketball team. He can get you a lot of minutes, make some big plays, but he can also get into foul trouble faster than anyone else on your squad.

Carbohydrate came up as a street baller who inspired the gameplay of many athletes all over the world. For years everyone, from little league coaches all the way to the pros, stressed how important carbohydrate was to performance. Whispers began that carbohydrate was the most important macronutrient on the team...and carbohydrate started to believe it. That's where things began to go wrong.

The overuse of carbohydrate led to up-and-down performance. His consistency and reliability was all over the place. There were sparks of high energy and electrifying gameplay, and then there were crashes where he was dragging back and forth on the court. The coach would've sat him out, but he believed that he needed him more than anyone else on the team to win. It wasn't until carbohydrate kept fouling out and getting called for technicals (one time it involved a Twinkie, a Gatorade, and chasing after the rival teams mascot— carbohydrate has been known to get a little bit hyperactive) that the coach noticed the other players really started stepping up. Without excessive carbohydrate in the mix, everyone got leaner, more consistent, and the inflammatory in-fighting within the organization went down. Carbohydrate was now able to step into his role as a team player and not have to carry the load that he was never built for. He's a big-time player, but when he's overworked, it's like a huge amount of weight gets added to the team.

When people see carbohydrate, they tend to just see the flashy stuff that he makes look "simple": cookies, candy, cakes, chips, bread, and pasta. But it's the complex side of carbohydrate that's overlooked...The leafy greens, the low glycemic fruits, and the other non-starchy vegetables that truly make carbohydrate special. These are the fundamentals and why carbohydrate is really on your team. Plus, carbohydrate can really make the game fun to play, too.

With all of the media attention going to the simple side of carbohydrate lately, it can get lost in the shuffle that many powerhouse vegetables are carb-dominant too! True enough, carbohydrate is the biggest driver of insulin and potential fat-storage, but the right type of carbohydrate gameplay can score you some big points in the fat-loss category.

Tip Drill

We've discussed the simple side of carbohydrate and the damage that can happen to your metabolic performance in previous sections. Too much, or the wrong types of, carbohydrates can blunt the effects of your satiety hormones, decrease insulin sensitivity, increase inflammation, and increase the storage of visceral fat. But, without adequate amounts of carbohydrates, many people can experience reduced levels of active thyroid hormone, elevated levels of cortisol, and reduced levels of testosterone. Plus, without the right types and amount of carbohydrate-dominant foods, we miss out on valuable fiber and resistant starch that supports the function of our microbiome. The real key here is to discover your body's own *carbohydrate tipping point.*

For all of us, there is an amount of carbohydrates we can eat that provides us with balanced energy, optimal hormone function, and consistent satiety that automatically supports fat loss. But there is a tipping point in carbohydrate consumption where, by surpassing it, we experience irregular energy levels, dysfunction in our hormones, increased hunger, and fat loss that is automatically downregulated. Basically, there's a point at which your carbohydrate intake crosses over from being supportive of fat *loss* to being supportive of fat *gain.*

What's so fascinating about this is that the tipping point occurs beyond the realm of conventional calorie management. As we've discussed earlier, simply shifting the ratio of carbohydrates, without proactively managing calories, can have remarkable impacts on fat loss. The aforementioned study from Chapter Two, published in *Cell Metabolism,* found that reducing carbs (under the test subjects' tipping point) improved their overall metabolism, reduced hepatic fat, and improved their liver function without proactively reducing calories. While another study we covered, cited in *The American Journal of Clinical Nutrition,* revealed that simply lowering the study participants' ratio of carbs and increasing their ratio of protein (without changing calorie intake) led to higher levels of satiety, a higher resting metabolic rate, and higher levels of fat oxidation.

Now, to take this a step further, a study conducted by researchers at Saint Louis University and published in the *International Journal of Obesity* sought to discover what happens with fat loss when you eat a high carbohydrate breakfast (bagel) versus a high protein/fat breakfast (eggs) when the calorie count of the meals stays the same. The researchers did have the study participants decrease their overall caloric intake by 1,000 calories a day in this study, but had different people use different macronutrient ratios for their first meal. Here's what they found after the eight-week study period...

The study participants in the lower carb breakfast group showed a 61 percent greater reduction in BMI, a 65 percent greater weight loss, a 34 percent greater reduction in waist circumference, and a 16 percent greater reduction in body fat percentage! This just trips me out. For so many years our society has been hyper-focused on cutting calories, but now the truth is emerging how powerful it is to simply make adjustments to your macronutrient ratio...including identifying your carbohydrate tipping point.

In a conversation I had with physician and fat-loss expert Dr. Jade Teta, he shared that he recommends that his patients initially drop their carb intake to 100 grams total for the day (sometimes a little more or a little less, depending on their lifestyle). From that starting point he encourages them to increase or decrease their intake based on two measures: fat loss results *and* monitoring of hunger, energy, and cravings. He stated that, "Paying close attention to these two measures helps you quickly dial in on your carbohydrate tipping point."

You want to reduce your carbs enough to support fat loss, but not so much that you have an increased appetite, lower levels of energy, and cravings so strong that if someone whispers the word *donut* in your ear, it makes the hairs on the back of your neck stand up. Eating smarter is feeling strong, energetic, and in control within your own body. Any diet that encourages you to struggle with those things is taking your power away from you.

The donut is not the problem. You can have the donut. But when the donut begins to Professor-Xavier your mind and control your thoughts, that's when you know something is off. You may need to adjust your carbohydrate ratio, the type of carbs you're eating, increase your protein and/or fat, or improve your micronutrient intake (which we'll get to shortly).

The bottom line is that finding your carbohydrate tipping point requires you to listen to your body's hormonal cues. These include hunger, energy level, and cravings as I stated, but also include mood, motivation, digestion, focus, and sleep quality. Dr. Teta reiterates, "The proper response should be no hunger between major meals, no cravings, and increased energy. You should also feel motivated and focused without anxiety and depression. Gas and bloating should not be present and sleep should normalize. And don't make the mistake of assuming these symptoms are not related to food intake."

Even within the context of a ketogenic diet (high fat, moderate to low protein, and very low carbohydrate approach), you need to be conscientious about adhering to your body's own carbohydrate tipping point. Every keto diet notes that going over your carbohydrate threshold will kick you out of ketosis (the state where your body is producing and running on ketones instead of glucose). But there are certain cells and processes in your body that can *only* use glucose. Research published in *Biochemistry* (5th Edition) asserts that each organ in your body has a unique metabolic profile. There's a diverse amount of energy required to support them (from your brain to your kidneys) and there's a diverse amount of glucose and/or ketones each organ can use. When glucose is low, we are hard-wired to make ketones (thanks to our amazing liver) that can run just about every system in our bodies exceptionally well. However, there are portions and processes in our brains, for example, that can only run on glucose. This can be supported by a sufficient intake of high-quality carbohydrates or, if need be, your body can make glucose out of protein (*gluconeogenesis*) using dietary sources of amino acids or using the amino acids that make up your muscle tissue.

Your body is incredibly versatile in its ability to burn different fuels (including stored body fat) when it's given the opportunity to do so. While talking with Mark Sisson, nutrition expert and author of *The Keto Reset Diet,* he shared with me that the goal is not necessarily to live in a ketogenic state, but to develop the *metabolic flexibility* for your body to be able to gracefully adapt to utilizing different fuels (glucose, ketones, and stored body fat) whenever the situation calls for it. There are times when your body can use a higher level of carbohydrates to support essential functions and performance *without* storing additional fat. And there are times that eating too many carbs will make you gain fat faster than the rise and fall of Gangnam Style.

The amount of carbs you need to support your health, happiness, and fat loss is unique to you. The important thing to note is that dialing back on your carbohydrate ratio, for most people in today's carboholic culture, is going to likely put you in a more metabolically advantaged position. It's funny how the macronutrient that is the most expendable rose to such a place of prominence and belief that it was the most important. In fact, a report by the U.S. Institute of Medicine's Food and Nutrition Board states, "The lower limit of dietary carbohydrate compatible with life apparently is zero, provided that adequate amounts of protein and fat are consumed." Unlike protein and fats, we can actually survive without carbohydrates. In times of scarcity of carb-based food, it's what our bodies were designed to do. But we now understand the valuable addition that certain plant-based, carbohydrate-rich foods bring to the table. Just because we can *survive* without carbohydrates doesn't mean that we can truly *thrive* without carbohydrates. Again, we want to aim for the right amount and types of carbohydrates for you. And here's another insight about how strangely diverse that can be.

What the Fructose?

In a discussion with *New York Times*–bestselling author and former research biochemist Robb Wolf, he shared some eye-opening data with me on the way different people respond to different sources of carbohydrates. The data he shared was from a paper titled "Personalized Nutrition by Prediction of Glycemic Responses," which appeared in the peer-reviewed journal *Cell*. The groundbreaking study revealed that a person's glycemic response (how much blood glucose increased for a given meal) appears to be influenced by various factors like genetics, current body composition, and (most interestingly) the composition of their microbiome. He said, "One of the most important findings of the study showed there was massive variation from person to person in how they reacted to various foods. Some foods that we'd normally assume would cause blood glucose problems were not problematic for some people, while foods normally thought of as 'good' caused some people to experience significant blood sugar increases."

For instance, one portion of the study gave test subjects a cookie to monitor their blood sugar response. At another time, they gave the same test subjects a banana (containing the same amount of carbohydrates as the cookie) and, again, monitored their blood sugar response. Clearly, since the banana is a natural food with fiber and other nutrients, it would have a lower blood sugar response for all participants than eating a freakin' cookie, right? Well, if you thought that, then in the words of the great Notorious B.I.G., "You're dead wrong."

Yes, some study participants had the glycemic response you'd suspect, high spike from the cookie, low to moderate change from the

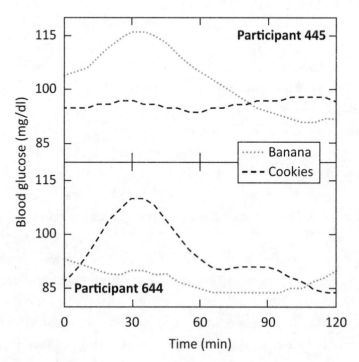

Variation in glycemic responses - Cell 2015

banana. But some study participants experienced the exact opposite! From the table you can see participant 445 had a negligible, dare I say "good" blood sugar response from eating the cookie, but eating the banana caused a major spike in blood sugar and a correlating "crash" that occurred shortly after. The variation in response to different foods was just mind-blowing. This reiterates that fact that *there is no one-size-fits-all diet,* and foods that resonate well with one person's body can be totally obstructive for someone else. Some of the researchers surmised that part of the large variation in food responses could also be an outgrowth of food sensitivities and intolerances. This points back to our discussion on the health of our microbiome, because as the test participants moved away from foods that continuously spiked their blood sugar, there were consistent changes toward a microbiome associated with leanness, low inflammation, and favorable glycemic control. Robb shared that eating a diet that doesn't chronically elevate blood sugar appears to "rehabilitate" our gut.

Now, this obviously doesn't mean that you should eat Cookie Crisp cereal for breakfast rather than a banana. But this does point to another interesting fact, which is: The sugar in fruit can be problematic for some people, too. Some experts assert that fruit can make you fat, while others say that fruit is supportive of losing fat. The truth is, it depends on you and your unique metabolism. What I can say without hesitation is that we definitely need to watch out for the big sugar fruits that are common today. As we touched on in the evolution of lettuce (from potential psychoactive narcotic to having the alkaloids bred out and now being as harmless as a baby kitten—unless, well, you're allergic to kittens and/or cuteness), much of today's fruit has been bred to contain less toxins, more calories, and more sugar. And, in some cases, a lot more.

Take for instance, the handy-dandy boomerang-shaped banana. A travel companion snack you can always count on, a pleasant addition to any smoothie, the literal centerpiece of a banana split, and the most common fruit used in sex education classes all over the world (that was definitely the weirdest day of eighth grade for me). The wild banana that humans began to cultivate upwards of 10,000 years ago barely resembles the modern hybridized banana that we all know today. The original bananas were smaller, contained a lot less sugar, and had large, hard seeds like the ones you see in the image. To get that sugar and starch you had to eat around and/or eat through a lot of seeds. This would slow you down substantially, give you more fats along with the banana (if you ate the seeds), and, let's face it, it would be a lot of work.

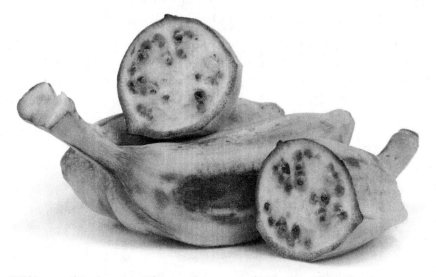

Wild banana of Southeast Asia (Photograph courtesy of Mohammed Choudhury)

So, we've bred the seeds out to the degree that you *might* see a few teeny, tiny, little impotent seeds. Yet, these seeds you might find in a banana today aren't even capable of reproducing on their own. Our conventional bananas can no longer grow without human intervention.

Today's banana is significantly higher in sugar, but it's also higher in several beneficial nutrients, too, like potassium, vitamin C, and resistant starch. As we discussed earlier, green, unripe bananas are a rich source of microbiome-supportive resistant starch. Green bananas actually contain up to 80 percent starch measured in dry weight. But during the ripening process, that starch is converted into sugars, and nearly all of the starch is gone once the banana is fully ripe.

In addition to bananas, many of our other favorite fruits that have been bred to be much bigger—like peaches, pineapples, mangoes, watermelons, grapes, and plums—have a combination of different types of sugar (including glucose and sucrose). But what makes fruit unique is that it's generally high in a sugar that's actually named after fruit itself, called *fructose,* or fruit sugar. We're not talking about the highly processed sweetener, high fructose corn syrup, which, according to research published in the journal *Pharmacology Biochemistry and Behavior,* is a major causative agent in visceral fat accumulation and leptin resistance. Hopefully everyone has gotten the memo by now that high fructose corn syrup is bad business. What we're talking about is the naturally occurring fructose in fruit that has risen to unnatural levels due to the intervention of humans.

As previously stated, many experts assert that fruit is pro-obesity due to its sugar and (specifically) fructose content. On the surface, it actually looks like fructose is a great form of sugar to eat since fructose doesn't hit your bloodstream and trigger the release of insulin like sucrose and glucose does. Because of this it actually has a *low* glycemic index. Well, at least from its immediate affects.

Fructose is slowed down because it, first, has to be processed in your liver (there's that amazing organ, again!), where 29 to 54 percent of the fructose you eat is converted into glucose. This glucose is then able to hit your bloodstream (like taking a different route home after work) and that's when insulin will be waiting at the door to say hello. Another big chunk of fructose will be converted in the liver into glycogen (your checking account), and a small percentage will be converted directly into fat (a process called *de novo lipogenesis*). According to research conducted by the National Institutes of Health, a sensible amount of fructose can actually spark the burning of more fuel, but overloading your liver with fructose can instigate more of your fat cells and increase their storage capacity.

The point is this: Fruit provides some remarkable benefits that are often not found in other categories of food. They can be helpful for your microbiome, for satiety, and also for supporting fat loss. A meta-analysis published in the journal *Obesity Reviews* cited the results of eight different studies that all found a statistically beneficial relationship between fruit and fat loss. Study participants who regularly ate fruit had lower levels of fat. But, the study acknowledged that the types and amounts of fruit need to be accounted for. Going overboard on sweet fruit (specifically) can definitely overburden your liver, stealthily decrease your insulin sensitivity, and increase your levels of body fat.

If you want to add half a ripe banana to your smoothie along with some healthy fats and protein, go for it. But snacking on a couple of bananas might not be the best idea for most people (particularly if you're not active and especially if your body responds negatively to it—i.e., a blood sugar spike then a crash). Whether you want to snack on some pineapple chunks, pop a handful of grapes, or nibble on a peach while sending someone a peach emoji, it's totally up to you. The best advice is simply to have smaller amounts of sweet fruit, moderate amounts of lower sugar fruits like berries, and big amounts of most fruits that were sent to the vegetable's office (which we'll talk about next).

For many people struggling with fat loss, the problem isn't that they're eating too many grapes, it's that they're likely eating too much processed food or grape-flavored soda. Fruit is not the enemy. But it's not a free-for-all either. Take advantage of fruit, but don't let it take advantage of you. Now, on to veggie headquarters to set a few things straight.

A Fruit in Vegetable's Clothing

All the way back in 1893, the Supreme Court had to decide whether a tomato should be classified as a vegetable or a fruit. The court was forced to decide if imported tomatoes should be taxed under the Tariff Act of 1883, which only applied to vegetables and not fruits. The court ruled in favor of classifying the tomato as a vegetable, not based on science, but based on the way people used it. Botanically speaking, a fruit is any food that grows from a plant (vine, bush, tree, etc.) and is the means by which that plant gets its seeds out into the world. Under that definition, tomatoes are clearly a fruit. But the use of the tomato is best summed up by journalist Miles Kington, who said, "Knowledge is knowing that a tomato is a fruit. Wisdom is not putting it in a fruit salad."

Knowledge tells us that several other nutritious fruits have found their way into the vegetable category. Cucumbers, peppers, pumpkins, squash, zucchini, eggplant, avocados, and olives are all fruits. But, thanks in part to the way that they are used from a culinary perspective (generally using these vegetable stand-ins in savory, salty, and spicy dishes), their "unsweet" tastes have culturally put them on team veggie.

Unlike the seed-bearing parts of a plant (the fruits), the parts of a plant that would be classified botanically as vegetables would be the roots, leaves, and stems. When we eat carrots, radishes, and beets, we're eating the roots of the plant. Leaves range from spinach to kale. And an example of a popular stem we eat is asparagus.

As a reminder, the vast majority of vegetables and fruits, alike, are carbohydrate-dominant foods. And even though carbs can be vilified, we need to be clear not to throw the baby carrots out with the bathwater. We've already touched on the benefits of intelligently including some fruits, but the family of vegetables (and fruits that commonly find themselves in the vegetable category) have some of the most potent effects on fat loss you're going to find.

A meta-analysis published in the journal *Nutrients* reviewed ten peer-reviewed studies to identify the impact that including more vegetables can have on metabolism. In several multiyear studies, here's what they found:

- Increasing vegetable consumption intrinsically increases the rate of fat loss.
- Increased intake of vegetables was found to be protective against weight gain and obesity.
- People who eat more than four servings of vegetables per day have the lowest risk for weight gain.
- For every serving of vegetables consumed each day, study participants had a 0.36-centimeter reduction in their waist circumference over the course of their study period.

This review shows clearly that not only are vegetables supportive of weight loss, but eating vegetables is actually protective against weight gain. A specific study published in the *Asia Pacific Journal of Clinical Nutrition* revealed that eating more vegetables can reduce the risk of gaining excess weight in a single year by 73 percent! The one thing most diets agree on is the generous inclusion of more vegetables, but they don't usually tell people why. Now you know why.

When we're talking about carbs, we want to make sure that we don't turn it into a dirty word like we did dietary fat. Carbs are important, particularly the carbs that come packaged up as vegetables.

And we've got one more important dimension of carbohydrate's game to look at, and that is its *timing*.

Clocking Carbohydrates

Earlier in our carb talk, we covered a study published in the *International Journal of Obesity* that found that eating a high carbohydrate breakfast versus a high protein/fat breakfast (with the calorie count of the meals being the same) led to drastically different fat loss results for the study participants. As a recap, over the course of the eight-week study period, people in the lower carb breakfast group showed a 61 percent greater reduction in BMI, a 65 percent greater weight loss, a 34 percent greater reduction in waist circumference, and a 16 percent greater reduction in body fat percentage. This study demonstrates another important point and a huge key to eating smarter: The timing of your carbohydrate consumption matters!

If your goal is fat loss, then loading up on carbs to start the day is probably not a good idea. The data shows that a higher ratio of carbs at your first meal tends to lead to storing more fat and having a bigger appetite. A study published in the peer-reviewed journal *Appetite* found that study participants eating a higher carb breakfast ended up being hungry again sooner after their meal than test subjects eating a lower carb breakfast.

If there's a time to bundle up on carbs, it's probably not during the first meal of the day. Simply shifting the time of day you eat your carb-centric foods can have noticeable effects on your metabolism. And please note, the carbohydrate source used in the aforementioned study in the *International Journal of Obesity* was a bagel. It was not a low glyce-mic fruit or non-starchy vegetables. When you calculate the net carbs and take into account the fiber, vitamins, minerals, and other microbi-ome supportive factors, having some smart carbs with breakfast is a huge benefit. But if you decide to have dessert for breakfast, then you're likely going to struggle.

What do I mean by dessert for breakfast? Well, many of us start our day by eating some cake. "Oh, no! I would never do such a thing." But what is a muffin? It's just a cake without frosting. What about a bagel? It's just cake that wasn't allowed to have sweets as a child, and it's rebel-ling by covering itself in cream cheese. Oh, and let's not forget about pancakes (my personal favorite). By changing the dimensions of it and making it flat, it suddenly becomes socially acceptable to order cake for breakfast. "These fried cakes are so thin. They're probably lower in calories. I'll just have three and pour a half cup of liquid sugar from that maple tree on it." Are any of these foods off-limits? Absolutely not. We'll talk more about that in the next one of our Three Fat Loss Essentials. You can upgrade the quality of these foods dramatically. You can also place your higher carbohydrate foods at a more beneficial spot in your day so that you don't go into a carb-coma while you're still trying to be productive. And, according to a fascinating study, shifting your carb-timing can actually improve fat loss.

A study published in the peer-reviewed journal *Obesity* took over-weight test subjects and put them on either a general reduced calorie diet *or* a reduced calorie diet where the majority of their carbohydrates (about 80 percent) were eaten at dinner. At the end of the six-month study, the study participants who ate most of their carbs at dinner lost more weight, had a greater reduction in waist circumference, and had an overall greater reduction of body fat mass compared to the conven-tional calorie-restricted dieters. Plus, the night-carbers also had greater improvements in their fasting blood sugar, better insulin sensitivity, improved cholesterol ratios, reduced inflammation (measured by CRP), and improved levels of leptin and adiponectin. In the well-suited words of Luke Cage, "Sweet Christmas!" How in the world could simply shifting the timing of macronutrients have such a pronounced effect? It actually seems illogical on the surface. But if you look a little deeper, it all makes sense.

Conventional wisdom would say eating more of your carbs and calories at night will make you store more fat. You're not doing anything to "burn them off." But that's looking at metabolism from an offensive perspective. But defense is what really wins championships.

Offensively, we eat carbs and calories, then we have to go into action to burn them off. But instead, by playing defense you'll put your metabolic players in position to stop the carbs and calories from scoring in the first place (i.e., slamming down more fat on your belly or backside).

From a basic defensive perspective, when you're not loading up on carbs to start the day, your metabolic defense shifts into gear to use your glycogen stores to power your body throughout the day. And having your carbs partitioned to the evening restocks your energy reserves *first* before spilling over into fat stores. As the analogy goes, if you drive your car around all day and the gas tank is being emptied, you need to fill it up for the next day. You've got adequate space to fill up on more carbohydrates as long as you don't overflow the tank like that crazy scene in *Zoolander*.

When you start your day with an abundance of carbohydrates and calories, then you are *forced* to play offense. This goes back to the hierarchy of energy utilization we talked about in Chapter Two. Generally speaking, your body will spend the cash on hand (glucose) first, then tap into your checking account (glycogen) which takes more work to access, and then (if need be) it will dip into your savings account (stored fat) for energy to carry out all the jobs it has to do. Fast-burning carbs for breakfast equals more cash on hand to spend, and far less need to dip into the savings account and burn fat. It's sort of like *LIFO*, which I learned about in my college accounting class. It stands for "Last In First Out," meaning that the last resources to come in, will be the first thing to be used. Why on earth would your body work hard to break down body fat when it's got all of these new carbohydrate resources that just came in?

Not only that, we now know that eating more carbs for breakfast can actually stimulate your appetite and make you hungrier, faster. The results: We eat again...there's more cash on hand...and the fat stays safely tucked away in savings.

Contrast that reality with playing championship-level defense. We start our day by eating fewer carbs (and fewer calories, in general—especially being that satiety is fueled by our increased intake of protein) and this enables us to dip into our reserves more quickly. We can hit our checking account and savings account and start burning fat faster if we don't have all of that cash on hand. The key here is that we are not starving ourselves (which would downregulate fat-burning hormones). We are nourished, energetic, and enabling our body to express its metabolic flexibility. Plus, by partitioning those carbs to later in the evening, it appears to make you even more satisfied and able to burn fat the next day.

A recent report published in the *British Journal of Nutrition* found that having a little more carbs at night reduced overweight study participant's appetites the next morning. And another study conducted by researchers at the Department of Nutrition, Food, and Exercise Sciences at Florida State University showed that the consumption of protein or carbs in the evening improved the resting metabolic rate of healthy test subjects the next morning.

To recap, without carbing up and overeating to start your day, your body will be able to utilize stored muscle glycogen, liver glycogen, and stored body fat *faster*. With more carbs and calories constantly coming in during the day, most folks hardly ever get to this step without exercising their face off to burn through those other reserves. If you're into exercising your face off, that's all good. But I want you to know that it's generally not the most effective or sustainable way to burn fat.

And this leads us to another point in timing our carbohydrate intake. Many people were taught to play offense when it comes to exercise, as well. Eat some carbs or even "carb load" before you work out. You're going to need that energy, right?! Again, I think we were really missing the point here. There are absolutely situations where knocking down some carbs before training is appropriate. If you're training for a competition, a sport, or just to get bigger, faster, and stronger, in general, then some pre-workout, and even intra-workout, carbs can be a welcome friend. But, if our goal is *fat loss,* then eating before your workout, particularly eating carbs, is kinda defeating the purpose.

The same hierarchy of energy usage applies here (for the most part) when it comes to exercise. If you eat carbs before you train, you've got to burn through those carbs first, then your stored glycogen, and then your body will start breaking down some fat. So many people have been taught to eat carbs before they work out, even though their goal is fat loss. They unfortunately end up trying to out-exercise what they just ate. But the truth is, trying to out-exercise your food is like trying to outrun a highly caffeinated cheetah. You'll never catch up with that approach.

In my days as a strength and conditioning coach in college, I saw a lot of crazy things at the gym. There were the people who spent more time lifting their phones than lifting weights, the super-sweaty guy who never cleaned the machine after he finished, the lady with way too much perfume on (seriously, what is she trying to hide?!). But one of the craziest things I would see was people downing bananas and cereal bars before working out. So many times, I'd see myself in slow motion... running and diving at them as they are lifting the bar to their mouth... and slapping it right out of their hand just in time. People would gather round me as I lay on the floor after the dive and say things like, "Did you see that? He dove right in front of those carbs for them. He's such a hero." And I'd say, "I'm no hero. I'm just a regular guy who's not afraid to stand up to bad advice." Then I'd faint a little, the scene would fade out, and a commercial for Snickers would come on. Of course, none of that ever happened...but I sure thought about it though.

There were always a lot of people in the gym, and in the moments when I was able to offer advice to folks struggling to lose fat who were sipping on Gatorade or chowing down on a carbolicious snack before exercising, I did. And time after time, simply shifting the scheduling of their carb intake, they saw improved results. Research published in the *Journal of the International Society of Sports Nutrition* showed that carbohydrate consumption *after* exercise was found to directly increase muscle glycogen resynthesis (replenishing muscle glycogen) rather than being stored as fat. The study also found that the inclusion of carbs and protein after resistance training triggered improvements in strength and body composition compared to a placebo.

Another study conducted by scientists from the Department of Medical Physiology at the University of Copenhagen in Denmark uncovered that there's a direct increase in muscle insulin sensitivity postexercise leading to a partitioning of carbs/glucose being shuttled into the muscles after working out (again, rather than being stored as fat). If fat loss is the goal, you want those carbs after you work out, not before it. Of course, we want to go for higher quality carb sources like fruit, sweet potatoes, etc. But if you're going to have a muffin, this is the time to have it. Those carbs you eat are far more likely to restock the store shelves of your muscles than to end up as body fat.

A Word on Fat-Burning and Exercise

Just to be clear, your body can actually switch gears and burn fat sooner (rather than glycogen) depending on the type of exercise you do. Low intensity exercise (like brisk walking) can prompt your body to use fat and bypass using glycogen stores. This sounds great (and it is), but doing intense exercise (like lifting weights and *high intensity interval training* [HIIT]) can burn even more overall calories and fat in less time. Through lifting weights or HIIT, your body will be prompted to burn through stored muscle glycogen on-site at the muscle first, then get to burning fat. However, the biggest benefit is the "afterburn" effect. A study published in the peer-reviewed journal *Physiological Reports* revealed that, compared to low intensity cardio, HIIT burns significantly more calories *after* the workout is over for the next several hours. This is due in large part to its positive impact on muscle tissue and fat loss–related hormones. The bottom line: It's smart to mix in different forms of exercise. But the most important form of exercise is the exercise that you'll actually do! Whether it's weight lifting, swimming, jogging, competitive sports, dancing, jumping on a trampoline, hiking, cycling, or anything else, doing what you actually enjoy transforms exercise from being a task into being something that brings you happiness.

As a point of clarity, this is a "hack" to include some simple sugars in your diet. But overdoing it is not very smart. Data published in the journal *Nutrients* found that going too hard with carbs post-workout can reduce your body's ability to burn maximum fat. Keep in mind, the test subjects in the study were taking upward of about 221 grams of carbs in the form of maltodextrin (which is a highly processed, rapidly absorbing form of sugar). So, the form and amount of carbohydrate intake was ridiculously abnormal. Nevertheless, even that amount of post-workout sugar didn't appear to stop potential benefits of exercise, but it definitely reduced them.

So, to reassert, the timing of your carbohydrate intake is another overlooked facet of nutrition that eating smarter brings to the forefront. When it comes to exercise, if you do feel like you can use a little carb hit before training, you always have the freedom to do so. I just encourage you to switch your pre-exercise fuel source to something that's protein-dominant (some high-quality BCAAs or protein powder would be good here) and see how you feel and perform. You might find that you never really needed the carbs. You might also consider working out in a fasted state (where you don't have food for at least a few hours before working out). Working out first thing in the morning can make this easy to achieve. But, what's most important, is that you do what's best for *you* where you are right now. Exercise is valuable, but what you eat far outweighs the impact of any exercise you could ever do. It is your food choices that literally determine what you're making your amazing body out of.

Carbs in the Spotlight

Love 'em or not, carbohydrates are grabbing the macronutrient spotlight right now. I want to make sure you have the full 30-for-30 background story on carbohydrate so that you can better understand how he's showing up as a player. The timing of carbs, the quality of carbs, and the carbohydrate tipping point all matter. But, most important, understanding how vital it is to proactively include more nutrient-dense, non-starchy vegetables is an absolute game-changer. These are the carbs that give you an unbelievable advantage in fat loss. Remember, the data clearly indicates that non-starchy vegetables (and fruits put into the vegetable category on the stats sheet) not only increase rates of fat loss, but they're also protective against fat *gain*.

If you can make sure that leafy greens and other non-starchy vegetables make up the majority of your plate at each of your meals (including breakfast), then you will be eating meals that support fat loss. Even when you have the more wild side of carbohydrates, make sure to have the fundamentally sound side of carbohydrates show up, too. Pizza? Cool. Have a big salad beforehand. Taco Tuesday? Have a big portion of sautéed veggies on the side along with them. I really like sautéed zucchini and/or squash paired up with my tacos. You will 1) get the fat-loss-supportive nutrients you need, 2) activate satiety-related hormones that protect you from overeating the lesser nutritious foods, and 3) enjoy yourself and have foods you like without sabotaging your success. Simply add. Stop trying to take away.

When it comes to food, we humans like the first part of elementary school math. We start with addition for a reason. You have one apple, and Billy gives you another apple, how many apples do you have? I've got two apples, now! Cut to a little later when you're learning about subtraction. You have one apple and Billy takes your apple, how many apples do you have? I don't know, but Billy better give me my freakin' apple back!

From here on out, strive to be more inclusive of fat-loss-supportive foods instead of being reclusive and hiding from foods you think are bad for you. There's a science to all of this that we'll get to later, and sometimes we even find out that things we believe to be bad for us are actually not bad at all. And nothing could be more true than when talking about the next one of our Big Three macronutrients, fat.

PUMP-FAKING FAT

Nothing can make someone look sillier than a good pump fake. And the pump fake that fat put on our society was one for the ages...

Most of the people in the league thought fat was a troublemaker.

They called him a dirty player, unstable, and a disrupter of the metabolic team. Fat was given the role of the bad guy. But he said nothing, kept his head down, and let his actions do the talking.

While carbohydrate and protein were showing up on Nutritional Sportscenter, fat wasn't making the highlights unless it was a story about him dissing a reporter for talking bad about him or when they put him on the *NOT* Top 10 list. But then something happened.

All the way back in the 2002 season, reporters from the Department of Epidemiology at the Harvard School of Public Health published a story about fat in *The American Journal of Medicine*. It was a meta-analysis of several studies on the impact fat was making. One of the biggest gripes about fat was that he was making the entire league fat. But then the story hit in this prestigious peer-reviewed journal with the headline: DIETARY FAT IS NOT A MAJOR DETERMINANT OF BODY FAT. It had the whole game shook.

All of these years had gone by with fat being dragged through the mud as a dirty player and bad teammate. But when the other teammates were interviewed and the stats were compiled, fat was found to make everything work *better* on the metabolic team. In fact, he was found to be a skilled player-coach that helped to manage things all the way from the brain to the muscles. Oh, and fat's pump fake *was* dirty. He made a lot of people look silly by appearing to do one thing, but ending up doing something totally different. And a big part of his misdirection had to do with his nametag.

Say My Name, Say My Name

Right out of the gate, fat was given a bad reputation because he had the same last name of an infamous coach everybody remembers named *body fat*. Body fat won a lot of titles the last few decades by taking up space and sabotaging teams' metabolisms, and people around the league couldn't take it anymore. Anybody with the last name fat was immediately ostracized and thrown under the bus…even if they weren't actually related!

Body fat and dietary fat are two totally different things. Yet, even hearing the word *fat,* people began lumping them together as one happy, heinous family. But in reality, they were as unrelated as Whoopi Goldberg would be from the wrestler Goldberg. Same name, two totally different backgrounds.

With our society's growing waistline and heart problems, we needed a dietary scapegoat. Prior to the name of dietary fat being vindicated in 2002, all the way back in 1978 (when fat was still a youngster in the nutritional world) a committee of the U.S. Senate led by George McGovern published the first "Dietary Goals for the United States" in order to reverse the epidemic of heart disease in the country. The diet recommended drastic reductions in dietary fat and a sharp increase in the consumption of whole grains. It was the official birth of the low-fat, high-carb diet for everyone. But the problem was that there wasn't any sound science to prove this would work. And guess what happened? In that 2002 meta-analysis from Harvard, researchers stated, "...within the United States, a substantial decline in the percentage of energy from fat during the last two decades has corresponded with a massive *increase* in the prevalence of obesity."

They called it...millions of people started eating less fat and more carbs and our body fat issues went from being a problem to an epidemic.

But the question is, how did it take so long to figure this out? And even though it's been many years since this information has come out, why has it still taken such a long time for people to accept that dietary fat isn't the bad guy? Well, to put it simply, it's a problem with semantics.

Semantics is a branch of linguistics that deals with the *meaning* of words. It's like the word *racket*. There's a tennis racket that Serena Williams used to dominate a record number of grand slams, then there's the racket that I hear every time my kids play the *High School Musical* soundtrack. Same word. Different meanings. When it comes to fat there's an issue with semantics, as well. We've programmed ourselves to believe that fat in food and fat on our bodies are the same thing. Because the word itself is so strong and feared, it was easy to lump them together in our minds. We began to think that *eating* fat in food would directly result in *seeing* more fat on our bodies. But, biochemically, it just doesn't work like that. It's akin to thinking that eating green beans will make you green, or eating blueberries will turn you blue. I know people who eat a ton of blueberries, but I've never seen them express any Smurf-like features.

As we've discussed earlier in the book, yes, eating an overabundance of any macronutrient can lead to excess storage of body fat. But, as you'll see, the right amount of healthy, real food–based dietary fats actually provides a huge advantage to your metabolism and fat loss. With this book I am advocating for a name change of dietary fat so that we can permanently stop all of the confusion. We can easily swap out dietary fat's name to dietary lipids, dietary oils, or some new made-up name like *fexies* (fat and sexies). Whatever name we change it to socially can help jettison the decades-long confusion over this subject matter. And another way we can go about healing our relationship with dietary fat is to understand more of its personality, so that's what we'll jump into next.

Who You Calling Fat?

Though dietary fat is jumbled together under one label, there are several different types of fat we need to know about. We'll be talking about these different fats throughout upcoming sections because of their wide-ranging benefits. So this will be just a brief synopsis.

The first thing to note is that our major categories of fats derive their names based on the formation of their chemical bonds. Fats are essentially like a LEGO arrangement of carbons and hydrogens, and that's pretty much it. All this fuss about fats and it's just these two chemicals scaring the crap out of everybody. But, just like everything in life, the way things are put together can lead to significantly different outcomes. And the way these LEGO blocks of carbon and hydrogen are put together changes their name and their effects on our bodies.

Saturated Fats

No fat has been fat shamed more than this category of nutrients. With saturated fats, every carbon "tail" is connected to other carbon atoms on either side through single bonds, and to as many hydrogen atoms as

Saturated

Unsaturated

Chemical structure: saturated fat vs. unsaturated fat

possible. Since it has as many hydrogen attachments as possible, it's considered to be *saturated* with hydrogen.

Because saturated fats are so uniform in their appearance and makeup, they can be tightly packed together like a bundle of ordinary drinking straws. This tightly packed arrangement makes them more stable and solid at room temperature.

Think saturated fat is bad for your heart? A meta-analysis of over 40 peer-reviewed studies published in *The American Journal of Clinical Nutrition* stated, "There is no significant evidence for concluding that dietary saturated fat is associated with an increased risk of coronary heart disease or cardiovascular disease." Yet, headlines continue to occasionally pop up claiming the opposite. In truth, most saturated fat–bashing studies are typically not taking into account the source nor type of saturated fat. Saturated fat in whole, real foods tends to be health-affirming, versus looking at what chemically isolated fats do in a laboratory. Yes, we need to take both into account, but we always need to remember that humans eat foods, not isolated nutrients.

In fact, a ten-year study including the data from over 135,000 participants from 18 different countries showed that not only did saturated fat not increase the risk of cardiovascular disease, people eating more fat (including saturated fat) actually lived longer!

And what about saturated fat's influence on our body composition? A recent study published in the journal *Metabolism* increased the ratio of dietary fats to about 50 percent of caloric intake in the diet of 144 overweight adults. With the higher fat intake, they had them consume one-third saturated fats, one-third monounsaturated fats, and one-third polyunsaturated fats, and at the end of the 16-week study period, here's what they found:

Study participants had significant decreases in body fat mass, increases in lean mass (muscle), and their blood levels of inflammatory cytokines fell substantially. Versus a placebo, test subjects who were also given a saturated fat supplement had inflammatory biomarkers drop even more. This is a far cry from the story we've been given about saturated fat (and fat in general). But there are still some fat nuances to address.

Within the family of saturated fats, there are also several different types. The most common saturated fats in the human diet can be broken down into groups of either long chain, medium chain, or short chain fats. The length of the chain is basically how many fat "straws" are packed into the bundle. Foods rich in long chain saturated fats (containing 12 to 22 carbon straws) include different types of animal fats (like those found in dairy and meat) as well as coconut fats, palm oil, and cocoa butter. Medium chain saturated fats (6 to 10 carbon straws) will be found in coconut fats, palm oil, and goat's milk. An interesting fact, caproic, caprylic, and capric acid are all medium chain fatty acids (MCFAs) that derive their name from the Latin root *capra,* meaning "female goat" (as these MCFAs are found in abundance in the milk). And finally, short chain fats (containing fewer than six carbons) are found in foods like butter, but primarily we receive them thanks to the action of our gut bacteria making them for us when we eat adequate fiber and prebiotics, as we discussed earlier in the book.

All of these dietary saturated fats are important and play significant roles in our health. But, particularly, it's the short chain and medium chain fats you want to be adamant about including/supporting in your diet. A study cited in the *European Journal of Clinical Nutrition* asserted that the inclusion of as little as 15 grams of MCFAs per day was enough to boost the study participants' rate of calorie burn by 5 percent! And, as you might recall, the short chain fat *propionate* was found to reduce inflammation and even help reduce visceral fat, according to research published in *BMJ*. Referring to saturated fats as "bad" is an oversimplification that we want to renounce for good. Too much of anything can get us into trouble, but missing out on adequate amounts of saturated fats can actually do more harm than good.

Monounsaturated Fats

Unsaturated fats differ from saturated fats in that they not only have single bonds connecting their carbon atoms, but they also have some double bonds, too. When the carbons are busy double-bonding to each other, that leaves no room for extra hydrogens to link up and join the party, so it's no longer fully saturated with hydrogen.

Remembering that our fats are packed together like bundles of drinking straws, a double bond is like a purposeful bend in the straw. I remember when bendy straws first came out. I had one along with my summer camp juice box. Straight straws would no longer cut it for me . . . I wanted to sip with my head upright like any sophisticated first grader would do. Straight straws just didn't hold any pizazz!

Monounsaturated fats have one bend in the straw, while polyunsaturated fats (which we'll talk about next) have many bends in the straw (this would be the equivalent of a crazy straw). Both of these types of fat pack some serious health benefits, as well. But there are some important caveats to pay attention to along the way. Since these unsaturated oils have more "bends," they are less stable. These bends enable the fats to remain liquid at room temperature, but this also makes the oils more fragile and easily damaged. If we select great food-based sources of these fats and treat them nicely when we prepare and store them, they will definitely return the favor. Let's take a look at some of the notable benefits of including more monounsaturated fats.

A meta-analysis of 24 studies found that a diet rich in monounsaturated fats was able to reduce blood glucose levels and improve insulin sensitivity better than a standard low fat–high carbohydrate diet for test subjects. Another study published in the *International Journal of Obesity and Related Metabolic Disorders* pitted a diet with a higher ratio of fats (specifically monounsaturated fats) head-to-head against a low fat–high carbohydrate diet for overweight test subjects for 18 months. The test subjects with the higher ratio of monounsaturated fats in their diet lost more weight, more body fat, and more inches off their waist than the low dietary fat group. In fact, the low-fat dieters gained in all those areas! Something else interesting about the study is that far more study participants who were allowed to eat more healthy fats on their program remained compliant and continued the diet. Whereas folks who were put on the low-fat diet dropped out of the study more often.

Some of the most popular sources of monounsaturated fats are olive oil, nuts and seeds (like almonds, Brazil nuts, cashews and pumpkin seeds), butter, pork, beef, duck, avocados, avocado oil, olives, and certain types of cheeses like cheddar and Colby. As we've been discussing the crucial theme of diversifying our nutrient sources, the same applies here with our fats. For years, I would have things like olive oil and different nuts and seeds, but I didn't pull the trigger on trying avocados until later in life. Avocados and guacamole just looked like some green, alien, weirdness to me. I was so foolish that I literally used to think that avocados and guacamole were one and the same thing. But guacamole is actually what happens to avocados when an angel gets their wings. It's the stuff of the heavens, and it's the first thing to be completely obliterated at any party. If you see an empty bowl amid an assortment of snacks at a party, that's where the guacamole was.

I actually want to give avocados some specific props here, since it's the food with the highest amount of fat that people commonly get from their produce section. With its ample amount of dietary fiber, excellent supply of vitamins and minerals, and impressive variety of dietary fats, this fat-filled food can actually fuel fat *loss* according to a new study published in the journal *Nutrients*. When study participants were instructed to replace some of their dietary carbohydrates with some avocado, they saw improved blood sugar levels, reduced levels of the hunger hormone ghrelin, higher levels of the satiety hormones PPY and GLP-1, and overall higher levels of subjective satisfaction and reduced hunger for longer periods of time. You special little wrinkly skinned fruit, you never cease to amaze me.

Thanks to the rise in popularity of the polyunsaturated fat omega-3, the omega class of fats have gotten a lot more attention in recent years. But what surprises me is how few people have been given the scoop on the monounsaturated fat omega-7.

Omega-7s are incredibly special in that they are known to be *lipokines*. Lipokines are hormone-like molecules that actually control what other fats are doing in your body! These omega-7s (also known as *palmitoleic acids*) have wide-ranging effects by linking up different organs and tissues to ensure optimal energy storage and utilization, meaning omega-7s have some serious influences on fat loss. For instance, data published in the journal *Lipids in Health and Disease* showed that the inclusion of more omega-7s increases weight loss, improves insulin sensitivity, and reduces levels of blood fats compared to a placebo. And what's really fascinating is that omega-7s were found to downregulate proinflammatory genes in white adipose tissue.

Another study conducted by my friend and colleague, *New York Times*–bestselling author Dr. Michael Roizen, is what initially put omega-7s on my radar in relationship to metabolism. His team at the Cleveland Clinic conducted a double-blind, randomized, placebo-controlled study to identify the effects (if any) of omega-7s in adult test subjects. At the end of just 30 days, test subjects utilizing omega-7s had significant reductions in inflammation (measured by CRP) and impressive reductions in triglycerides as well. Dr. Roizen noted that the source of omega-7s, as with any of these fats, really matters a lot.

Some of the best food sources of omega-7s are wild-caught cold water fish (like salmon, sea bass, and sardines), avocados, macadamia nuts, macadamia nut oil, and sea buckthorn berry oil. (Note however that the palmitic acid content in these foods—especially the macadamia and sea buckthorn oils—appears to be an antagonist of omega-7s that reduces their benefits.) You can also find supplemental forms of omega-7s but, according to Dr. Roizen, it's important to make sure they are high-quality purified fish sources to make sure the antagonist (palmitic acid) is removed to get the most out of it.

Next up, we have omega-9s, or oleic acid, which is the most common form of monounsaturated fats in a healthy diet. Omega-9s are one of the reasons that olive oil is touted as such a health-affirming oil, and the research definitely supports this. A multiyear study published in the *European Journal of Clinical Nutrition* found that study participants with a high intake of olive oil lost significantly more weight than participants on a conventional low-fat diet. A separate double-blind, placebo-controlled trial had overweight test subjects consume a breakfast that contained a little more than 1½ tablespoons of extra virgin olive oil or 1½ tablespoons of soybean oil as part of an overall reduced-calorie diet. At the end of the study they found that test subjects given the extra virgin olive oil lost 80 percent more body fat!

Now, before anyone runs out and starts guzzling olive oil, there are a couple of important caveats. Being that olive oil is high in unsaturated fats, it's going to be more susceptible to oxidation and heat damage. You may have noticed that most olive oils are sold in dark glass bottles, which is to help protect the oil from going rancid. A 2012 study titled "The Effect of Storage Conditions on Extra Virgin Olive Oil Quality" found that exposure to light can damage the oils. So, seriously, please don't buy olive oil bottled in clear containers! Part of olive oil's photosensitivity appears to be due to its chlorophyll content. We discussed the eye-opening benefits of chlorophyll earlier, and chlorophyll is actually one of the main pigments found in high-quality olive oil. The monounsaturated fat and chlorophyll combo are safely protected in dark glass…and preferably, it'll be stored in a cool location, too. This is because olive oil is heat sensitive, contrary to popular belief. Yes, it can be used for cooking, and it's a helluva lot better for you than cooking with so-called vegetable oils, but it should ideally only be used for low to low-moderate temperature cooking because the oils are more fragile and susceptible to oxidation. The rich concentration of antioxidants in olive oil is what enables it to be heated and protected to a certain degree. But for anything going to a moderate to high heat, you'd be better off using a more saturated fat that's more stable (coconut oil, butter, ghee, etc.).

A great way to include more extra virgin olive oil in your diet is to use it for fresh salad dressings and as a "finisher" to different dishes (where you drizzle some olive oil on top of the dish after it's finished cooking). Again, olive oil is a great source of omega-9 fats, but other rich sources include avocado oil, macadamia nuts, almonds, and sunflower seeds.

Polyunsaturated Fats

The prefix *poly* means "many," so, going back to the fat straws analogy, these unsaturated fats equate to having *many* bends in the straws. As a reminder, the more bends, the more unstable the oils will be. There are some great benefits from foods high in polyunsaturated fats, but we've got to treat them like the sensitive nutrients they are.

Polyunsaturated fats, or PUFAs, are generally found alongside other dietary fats in foods like nuts, seeds, fish, beef, and various plant-based oils. The crown jewels of the PUFA family are the essential fatty acids omega-3 and omega-6. These vital nutrients are called *essential* because your body cannot make them and they must be procured from your diet.

Omega-3s have definitely emerged as the biggest star in this ensemble cast of dietary fats. As noted earlier, research cited in the *European Journal of Clinical Nutrition* revealed that omega-3 fatty acids have anti-obesity effects and improve levels of adiponectin (helping to regulate appetite). But what they're really known for is the powerful ability to protect your body against the fat-inducing effects of inflammation. Research published in *The American Journal of Clinical Nutrition* found that omega-3 fatty acids have potent anti-inflammatory properties that can be therapeutic against several acute and chronic inflammatory conditions.

One of the most popular forms of concentrated omega-3s is high-quality fish oil. And the data here is pretty amazing. A recent study published in the journal *PLOS ONE* found that when test subjects took 3 grams of fish oil per day for 12 weeks, their metabolic rates increased by around 14 percent! This was the equivalent of burning about 200 extra calories per day simply from using this food-based supplement. In addition, a meta-analysis of 21 studies found that participants taking fish oil were able to reduce belly fat and improve their hip-to-waist ratio more effectively than participants not taking it.

Now, this is a very important point: The specific types of omega-3s you'll find in fish oil are what makes them so effective. They are forms of omega-3s called *docosahexaenoic acid* (DHA) and *eicosapentaenoic acid* (EPA). These are the omega-3s you'll get from animal sources. While the primary omega-3s you'll find in plant sources is *alpha-linolenic acid* (ALA). The data is pretty clear that ALA isn't nearly as effective as DHA and EPA. The good news is that your body can convert some of the ALA you consume into DHA and EPA if you're taking a vegan approach or don't like seafood (or other dense sources of bioavailable omega-3s). The not-so-good-news is that a tremendous amount of it is lost in the conversion process. Data cited in the journal *Applied Physiology, Nutrition, and Metabolism* found that only about 5 percent of ALA gets converted into EPA and less than 1 percent of ALA get converted into DHA. Factors like age, genetics, and the health of your microbiome can shift these numbers a bit, but not by a significant degree.

Though ALA is not touted for its fat loss benefits, it still has value in being protective of your heart and nervous system. ALA is found in foods like flaxseeds, flaxseed oil, chia seeds, walnuts, kale, purslane, hemp seeds, hemp oil, as well as some animal fats. To reprise one of our main themes, diversity in your omega sources is important too. It's wonderful to include different foods rich in ALA, but it's essential to get in some dense sources of DHA and EPA as well. Some of the best food sources of these omega-3s are fatty fish like mackerel, salmon, sardines and anchovies, grass-fed beef, egg yolks, and, of course, fish oil. An additional way to get them if you're not inspired to utilize fish and/or fish oil is to get it from where the fish get it from, which is by consuming algae. There are supplements with concentrated amounts of omega-3s in the form of algae oil. Algae oils have not been analyzed nearly to the degree that fish oil has as of yet, but new studies are constantly being done. As always, I'll keep my recommendations updated for you in the Eat Smarter Bonus Resources at eatsmarterbook.com /bonus.

Next up in the omega family are the omega-6s. This essential fatty acid's primary role is in being used as energy. It also works along with the other omega fats to support proper function of several organs in your body. As with omega-3s, there are many different types of omega-6s that have very different impacts on our bodies.

Gamma-linolenic acid (GLA) is an omega-6 fatty acid found in oils like evening primrose oil, borage oil, hemp oil, and in lesser amounts in foods like hemp seeds and spirulina. Several studies boast the effectiveness of GLA on helping to reduce pain. But, as far as benefiting fat loss, we have to look to its sibling omega-6 fatty acid, CLA.

We've already noted CLA (or *conjugated linoleic acid*) several times for some of its impressive attributes regarding metabolism. Another study cited in *The Journal of Nutrition* demonstrated that test subjects consuming CLA (versus a placebo of olive oil—which is beneficial in its own regard) lost significantly more body fat mass over the course of the 12-week study. CLA is found in notable amounts in beef, lamb, milk, and yogurt, but where it really shines is in grass-fed butter.

Butter is another food eaten by humans for thousands of years that fell out of favor due to the haphazard war on dietary fats. What makes butter so advantageous is its diversity of fats, its limited number of potential allergens (since the milk sugars and proteins are removed), and its stability at different temperatures. We've noted butter for being a viable source of short chain fats and monounsaturated fats, but what makes butter stand out is its rich concentration of CLA and its influence on metabolism.

In fact, in a surprising meta-analysis that included more than 630,000 study participants, and published in the peer-reviewed journal *PLOS ONE,* it was found that for each tablespoon of butter included in participants' daily diet they saw an additional 4 percent reduction in their risk for type 2 diabetes. Plus, a new randomized, double-blind study found that the CLA in butter is able to reduce levels of several proteins involved in inflammation, including tumor necrosis factor and C-reactive protein. If you choose to include butter in your fat-loss protocol, it's important to keep the data in mind from the scientists at the University of Wisconsin–Madison indicating that grass-fed butter contains up to 500 percent more CLA than conventional grain-fed butter.

Next up on our list of omega-6 siblings is the big brother, linoleic acid. The majority of dietary omega-6s are in the form of linoleic acid. But the stranger thing about linoleic acid is that it seems to be an upside-down version of omega-3s. Instead of being anti-inflammatory, omega-6 linoleic acids appear to be *pro*-inflammatory. This phenomenon may be true, but it's not in the conventional sense that people have come to believe.

Many experts assert that linoleic acid is inherently inflammatory and increases the risk of chronic illness in and of itself. But a systematic review of multiple trials published in the *Journal of the Academy of Nutrition and Dietetics* uncovered that there's virtually no evidence from randomized, controlled intervention studies showing that the consumption of linoleic acid in the diet increases the concentration of inflammatory biomarkers. Yet, there's a much deeper story here when it comes to omega-6s and inflammation.

If you recall from an earlier discussion, inflammation is not a "bad" thing. It's actually essential for life and for supporting many processes in our bodies. Take our immune system, for example. When our immune system mounts a defense against a pathogen or sends in support to protect a wound, inflammation is present as protection, and that's where you'll find some omega-6s in the mix.

Now, the problem is when inflammation gets out of control, and, dietarily speaking, when linoleic acids get out of control. The average diet in today's modern society consists of an absurd amount of omega-6 linoleic acids, largely due to the inclusion of very volatile plant-based "vegetable oils." And the term *vegetable oil,* itself, is a misnomer. It's not broccoli oil! It's not kale oil! What it really consists of are industrial seed oils from corn, cottonseed, safflower seeds, rapeseeds, and soybean oil. All of them are processed at extremely high temperatures and must be refined, bleached, and deodorized before they are suitable for human consumption. Remember how polyunsaturated fats (many "bends") are the most unstable and sensitive of all the fats? Well, what do you think happens to these omega-6s when they're treated like this? In short, they become oxidized, corrupted, and, according to research published in *Inhalation Toxicology,* even inhaling the smell of them while cooking can damage your DNA. WTF?!

The exposure we'd get to linoleic acids in natural foods throughout human evolution isn't the issue at all. The data shows that humans

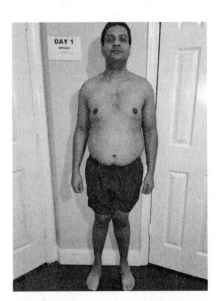 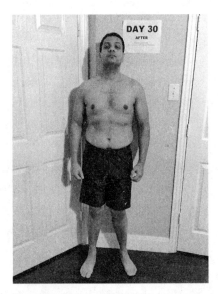

I have always seen myself as an unhealthy and overweight person. This caused me to grow up as a fat-phobe, avoiding dietary fats like the plague, instead opting for high-carbohydrate diets. This never worked and my weight continued to climb. Having grown up in the low-fat era it was unbelievable to me that eating fat could make me thinner. However, I was desperate to try anything, and I gave it a shot (increasing my intake of healthy fats). What followed was a miracle.

I started to make progress once again—the scale started showing lower numbers and my clothes fit better…and I had lost twelve pounds. I am happy that the lessons learned from Shawn will guide me towards a lifetime of health, success, and a positive self-image. Thanks Shawn and may God bless you.

would have consumed a ratio of about 3:1 omega-6s to omega-3s, respectively (from sources like nuts, seeds, and various meats). Now, thanks in large part to our consumption of these industrialized vegetable oils (primarily in cooking and processed foods), that ratio is at approximately 17:1 on average, according to data cited in the journal *Biomedicine and Pharmacotherapy*. What's even more alarming is that some segments of the U.S. population are getting 50:1 omega-6s to omega-3s, and that polarity continues to keep climbing.

A diet with a balance of omega-6s and omega-3s reduces inflammation, but a diet with an excessively heavy ratio of omega-6s is pro-inflammatory, and pro-obesity as well. A recent study published in the journal *Nutrients* found that a large increase in the ratio of omega-6s in the diet compared to omega-3s directly increases our risk for obesity. Another study found that an imbalanced omega-6 to omega-3 ratio can lead to dysfunction of our hunger-related hormones and increase fat storage. Even with caloric intake being the same, the researchers found that a diet higher in omega-6s led to more weight gain than a diet with a more favorable ratio of omega-6s to omega-3s.

The bottom line is, with the inclusion of more omega-6 linoleic acid foods, we need to be adamant about getting in plenty of omega-3 fats as well. And since we've established that polyunsaturated fats are the extra-sensitive member of the dietary fats boy band (you've got to have at least one to make the formula work), we need to be mindful in how we treat them. Cooking polyunsaturated fats at high heat will cause their delicate omega fats to quit the group and write emotional street songs about how you did them wrong and now they want you to gain weight (Drake would make a great ghostwriter on this). With that said, cooking with so-called "vegetable oil" is just a bad idea. And, have you ever noticed that bottles of concentrated polyunsaturated fats like flaxseed oil and hemp seed oil are in the refrigerated section of the store? Some folks got the memo that those oils are *that* sensitive, while other folks are unknowingly still cooking with canola oil that's damaging their DNA and depressing the function of their metabolism. Hopefully, we can shift our demand and make eating smarter the norm, and put an end to companies having those toxic oils on store shelves for unsuspecting families.

Even a report published in the journal *BMJ: Open Heart* found that these vegetable oils can be a major culprit behind organ failure, cardiac arrest, and sudden death. The creation of industrialized vegetable oil is clearly not one of our society's greatest innovations. But the good news is that we get to decide which fats and oils we use in food preparation and food purchases for ourselves and our loved ones.

Fat Words to Live By

In covering the nuances of this powerful Big Three macronutrient we call fat, I want to encourage you to be proactive at getting plenty of healthy fats into your meals each day. You can now be confidently empowered to eat high-quality fats and see improved results in fat *loss,* like what was demonstrated in a landmark study published in *The New England Journal of Medicine*. Researchers took 132 people (many of whom had metabolic syndrome or type 2 diabetes) and split them into either a higher-fat/lower-carb group or a lower-fat/higher-carb group for a six-month study period. At the end of the study, the researchers found that the higher-fat/lower-carb group lost an average of 12.8 pounds, while the lower-fat/higher-carb group lost an average of only 4.2 pounds. Even though their caloric intake was the same, shifting the ratio of their macronutrients to include more fats resulted in losing three times as much weight!

And fat doesn't just affect the fat most people are trying to lose . . . it also affects our valuable brown fat that gives us another metabolic advantage. A study cited in *The Journal of Nutrition* found that the inclusion of more fat, specifically essential fatty acids, has the potential to increase the amount and activity of our brown adipose tissue. As you recall from Chapter One, this is a type of fat that *burns* fat. And this is yet another way that the essential fatty acids we covered in this section can help you optimize your body and your health.

POWERFUL MACROS THAT ROUND OUT YOUR STARTING FIVE

Though they are often overlooked in the conversation about fat loss, you can't have a complete roster without the other two members of your macronutrient Starting Five. Here we will hit some important points for these two fluid players so that you can be empowered in using them to win your fat-loss game.

Alcohol Alley-Oop

When it comes to controversy, no one is more acclimated to creating drama than alcohol. The interesting thing about alcohol is that he's incredibly energetic. In fact, when alcohol is in the game, he immediately takes precedence over everyone else and gets burned for fuel *first*. The burning of body fat, glucose, or other dietary macros that may be in the mix comes to a halt when alcohol steps on the court. This is because alcohol is a calorically dense compound that can provide large amounts of bioavailable energy. But he's also very toxic to the system, and cannot be stored as energy in the body like proteins, carbs, and fat can. So, when he's tapped into the game, he goes hard and fast, and doesn't care who stands in the way. Other players might try and shoot their shot, but alcohol starts grabbing everything out of the air like it was an alley-oop, even though nobody wanted him to.

Back in Chapter One, we noted how each gram of protein contains 4 calories, each gram of carbohydrate contains 4 calories, and each gram of fat contains 9 calories. Well, alcohol is coming in ranked at the higher end of calorie density at 7 calories per gram. The shining difference here is that it's in liquid form without any other accompanying nutrients that can benefit your metabolism (like omega-3–rich oils, for example). This is why alcohol consumption is widely regarded as "empty calories." But, again, these calories don't get stored...so how in the world can getting your sip on cause drama for your metabolism? Part one is how it stops the burning of stored fat, but part two is how it affects your other systems.

Alcohol is yet another thing that's been utilized by humans for thousands of years. True enough, it's likely contributed to more fights, table dances, and adult bed-wetting than any other nutrient, but it can't be all that bad, right?

Well, if you look openly at the data, you see some pretty interesting things manifest. A study published in the *Journal of the American College of Cardiology* analyzed the data of over 333,000 participants for eight years and found that light to moderate drinkers (approximately two or less drinks per day for men and one drink per day for women) were about 20 percent less likely to die from any cause during the study period (compared to non-drinkers). The study did note that several other lifestyle factors weren't taken into account, and that there wasn't a specification for people who were drinkers and became nondrinkers or nondrinkers who began drinking. With that in mind, the researchers affirmed that lifelong nondrinkers "should not start drinking for health reasons only, but should be encouraged to adopt healthy lifestyles (like regular exercise and not smoking)."

That study was fascinating enough, but what was really eye-opening was when the researchers noted that there is a drastic *increase* in risk of death from all causes in people who are heavy drinkers (more than three drinks per day for men and more than two drinks per day for women). The study authors stated that, "A balance between beneficial and detrimental effects of alcohol consumption on health should be considered when making individual or population-wide recommendations." They added, "But the reduction of harmful or high consumption of alcohol remains necessary and essential." Alcohol consumption appears to be a little like that movie *A Thin Line Between Love and Hate*. A little bit might get some benefits, but too much can have you waking up to a stranger cooking breakfast in your kitchen.

Now, what about the impact that alcohol has on weight and body fat? First of all, a meta-analysis published in the journal *Current Obesity Reports* deduced that many studies show light to moderate alcohol intake—again, at most two drinks a day for men, one for women—does not seem to be associated with obesity risk in a short-term follow-up period. Heavy drinking, on the other hand, was clearly linked to an increased risk of obesity and the accumulation of more visceral fat. But even light to moderate drinking *long-term* raised some serious concerns.

Since alcohol is quickly burned as fuel, it takes a sneaky route to influencing weight and body fat. The researchers found that frequent alcohol consumption could lead to something referred to as *fat sparing,* where fatty acid oxidation is suppressed. In other words, fats are being spared from being burned as fuel more often, leading to statistically higher body fat long-term.

Another thing the meta-analysis noted, which was highlighted in the journal *Clinical Endocrinology,* was that even a moderate intake of alcohol can have an inhibitory effect on leptin. This manifests with several studies showing folks tend to eat more and make poorer food choices when they're drinking.

That lowered inhibition is part of the luster that comes along with drinking. But most of us don't think about it in regard to our food choices. I don't know about you, but I've seen more people stroll into White Castle for some sliders after drinking than at any other time in their lives. When it comes to fat loss, it's not that alcohol is off-limits, but I feel we need to be reminded that it's one of the world's most powerful psychoactive drugs. I think we don't put it in that category consciously because 1) it's not something you purchase from a doctor or a dealer, 2) it's socially acceptable to consume it in public, and 3) how bad can a drink named *Sand in the Crack* be for you anyway? (That's a mixture of rum, pineapple juice, and cranberry juice, if you were wondering.)

And this leads to the next point: The form of alcohol you're drinking matters. Just like other macronutrients, how it's prepared and served can make a world of difference to your waistline. Let's just be honest, the alcoholic beverages that have added sugars from soda and juices are really just adult Kool-Aid. Combining alcohol *and* sugar is a surefire way to negatively impact your metabolism.

Does this mean you can't drink alcohol if you want to support fat loss? Of course not! You can still get your sip on, but this is a very sensitive area without a lot of wiggle room. Even a little too much alcohol can lead to extra fat storage—and that amount depends on your genetics, gender, age, gut bacteria balance, current body fat levels, and several other factors that make up your metabolic fingerprint. For example, a study from the University of Pennsylvania School of Nursing found that people who were already overweight and consuming alcohol had a more difficult time losing weight than those who were nondrinkers. The study also noted that people tend to underestimate their drinking, which is another important thing that might set off a lightbulb moment for you. There are often no serving sizes on glasses of alcohol and mixed drinks. You've got to be great at eye-balling and sensing it. But the problem is, the more we drink, the more our eyeballs and senses start to forget who they even belong to.

Most of the touted benefits of alcohol come from the world of red wine. It's where you find the antioxidants and resveratrol! But, let's keep it real. Hardly anyone is drinking wine for the health benefits. "I heard antioxidants can help you live longer...well I'm trying to live to be 600 years old, so let's polish off another bottle." Yes, red wine has some noted benefits, but let's not toss it in the category of a health food. If you enjoy wine or other alcoholic beverages, I simply encourage you to seek out better quality (avoiding pesticides and other allergens), be mindful of how much and how often you drink, and if you're not seeing the results you want (even with a reduced-calorie diet), the alcohol may be the thing that's holding you back. And if you're wondering why, it could also be due to your microbiome.

A study cited in the *American Journal of Physiology* found that microbiome dysbiosis is significantly more prevalent in heavy alcohol drinkers. The researchers discovered that heavy drinkers have substantially lower levels of metabolism-supportive bacteroidetes and much higher levels of pathogenic bacteria. The scientists stated, "Alcohol use is correlated with decreased connectivity of the microbial network, and this alteration is seen even after an extended period of sobriety."

A small exception to this may be, again, found in red wine. Research published in *The American Journal of Clinical Nutrition* showed that study participants drinking about 1½ glasses of red wine a day for 20 days actually increased their ratio of friendly bacteria and lowered their levels of pathogenic bacteria.

Now, before anyone runs out and cracks open another bottle, I want to reiterate how important it is to be mindful with alcohol use in regard to fat loss and your health overall. Additional concerns regarding addiction, reduced cognitive function, and increased likelihood of liver damage (as you know, your liver plays a big role in fat loss and it bears the burden of processing the alcohol to protect your organs from toxicity) puts up a huge warning sign that should encourage you to pay more attention to its effects on your body. Eat, drink, and be merry… but if fat loss is your goal, you're going to want to drink ample amounts of our next powerhouse macro.

Winning Water

The most underrated member of your macronutrient Starting Five is *water*. He doesn't get a lot of acknowledgment, in fact, he's often taken for granted. But one thing that water knows how to do is win when it comes to fat loss.

Water is not talked about much in the macronutrient conversation because it's considered to be a macronutrient that doesn't provide any energy. But that's not completely accurate.

Saying that water doesn't provide energy is looking at metabolism through the lens of calories again. We've already broken down how flawed caloric tunnel vision can be earlier in the book. And the metabolic power that water provides is another example of how we need to expand our thinking.

Simply drinking water can have the metabolic impact of powerful fat-loss hormones like glucagon and HGH. A peer-reviewed study published in the journal *Obesity* found that drinking adequate amounts of water can literally trigger the release of stored body fat (i.e., lipolysis)! And if that didn't perk your ears up enough, another study published in *The Journal of Clinical Endocrinology and Metabolism* found that drinking water can also increase your metabolic rate through a process called *water-induced thermogenesis*.

The researchers discovered that by drinking about 17 ounces of water (within a couple of minutes) you can temporarily boost your metabolic rate by 30 percent! The increase was found to occur within 10 minutes and reach a maximum after 30 to 40 minutes. The total thermogenic calorie burn is around 25 calories. So, doing this three or four times a day can help folks burn an additional 75 to 100 calories.

Now, to be very clear about this, simply drinking more water (which is calorie-free) triggers your body to burn *more* calories. If only looking at this from a calorie perspective, that's pretty amazing (and actually explains why "drink plenty of water" really works for weight loss). But we know the fat-loss story is much deeper than calories, so let's dive into some of the other ways that water impacts your system.

Here's a list of just some of the things water is responsible for in your body:

- Maintenance of your DNA
- Facilitating reactions in your mitochondria (where fat is burned!)
- Maintaining the integrity of your blood (your blood is over 90 percent water and it's used to transfer many of the nutrients, oxygen, and immune cells throughout your body, and to assist in waste removal)
- Creating lymph fluid (to support your immune system and waste removal)
- Building fluids for your digestive tract and digestive secretions
- Regulating body temperature
- Creating the cerebrospinal fluid of your central nervous system
- Making the synovial fluid of your joints and discs

There are two really important things I want you to know. First of all, your body uses pathways built on water to transmit your hormones and neurotransmitters throughout your entire body. Water literally enables communication between all of your cells, tissues, and organs. Secondly, probably the most important thing that water helps to create in your body is *your brain*. We'll talk more about this in the next section, but just note that your brain (as we've discussed) is a huge player in regulating your metabolism. In fact, your hypothalamus, located in that amazing brain of yours, is considered to be the master regulator of your hormones, as we touched on in Chapter Two. It helps regulate your hunger, influences thyroid function, plus a whole lot more. And two major things that damage your hypothalamic function are 1) inflammation and 2) dehydration.

What I'm really striving to communicate here is that *none of the processes of metabolism can take place without the presence of water.* It is truly that important. Simply drinking water provides an immediate boost to your metabolism because it makes everything work better. Millions of people who are chronically dehydrated have put themselves at a metabolic disadvantage and don't even know it. A big part of eating smarter is to ensure you're getting the right amount of hydration for *you*.

So how much water should we be drinking? Well, in our culture of "some is good, more must be better," some folks will see this as a cue to go chug-a-lugging a few gallons of water a day. The problem with that is drinking too much water gives you diminishing returns and can be problematic for your metabolism, too. So, when it comes to hydration there are a few basic principles to follow.

Liquid Intelligence

It's important to know that the type of water you drink matters. Now, you might be thinking, "What does he mean by type of water?" Well, water is not just H_2O like we were taught in school...in fact, you don't find ordinary H_2O anywhere in nature, at all. Water is known as "the universal solvent" because it's able to combine with and dissolve more substances than any other liquid on earth. Wherever water goes, whether it's through the air, the ground, or through our bodies, it integrates with and takes along valuable chemicals, minerals, and nutrients. Water isn't just H_2O, it's H_2O with other things dissolved in it. And the things dissolved in it help determine how it hydrates or *dehydrates* your cells.

It's a really strange phenomenon, but you're probably well aware that drinking too much ocean water can straight up kill you. This is because the excessive salt/mineral content of that water prevents it from traveling into your cells when you drink it. Instead, that water stays quarantined in your extracellular fluid and (because of osmosis) the water you *do* have in your cells is leached out in an attempt to reduce the concentration of minerals outside of the cells. So, even though you may be drinking water, the excess mineral content makes your cells dehydrated, and this can be life-threatening.

Water carries a unique form of intelligence. In nature, water is always moving from a place of less concentrated solution (where there's more water and less minerals) to a place of more concentrated solution (where there's more minerals and less water). Water is driven to go where it's needed. That's why, on the other side, not having enough minerals/salts in your water can hurt you, too. Remember, in nature, you won't find blank H_2O anywhere. Humans evolved drinking H_2O with minerals/salts dissolved in it. Albeit, in small amounts, but those small amounts matter!

Chugging down distilled water or water that's had all of the minerals filtered out of it creates a situation where, now, the higher concentration of minerals is *inside* the cell. So, water keeps getting pulled from the extracellular fluid into the cell in droves. Your extracellular fluid is now being dehydrated, and as you keep chugging this blank water trying to address your thirst, all the water being pulled into the cell can potentially make some of your cells explode! Not a very attractive situation, but you could confidently say that your cells are the bomb.

Here's the bottom line: You need water that has *some* minerals in it. If you use a water filtration system like reverse osmosis or distillation, you simply need to add some minerals/salts to the water that you're going to drink to give it some structure. This could be in the form of ionic mineral drops or high-quality salts. Either way, that's one method of literally "charging up" your water. Another way is through adding some fresh fruits or veggies to the water (like lemon, lime, mint, etc.). These plants provide minerals and electrons to the water that gives it a charge and structure as well. These minerals are in a natural, low concentration, so they inherently make it more hydrating. Feeling a little thirsty yet?

And speaking of natural concentrations of minerals, natural spring water is a great resource for structured water with a (generally) ideal mineral content. Water coming from a spring has gone through the earth's hydrological cycle (the earth, itself, is sort of like a giant water filter) and this has been the most valued commodity in human evolution. Prior to recent times where humans could "treat" our own water, people moved and settled where the springs were. Eventually, we learned how to bypass looking for springs and dig down into where the spring water comes from, which are these underground lakes called *aquifers* to procure our water. And now, with a population of billions of people on the planet, we've found more innovative ways to provide safe drinking water all over the world.

Chemical Drip

If you're drinking from municipal tap water, you might want to know about a report published by the Associated Press that found nearly 41 million Americans have been consuming tainted pharmaceutical chemicals in their water. From antidepressants to pain relievers to hormone replacement medications, 56 different pharmaceutical chemicals were found in water supplies ranging from southern California all the way to northern New Jersey. The researchers noted that these chemicals were in trace amounts, but they were present, nevertheless.

If you're curious how this happens (and without getting too deep into the murky waters), as humans have been consuming these drugs in recent years, their metabolic byproducts (aka when people poop and pee them out) are finding their way back into the water supply. Even though our waste water (coming from toilets, sinks, tubs, etc.) is heavily treated, we don't currently have systems that effectively eliminate all of the new chemicals and drugs that are being consumed. And as our wastewater is treated and released into our rivers and oceans, it eventually makes its way back into our water system indirectly, or it's used *directly* as additional water for agricultural and landscape irrigation, industrial processes, toilet flushing, replenishing groundwater basins, and even for drinking water. In fact, some water experts assert that recycled wastewater is totally safe to drink. And they believe that it's part of a solution to solve our growing need for clean water sources. The craziest part is, people seem to like it.

Researchers at the University of California–Riverside and Santa Barbara City College found that, in a blind taste test, more people preferred the taste of recycled waste tap water over conventional tap water. For the study, published in the journal *Appetite,* researchers gave bottled water, recycled wastewater from the tap, and conventional groundwater tap water to 143 participants and asked them to rate the waters without knowing where they came from. Most of them picked the recycled wastewater—they call it "toilet to tap."

I don't know about you, but suddenly I'm not as thirsty anymore. Seriously speaking, this is not a common practice in municipalities *yet,* but I'm just letting you know that if you are drinking tap water, it's probably a good idea to get a strong enough filter to remove more of the suspicious things that aren't currently being accounted for. In truth, if you don't use a water filter, you *become* the filter.

Reverse osmosis (RO) systems work well, as it pushes water through a very tight membrane (approximately .0001 micron—compared to a bacteria which is .4 micron and many drug residues and pesticides that are comparable in size), so it gets rid of a lot of stuff. But, remember, whether it's RO or distillation, you need to add some minerals back to that water. Alkalizing machines don't address these pharmaceutical chemicals at all. You'll just be drinking alkaline water with a zest of Tylenol. Not a biggie. Or is it?

What we really need to understand is that these things intrinsically affect our cells, affect our hormones, and affect our metabolism in subtle, but real, ways. Yes, we absolutely need to be adamant about our hydration. But choosing reputable spring water sources, well water, or RO water or distilled water that has been remineralized is key to doing this in a safer, smarter way.

How Much Do We Need?

The most important marker for how much water we need to drink is to listen to your body. This can be easier said than done today with all of the external distractions, stress, and faulty things going on with our hormones and neurotransmitters to begin with. So, if you know that things are not completely "online" yet with your body's communication of thirst and water needs, use this simple barometer.

The standard recommendation to drink eight 8-ounce glasses of water per day doesn't take into account our different heights, weights, activity levels, or current states of health. There's no hard science on how much water each of us needs, but what we do know is that most people aren't drinking enough. That said, I like to use a simple formula as a baseline while folks are working toward getting that accurate cellular communication rebooted. Simply take your body weight in pounds and divide that number in half. The number that you come up with is the number of ounces you need to target each day. So, if someone is 150 pounds, divide that in half to get 75. So, 75 ounces is the target for that person. Generally, if someone is 200+ pounds, I simply make 100 ounces the baseline. We don't need to go much higher than that and make drinking water and peeing a part-time job.

So, use this formula as a baseline and adjust depending on your activity level and environmental exposures. If you're more active, sweating, or dealing with some acute or chronic health issues, generally speaking, a little more water is going to be helpful.

I've found that the two best ways to ensure that you're drinking enough water are:

1. **Take an "inner bath" to start your day.** While we are asleep, our bodies undertake hundreds of different processes to repair damaged tissues, fortify our immune system, eliminate old cells, and more. All of this results in a tremendous amount of metabolic waste products that need to be removed. Drinking water when you wake up literally helps to flush these things out (or you'll risk them slowing your metabolism down like a hormonal clog). And, just logically speaking, your hydration levels are lower due to the sheer amount of time you've gone without water while you're asleep for several hours. When you wake up, your body needs water first. Not coffee. Not SunnyD. Water.

   a. Plus, you'll also receive that metabolic boost via water-induced thermogenesis that we talked about earlier. This helps to put your metabolic systems in the "ON" position to start the day. It's a huge advantage, and it's a great opportunity to get in a nice chunk of your hydration needs before the busyness of the day sets in. I recommend drinking 16 to 30 ounces of water within the first 10 minutes of waking up. This is what constitutes as taking your inner bath. We generally take an outer bath or shower to get ourselves ready for the day, but isn't the inside even more important?

2. **Keep it on hand at all times.** The #1 way to ensure you're drinking enough water is simply to have it with you. You can't drink it if you don't have it. So, keep it close by. You're Batman, your bottle is Robin. You're Lucy, your bottle is Ethel. You're Will Smith, your bottle is Carlton. I don't want to see you without each other. And, today, it's easier than ever.

   b. There are several incredible bottles that keep your water safe and secure that are easy to travel with. Plus, many computer bags, book bags, and purses have special compartments made for your bottle. And get a bottle that you like! Something that you like to see and hold. I don't care if it's a bottle branded with the place where you went on vacation, a bottle that's your favorite color, or a bottle with a picture of the Power Rangers on it. It's just a good idea to get something you like. It's *your* bottle, your health provider, your trusted sidekick.

   c. Stainless steel is great (and keeps your water cooler, longer) and there's also fancy glass bottles (use with caution, obviously), and several other options. The only thing I'd say to steer clear of is plastic if at all possible. Just to be clear, pouring into and drinking out of a plastic cup or using a BPA-free plastic bottle for the day is not a major concern. It's when water is stored and sitting in plastics for a long time or in excessive light or heat that problems can start to arise (see "BPA: Myth or Menace?" for more). But regardless of the type of bottle you choose, remember to keep it close by or you might find yourself in an unwelcome thirst trap.

BPA: Myth or Menace?

Have you ever left a plastic water bottle sitting in your car or around your house in the sun for a while, and then taken a sip only to find out that you can actually taste the plastic? It's not just in your head. Conventional plastics don't biodegrade, they *photodegrade,* meaning that exposure to light breaks them down. As you'll recall, water is known as the universal solvent, so when those plastic compounds break down into your water, you are effectively making yourself a nice plastic tea. Now, this wouldn't be such a big deal if it weren't for the data affirming that compounds in plastic, namely *bisphenol-A* (BPA) is a noted xenoestrogen. A xenoestrogen is a foreign estrogenic compound that's able to mimic estrogen in our bodies. According to data published in *Frontiers in Bioscience,* xenoestrogens like BPA are able to bond to estrogen receptor sites in our body and disrupt the function of our endocrine system.

Complete photodegradation of plastics takes many, many lifetimes, so there's likely not crazy amounts in an average bottle of water you buy at the store. But even small amounts have been found to be harmful to humans. The safety of BPA has been debated for several years, with legal doses found in many packaged foods and beverages reported as having "no significant effects." Yet, a meta-analysis of over 100 studies published in the peer-reviewed journal *Environmental Research* found significant detrimental effects of BPA at even low exposures.

Issues connected to BPA exposure range from infertility to obesity, and more. A study published in *Fertility and Sterility* found that men with detectable levels of BPA in their system were three to four times more likely to have a low sperm concentration and low sperm count, while a study cited in *Environmental Health Perspectives* discovered that women undergoing fertility treatments who had higher levels of detectable BPA were up to two times less likely to become pregnant. Again, be reminded that this is correlation, not causation. But with science, our goal is to have enough evidence for us all to conclude that something is connected. And speaking of more evidence, a study published in *The Journal of Clinical Endocrinology and Metabolism* found that people with the highest percentage of BPA in their system were at least 50 percent more likely to be overweight or obese.

Part of the connection with BPA is likely due to the fact that more overweight and obese folks statistically eat more packaged food. BPA isn't just in your water bottles, it's also in food packaging...including on the inside of many canned foods. BPA is found in the epoxy resin that's used to coat the inside of cans to help prevent erosion. A randomized study conducted by researchers at the Harvard School of Public Health had folks either eat fresh-made soup or canned soup for five days. They found that the urine levels of BPA were 1,221 percent higher in those who ate the canned soup. In the words of C+C Music Factory, these are "things that make you go hmmmm..."

Is going BPA-free enough? Well, it's probably a good idea. But I want you to be aware that there are other concerning compounds in our conventional bottles (for juice, soda, water, etc.) and food packaging, like bisphenol-S (BPS) and bisphenol-F (BPF). A report cited in *Environmental Health Perspectives* stated, "Based on the current literature, BPS and BPF are as hormonally active as BPA, and they have endocrine-disrupting effects."

When it comes to fat loss, supporting our endocrine system and hormones is of the utmost importance. Compared to your body's overall need for healthy food and water, BPA may be a small thing in the grand scheme of things. But our goal is to stack conditions in your favor to make the results you want inevitable. If I plan accordingly, I'll choose to have water that's not stored in plastic. But if I'm in a situation where water bottled in plastic is the only option available (during a long flight, for example), I'm going to drink that water rather than dehydrating myself. And I'll upgrade my water source the next time I get a chance to. The sum and summary is to simply skip the BPA whenever possible, but the most important thing is that you continue to stay hydrated!

Up until now, water has played the background as the little-respected macronutrient. In fact, most people are focused on the newest, hottest eating trend and overlook how much of a talent water truly is. Leonardo da Vinci said, "Water is the driving force of all nature." Remember its power, and use it to your advantage, because it's critical to having the health, energy, and body composition you want to have!

THE DREAM TEAM

So, there we have the five macros in your nutritional starting lineup! As a reminder, no matter what diet framework you subscribe to, minding your macros is one of the three key elements to achieving long-term success.

If any of these foods jump out at you as something you want to incorporate, but you find yourself wondering how to make them, no worries. We've got several recipes that incorporate many of them in the recipe section.

Up next, we've got the final one of your Three Fat Loss Essentials, so let's get this thing locked down!

CHAPTER FIVE

Fat Loss Essential #3: Optimize Hormone Function

When the stomach is full, the heart is glad.

~*Dutch proverb*

From insulin to glucagon and from ghrelin to leptin, we've taken a trip into the vast universe of our hormones to truly uncover what's controlling our metabolic solar system. As you've learned, our hormones play a major role in what our bodies actually do with the food that we eat. So the question then arises, how do we better support our hormones to launch us toward the results that we want?

In this chapter we're going to defy gravity and uncover the specific things that will optimize your hormone function. So, buckle up and focus in as we reveal these hormonal *Guardians of the Galaxy.*

SMALL BUT MIGHTY

In the last chapter we broke down the critical importance of minding your macronutrients. Yes, your macros are clearly important, but it's the *micronutrients* that, in many ways, control what the macronutrients are able to do.

There's been such a barrier to the public getting this information because most nutrition experts are so hyper-focused on macronutrients that they don't give a lot of credence to the impact of micronutrients. In many ways, they think they're cute but unnecessary. Like when I was about to turn 18 years old and head to college and my grandma gave me a birthday card with $10 in it. But she also added a small note that said, "Don't tell your grandpa," like she secretly gave me a family fortune or something. I promise, that little $10 wasn't going to change my life one bit. The sentiment was super cute, but unnecessary.

But micronutrients aren't just a sweet little side note. They are *extremely* necessary for your hormonal function and much more. For instance, remember the energy power plants in our cells called *mitochondria* (where fat is actually burned)? In a conversation with bestselling author and physician Dr. Terry Wahls, she shared with me: "When our mitochondria are unhealthy, they don't produce as much ATP as our cells need to be robust and healthy... Our energy levels (and burning of stored fat) are critically dependent on having vigorous mitochondria." She said that our mitochondria desperately need micronutrients like B vitamins, sulfur, and magnesium to function effectively.

In fact, magnesium is literally *required* to make new mitochondria! Magnesium is used as an enzyme cofactor that enables our mitochondria to make copies of itself. If your magnesium levels are low, then you're automatically going to have a difficult time making new mitochondria (and your metabolism will suffer as a result). Simply ensuring that you're getting enough of this essential mineral can help to support your mitochondria's ability to burn fat and help optimize your hormones as well. The problem is that at least 56 percent of the U.S. population is deficient in magnesium.

A meta-analysis published in the *Journal of Internal Medicine* reviewed the data of nearly 300,000 people and found that the consumption of magnesium-rich foods (like spinach, almonds, and avocados) significantly reduces the risk of insulin resistance and type 2 diabetes. As we discussed earlier in the book, intelligently managing the hormone insulin is a huge key in our fat-loss equation. And another peer-reviewed study found that test subjects with optimal levels of magnesium consistently had lower levels of abdominal fat and a lower body mass index. This is just one little micronutrient, yet it can have a mighty impact! Keep in mind, there are many other powerful micronutrients that help to fortify your metabolism. So, before we go any further, let's get clear on what our micronutrients really are.

Micronutrients are essentially all of the other nutritive factors found in food besides the core five macronutrients. This means there are literally *hundreds* of different micronutrients that play a role in human health and metabolism. In short, micronutrients include all of the vitamins, minerals, trace minerals, antioxidants, enzymes, polyphenols, carotenoids, and more. Modern science has identified many of these micronutrients already, but we still have a lot more to discover.

This is what makes food so special when it comes to obtaining these vital micronutrients. Real food doesn't have just one isolated nutrient, it has an abundance of micronutrients along with cofactors and biopotentiators that make them work better in our bodies. Synthetic, man-made supplements and processed "fortified" foods simply can't do what real food can. And this brings us to one of the most important principles in eating smarter. Your hormones aren't only controlled by your macro- and micronutrient intake. They're also controlled by your genes.

KEEP IT REAL

Did you know that food deeply impacts your genetic expression? There's an entire blossoming field of science called *nutrigenomics* that is dedicated to the study of how *what we eat determines what our genes are doing*. Your genes contain the information that determines everything about you: things that are considered static like eye color and height, as well as things that can be modulated like body fat, insulin sensitivity, and the expression of illnesses.

Your genes essentially control what type of "copies" are being printed out of yourself. We all have genes that provide the expression of health, energy, and vitality. But we also have genes that code for various diseases, enervation, and atrophy. We once believed that our genes controlled our fate, and that was the end of the story. If you've got genes for obesity, heart disease, arthritis, etc., you'd better stand in line, because it's headed your way! Thankfully, within recent decades, *epigenetics* has risen to the top as a primary discipline helping us to better understand our genes and put more power into our hands.

As humans, we collectively have 25,000 to 35,000 genes that we all share. But what makes us so diverse (in our appearance, personality, and most relevant to us, our levels of health and fitness) is that each of our genes has hundreds or even *thousands* of different potential expressions. Epigenetics teaches us that countless things can influence what our genes are doing from moment to moment. Epigenetics has revealed that environmental factors like stress, level of activity, and, of course, what we eat, can have a huge influence on whether or not certain gene variations are being expressed.

For example, essentially every human has one of the genes largely linked to obesity called the *fat mass and obesity-associated gene* (FTO gene), yet many of the people carrying the gene are fit and healthy, and the hallmark expression of the gene has not manifested. The FTO gene plays a role in controlling hormones that regulate feeding behavior and energy expenditure. So, if this gene is expressed, it can seem as though your body is working against you. This is why shaming people and judging people for their weight challenges is often misguided. People judge others as if they have no discipline and no determination when, in fact, they are often working as hard or harder than others to achieve the health results they want.

I come from a family of significantly overweight or obese folks. And I was always the skinny kid in my family. But, with enough poor epigenetic influences, my fat genes kicked in with a vengeance, and within a couple of years of the breakdown of my health in my 20s, I could hardly recognize myself in the mirror.

This is why it's so vital to stack conditions in your favor to not just support fat loss, but to support the healthy expression of your genes. This is truly what controls everything.

With that said, every bite of food we eat literally affects our genetic expression. And just from a logical perspective, what do you think has a more positive influence on your genes, foods that humans have been eating for thousands of years, or processed, food-like products that a food scientist created last week? Eating real food isn't a matter of popularity. It's a matter of controlling your genetic fate.

The big issue is that real food has a publicity problem today. And that has a lot to do with framing and public perception. There's a common belief that healthy food doesn't taste good. I remember one time my family was getting together for a barbecue and a family member said to me, "I don't want any of that organic stuff." Oh, you mean the food without pesticides, herbicides, rodenticides, and artificial flavors, colors, and preservatives? Oh, yeah. That's actually called *food*. I know the label *organic* can throw people off (even though it's loosely used in many regards). But, in general, it just means that there are less chemicals in the mix that can cause your genes to throw a hissy fit.

Another issue that has normalized eating processed foods are all of the celebrity endorsements. From cereal to soda to fast food, the people that most folks look up to are telling them to consume things that are harmful to them. It's a sad state of affairs, but rather than ragging on the celebrities who are just trying to make a living and often don't realize the impact of the foods they're endorsing, I'd rather see more celebrities standing up and advocating healthy food. No one is glamorizing real food. But what if they were? What if Arnold Schwarzenegger was like, "Aaaaah! Get to tha choppa so we can go to the farmers market!" Or Samuel L. Jackson was on TV telling you to, "eat your Brussels sprouts mutha%#@&$!"

I know it sounds crazy, but I think it might help to balance out the power. And all of us, celebrity or not, can endorse real food in our own ways. In doing so, we can empower more people to get access to the things that help them tap into their highest genetic potential and become the best version of themselves.

And there's one more simple principle that can help you do that. I call it the 80+ Rule. My approach is to encourage people to simply target 80+ percent whole, real foods daily. As stated, time-tested foods naturally have a familiar interaction with our genes versus today's overconsumption of heavily processed foods. Certain whole foods are better than others when it comes to fat loss, and not all whole food–based, processed foods are bad.

Part of what makes my approach so different and effective is that no food is really off-limits. Eating a can of beans might bring about WWIII in your bathroom afterward, but if that's all we've got to eat during a zombie apocalypse, then pass me a can opener and some toilet paper, because I'm going to live to fight another day! But, on a daily basis, where I get to *choose* to eat foods that taste good and actually feel good in my body, then that can of baked beans can stay on the shelf, and I can stay out of the nearest porta potty.

What I'm really trying to express is that every food has its value, though some foods are far more valuable and health-supporting than others. Nothing is forbidden, but we need to understand that there's a spectrum ranging from whole turkey to turkey casserole to turkey-and-cheese Hot Pocket. Minimal processing and cooking of the turkey with other natural ingredients still keeps it in the context of real food. But at some point, with all of the additional processing and artificial ingredients, it transforms from a wholesome food into something that makes you feel like you need to take a shower afterward.

Everything is an option, just ensure that 80+ percent of your food each day is from real foods that you can actually still recognize where they came from. Whole foods including veggies, fruits, meats (if you're not vegetarian or vegan), as well as eggs and dairy (if those foods fit for you based on what you've learned in previous chapters), nuts, seeds, herbs, and spices. These all round out the bank of real food...and this gives us literally tens of thousands of foods to choose from!

Then with our remaining 20 percent (or less) of our diet, we can enjoy other high-quality food-based things like organic protein powder, sprouted grain bread (if it resonates with your body), unsweetened nut or seed milks, and a wide variety of snacks and treats. You might not have been given permission to put *high-quality* and *treats* in the same sentence before, but simply by upgrading the ingredients you can make and have treats that provide metabolism-supporting nutrients while giving you the treat experience you may desire.

With all of this in mind, and our 80+ Rule in hand, let's talk about some of the foods that fit the bill!

LOOKING GOOD IN THOSE GENES

To recap the importance of real foods packed with bioavailable micronutrients, research published in the peer-reviewed journal *Environmental Health Perspectives* reiterated that micronutrients like vitamins, minerals, and carotenoids regulate gene expression in diverse ways. The study stated, "Many of the micronutrients and bioreactive chemicals in foods are directly involved in metabolic reactions that determine everything from hormonal balances and immune competence to detoxification processes and the utilization of macronutrients for fuel and growth."

And always remember this statement: Chronic micronutrient deficiency leads to chronic overeating. One of the biggest driving forces of our hunger is to seek out and ingest key micronutrients that enable the function of every cell and organ in our bodies. If we are deficient in minerals like zinc (which is needed for DNA synthesis and immune function), iron (needed to build our blood), and potassium (needed to maintain proper fluid balance and muscle function), this can trigger increased appetite as a primal mechanism to seek out these nutrients to help you survive. Though your body is calling out for nutrient-rich food in the form of increased hunger, in today's world we can head to the refrigerator or cabinet or fast food place and grab any number of highly processed foods that are devoid of the nutrients we really need. Yes, we get some calories and substance in our bellies, but our appetite will continue to rage on over and over again until we give our bodies the micronutrients it really needs. Without micronutrients, macronutrients can't even do their jobs. And, as far as fat loss, micronutrients need to be present for fat-burning enzymes like hormone-sensitive lipase to unlock fat stores and get rid of them for good.

Though no food is a magic bullet to optimal gene expression and fat loss, including more of these foods (and other foods you're learning more about in *Eat Smarter*) helps stack conditions in your favor to make your success unstoppable. Here are some of the most micronutrient-dense foods that support a favorable genetic expression and positively influence your hormones.

Fit Fruits

We've talked about various fruits throughout the book in terms of their benefits to our microbiome, protection against weight gain, and much more. Here's some additional information on a couple of fruits that provide some pretty sweet advantages for your metabolism.

Blueberries

Researchers at the University of Michigan published data finding that blueberry intake can potentially affect genes related to fat burning. The unsung hero of many smoothies and fruit salads, these little berries are a powerhouse source of the micronutrients vitamin C, vitamin K, manganese, and inflammation-fighting antioxidants. Plus, the flavonoids found in blueberries were found to be protective against weight gain, according to scientists at Harvard University. As an added bonus, it was also uncovered that having a serving of blueberries (and/or strawberries) three times per week can reduce your risk of having a heart attack by 34 percent. If it's good for fat loss, it's probably good for your heart, too!

If we look at the direct impact that blueberries can have on your hormones, a study published in *The Journal of Nutrition* showed that the consumption of blueberries was able to reduce insulin resistance in study participants. Keep in mind, a consistent sign of insulin resistance is carrying more body fat around the midsection. Anything we can do to improve insulin sensitivity is going to be a welcome friend for our waistline.

Fresh or frozen organic blueberries are a great choice, and wild harvested blueberries are even better (thanks to their higher level of micronutrients). Growing up, the closest thing I got to a blueberry was in my Hostess mini muffins. So, when I first had some fresh blueberries, I was surprised at the diversity in their flavor, ranging from sweet to sour. Today, it's one of my favorite snacks to grab, and definitely one of my all-time favorites to add fiber and powerhouse antioxidants to my smoothies. Remember: A half-cup of berries a day can help keep your fat genes at bay!

Cherries

Cherries are associated with desserts (a cherry on top), cocktails, and even car fresheners. But I don't think a lot of people actually eat fresh cherries, because they don't know how remarkable they are. According to data published in the *International Journal of Food Sciences and Nutrition,* micronutrients called *anthocyanins* found in cherries have the potential to literally shrink fat cells! The researchers also noted that these cherry anthocyanins are able to reduce the expression of genes associated with inflammation.

Both sweet cherries and tart cherries carry similar benefits. But tart cherries, specifically, according to physician and *New York Times*–bestselling author Dr. William Li, have *antiangiogenesis* effects that actually help cut off the blood supply to fat cells. Dr. Li is the founder of the Angiogenesis Foundation and is well noted for his research in cancer therapies. He shared with me that fat cells, like cancer cells, need a nutrient supply to grow. Angiogenesis is the creation of new blood vessels that supply those nutrients. The inclusion of selective antiangiogenic foods like cherries can help reduce adiposity in conjunction with other micronutrient-rich foods that help support metabolism.

Seeds of Life

Nuts and seeds are often paired together in nutritional conversations, which makes sense since they're actually quite identical in their benefits. They're both typically great sources of fiber, healthy fats, and packed with micronutrients. But even though they are similar, there are some interesting differences.

Technically, nuts are the hard-shelled "fruit" of certain plants. Contained within the hard shell itself is a dry fruit and one or two seeds. The distinctive thing about nuts is that the shell doesn't just separate when the fruit is ready to eat. It must be practically pried off (i.e., have your nut cracker handy or you're not getting any). True nuts include chestnuts, acorns, and hazelnuts. Seeds, on the other hand, are an edible small plant that's enclosed in a seed coat (which is stored food to nourish the plant as it grows). Some seeds need their exterior husk removed before eating, but some do not. There are many seeds in fruits that most folks have top-of-mind, like apple seeds, watermelon seeds, and pumpkin seeds. But leaning on the definition of what a seed is, miscategorized nuts like almonds and even chocolate (cacao) "beans" are in the seed family. Here's some powerhouse information on these two seeds that can help bring your metabolism more life!

Chocolate

Growing up, when I thought of chocolate I thought of Hershey's candy bars or those heart-shaped boxes of chocolate you get on Valentine's Day, when I played a little game of chocolate Russian roulette.

> Me staring at a box of "assorted" chocolates: OK, depending on which chocolate I choose, I can be biting into something delicious or something that tastes like toothpaste.

Earlier in the book when talking about the surprising benefits of cocoa as a prebiotic, we helped make the distinction between the origins of chocolate (cacao) and its twisted sisters (candy bars, chocolate-flavored candies, etc.) that we see on many store shelves today. In the aforementioned study published in *The American Journal of Clinical Nutrition,* participants consuming a sugar-free cocoa flavanol drink for four weeks significantly increased their ratio of beneficial gut flora, while significantly *decreasing* their counts of clostridia (a class of firmicutes associated with fat gain). But chocolate also has some other interesting impacts on metabolism you should know about.

A fascinating study published in the *International Archives of Medicine* put two groups of test subjects on a low-carb diet. One group was instructed to eat a low-carb diet and to consume an additional serving of 1.5 ounces of chocolate with 81 percent cacao content each day, while the other group was instructed to maintain the low-carb diet without the chocolate. At the end of the multi-week study, the researchers discovered that study participants who included chocolate in their diet lost 10 percent more weight! And they found that their weight loss was "easier" with less challenges adhering to the low-carb diet. Hot chocolate, indeed.

The crushed pieces of the cacao beans themselves (called *cacao nibs*) are a remarkable source of micronutrients. They're rich in magnesium (you know how important magnesium is), iron, and copper. As an aside on copper, researchers at the Department of Energy's Lawrence Berkeley National Laboratory at the University of California–Berkeley recently confirmed that copper plays a key role in metabolizing fat. This furthers the need to understand the value of eating a variety of foods rich in micronutrients. Through food, you can receive the right amount of these nutrients with additional cofactors that make them work better in your body, plus better help to prevent overconsumption and toxicity (even from helpful nutrients like copper). Synthetic supplements simply don't work the same way. Food first is the golden rule. And high-quality chocolate is one of the foods delivering the goods.

Almonds

A study cited in the *Journal of Research in Medical Sciences* put study participants on matching reduced-calorie diets for three months, with one interesting difference: One group included almonds in their diet, while the other group did not. After the data was compiled at the end of the study, the folks who included almonds in their diet lost *twice* as much weight and had a greater reduction in their hip-to-waist ratio than those in the almond-free group! The researchers found a greater improvement in insulin sensitivity and the satiety hormone GLP-1 in the almond group. Almonds are a great source of the micronutrients magnesium, calcium, copper, B-vitamins, and vitamin E. As we've discussed in earlier chapters, many of the foods in the nuts and seeds family pack some serious power when it comes to supporting metabolism. One-fourth cup of raw almonds (split into two different times of the day) was used in this study. But mixing and matching and getting a wide variety of nuts and seeds can definitely be a part of your approach to eating smarter.

So Eggcited

When it comes to micronutrient density and managing satiety hormones, there are few foods that fit the bill like eggs do. But, surprisingly, our egg awareness is often limited here in the U.S. There are so many egg options to try, so we'll start with the chicken egg (the one that most folks think of) and then we'll take flight to another form of eggs from there.

Chicken Eggs

Humans have figured out more ways to cook eggs than ways to store our electronic data. (Seriously...floppy discs were the bane of my existence. I still can't believe I lost that entire essay on why I thought recess should be extended into high school.) Hard-boiled, scrambled, over easy, frittata'd...the list goes on and on. Whichever way a person might like their eggs, the important thing is that they're likely cracking open some additional fat-loss benefits. Research published in the journal *Nutrients* found that study participants who ate two eggs per day (versus a calorically equal amount of oatmeal) had lower levels of the hunger hormone ghrelin between meals. Subjectively, the people eating eggs reported fewer cravings throughout the day as well.

Eggs (and specifically the egg yolks) are an impressive source of B-vitamins (including energy-important vitamin B12), choline, zinc, and vitamin D. By the way, vitamin D functions as a powerful hormone in our bodies and influences processes related to our immune system, defense against cancer, managing blood sugar and, of course, fat loss. Recent data published in *The American Journal of Clinical Nutrition* revealed that women with optimal levels of vitamin D lost more weight, lost nearly twice as much body fat, and lost an average of 4 more inches from their waist over the course of the one-year study period. A healthy amount of sunlight exposure is important for improving our vitamin D levels, but dietary food sources are important, too. And an even greater source of vitamin D can be found in our next eggcellent food.

Duck Eggs

In our culture, when we think of eggs, we generally think of chicken eggs. But many cultures around the world prize the benefits of eggs like quail eggs, turkey eggs, and duck eggs. Duck eggs, in particular, are growing in popularity in the U.S. due to their higher ratio of anti-inflammatory omega-3 fatty acids than their chicken egg counterparts. Duck eggs also have upward of six times more vitamin D than chicken eggs!

Something particularly noteworthy about duck eggs was highlighted in a study published in the *Journal of Agricultural and Food Chemistry*, which found that amino acids in duck eggs are able to significantly increase your body's absorption and utilization of calcium. It doesn't just matter that a nutrient is in a food, but whether or not your body can readily use it. This speaks, again, to the power of real food to effectively communicate with your cells to bring about better health outcomes.

Calcium is another nutrient involved in the fat-loss conversation, as seen in a study cited in the journal *Obesity Reviews*. The study put test subjects on an exercise program and reduced-calorie diet that was either low in calcium (500 milligrams per day) or adequate in calcium (1,400 milligrams per day). At the end of the study, the researchers found that participants taking in adequate levels of calcium burned up to 30 percent more fat. Calcium isn't just about bone health, and some of the best sources of bioavailable calcium are not the things you hear about in the media. Spinach, sesame seeds, and fatty fish are all great sources of calcium. Which leads us to our next category of micronutrient-dense, fat-loss foods.

Under the Sea

Many scientists would assert that all of the life on our planet could be traced back to origins in our oceans and seas. It's only fitting that within these waters are some of the most valuable nutrients that support our health and well-being. And the good news is that you don't have to be a merman to appreciate and access some of the fat-burning foods you're about to learn about. So, in the melodic words of Sebastian the crab, let's see what's shaking "Under the Sea!"

Lean and Fatty Fish

A study published in the International *Journal of Obesity* put test subjects on a reduced calorie diet that either included salmon (fatty fish), cod (lean fish), or no fish. Even though the macronutrient content of all the diets was the same, simply including three 5-ounce servings of either type of fish per week resulted in male study participants losing over 2 additional pounds within four weeks. Again, same amount of calories, same macronutrient ratio, but including fish did something extra for their metabolism.

To add to that, in the previous chapter we discussed how healthy fat-rich fish are a great source of essential fatty acids DHA and EPA. Well, a recent study conducted by Japanese researchers found that these fatty acids are capable of suppressing the growth of body fat, even with the inclusion of low-quality foodstuffs in the diet like high fructose corn syrup.

Wild-caught fish is also a great source of the micronutrients vitamin B12, iodine, and potassium. Another study published in *The Journal of Nutrition* found that the inclusion of lean, white fish (such as halibut) helps optimize satiety hormones and can be significantly more satiating than other dense protein foods. Other examples of lean fish like halibut and cod are red snapper, tilapia, and sole.

Sea Veggies

Our oceans are home to some of the last truly wild foods that humans regularly consume. And this category might seem a little strange, but while modern folks are trying to find Nemo, our ancestors were trying to find some seaweeds to munch on.

The benefits you're about to discover are pretty mind-blowing, but many cultures have prized the benefits of seaweeds (lovingly referred to as sea veggies) for centuries. Records show that for over 2,000 years, seaweeds have been used as a supportive food in the Japanese diet. And as far back as 300 BC in China, a writer named Chi Han documented the benefits and wrote a book about the importance of seaweeds.

In Europe, Mediterranean seaweeds were used as medicine during the times of the great Greek and Roman empires. In Hawaii and the islands of the South Pacific, 60 to 70 species of seaweed were used for food, medicine, and ceremonies. Today, more and more sea veggies are showing up on store shelves in the U.S. due to their unique health attributes and incredible concentration of micronutrients. The first to jump onto my radar about a decade and a half ago was kelp, which could easily be crowned the King Triton of the class.

Kelp is most noted for being one of the best natural sources of iodine. Going back to our relationship to fat loss, iodine is required to make the thyroid hormones T3 and T4. You only need a small amount of iodine in your diet, but current estimates show that approximately 40 percent of people worldwide are deficient in iodine. To dig a little deeper into kelp's fat-loss benefits, it's also one of the very best sources of bioavailable calcium. According to UCSF Medical Center, kelp has more calcium than just about all other vegetables and, gram-for-gram, kelp can contain over five times more calcium than milk. As we noted, calcium is a micronutrient that supports a healthy metabolic rate, but another way it impacts fat loss was highlighted in a study published in the *International Journal of Obesity* when scientists discovered that adequate calcium intake can downregulate enzymes that create fat *and* it's able to decrease levels of triglycerides. Pretty impressive. And that's just for starters!

One of the most fascinating micronutrients found in sea veggies like wakame, hijiki, and kelp is a carotenoid called *fucoxanthin*. Research cited in the journal *Food Science and Human Wellness* asserts that sea-weeds have anti-obesity effects that can improve metabolic rate and increase satiety. Specifically, seaweed's fucoxanthin was found to boost the activity of *uncoupling protein 1* (UCP1), which enhances the activity of brown adipose tissue, while simultaneously supporting the reduction of white adipose tissue from the waistline.

Other sea veggies include dulse, arame, sea lettuce, nori, and many others. Rich in potassium, magnesium, selenium, zinc, B-vitamins, and an abundance of other nutrients, this category of foods might just be the most micronutrient-dense foods on the planet.

You can purchase whole, dried sea veggies, granulated flakes of seaweeds like kelp and dulse, and even find them in ground powder. They have a salty taste that makes them a great addition to salads and entrées like chicken and fish. The most common place the average person encounters sea veggies is through the seaweed nori used to roll up their favorite sushi. There are several ways to add some sea veggies to your diet, and three to four servings a week would be an excellent place to drop your anchor.

Get Your Sip On

The liquid format is an incredibly fast method for delivering a lot of nutrients to your system or (in the case of sugary drinks like soda and fruit juice) a lot of problems. If you want to get your sip on while pro-viding your body with an abundance of fat-loss supporting nutrients, check out the surprising details on these.

Coffee

Coffee is a thing I swore off very early in life. I watched my grandpar-ents sip on coffee every morning and it seemed like they were really enjoying it. So, at the age of about 6, I took my first sip. As soon as it touched my tongue, I thought 1) there must be something wrong with my grandparents for enjoying something this nasty, and 2) I will NEVER drink this stuff again in my life.

After I got over the initial repulsion experienced by my mac and cheese trained palate, I saw that it made my grandmother happy to make her and my grandfather coffee, so for Christmas that year, I took the $8 that I'd saved up and bought my grandmother a miniature container of Folgers (which was her favorite) with a stickable bow placed right on top. On Christmas morning, I hid it behind my back and walked over to her. I pulled the tiny container of coffee from behind me and held it up high so she could see it. I have to tell you, I don't think I've ever received a bigger hug in my life. I thought, "Wow, she must really love coffee!" But what really sparked that hug was the fact that I paid attention to what she liked and gave her something that had meaning. She kept that container of coffee, bow and all, tucked away unopened until she passed away when I was in my late 20s.

So, my first experience of coffee was bittersweet. It held a special connection for me, but I still wasn't about to drink the stuff myself. You see, not only did I not enjoy having things I thought were gross (coffee), but coffee had always been controversial in the health space as well. It had two strikes against it for me already. And then my wife stepped up to the plate and provided me with a moment of revelation.

We'd been together for over ten years at this point. Since we met in college, we'd experienced so much together…but I never, once, saw her drink coffee either. Then one day we received a care package from a friend that included some organic coffee and teas. I, of course, went with the teas, while my wife decided to give the coffee a shot. As each day passed, she continued to ask me to make her the coffee in the morning while I was making my tea. Until eventually I became her own personal barista.

About a year went by, and I could see the same level of happiness on my wife's face when I handed her the cup that I once saw in my grandparents. I finally decided to ask her why she liked it so much, and she said that it tasted good and she liked the way it made her feel. Tasted good?! Not from what I remember! But, I decided that after all of these years, it's time to give it a new taste test.

In addition, I kept coming across peer-reviewed evidence touting the remarkable benefits of coffee. Even though it appeared to be debatable on the surface, the positive evidence became too much for me to ignore... especially when it came to fat loss. For instance, a study published in the journal *Nutrition* found that light to moderate coffee drinkers (one to four cups per day) had the lowest amounts of visceral fat compared to non-coffee drinkers and heavy coffee drinkers. This was after adjusting for an array of other lifestyle factors that included exercise, alcohol consumption, and smoking. Drinking coffee has a clear U-shaped curve of benefits with a couple cups a day being good for your waistline.

Since I'm always asking "how does this actually work?," I dug deeper and found that some of the compounds in coffee have surprising influences on certain hormones. As you'll recall, the hormone adiponectin has the ability to basically eject body fat from the viscera (belly fat region) and move it toward the subcutaneous fat region. Adiponectin has also been found to support fat loss *without* increasing appetite. Well, researchers at Harvard Medical School discovered that test subjects who regularly drink coffee have higher levels of adiponectin and lower levels of inflammatory biomarkers. In fact, not only does this affect fat loss, but scientists at Stanford University recently deduced that the caffeine in coffee is able to defend the body against age-related inflammation. Their research revealed that light to moderate coffee drinkers live longer and more healthfully thanks, in part, to the protection caffeine provides by suppressing genes related to inflammation. Nutrigenomics in its freshly brewed glory.

Continuing in the fat-loss lane, research cited in *The American Journal of Clinical Nutrition* found that the caffeine in coffee can increase our metabolic rate by 3 to 11 percent, and most of the increase in metabolism is caused directly by an increase in the burning of fat. The interesting thing about caffeine is that it works sort of like exercise in that it triggers the release of catecholamines (including adrenaline) that spark the release of stored fat to be used for fuel. Adrenaline can bypass the typical body bank account process and grab those fat security deposits much faster. As you might remember from our earlier discussion on hormones, researchers at the University of Missouri School of Medicine found that fat cells have receptors that bind with adrenaline, which signals adipocytes to release stored fat into the system to use for energy. This is yet another way coffee encourages fat loss in small to moderate amounts. But, too much can downregulate the communication and you'll see diminishing returns in the benefits.

Another fascinating connection between coffee and metabolism is highlighted in a brand-new study featured in the journal *Scientific Reports*. Scientists from the School of Medicine at the University of Nottingham discovered that coffee may be able to influence the activity of your brown adipose tissue. As we discussed in Chapter One, there are certain lifestyle factors that can trigger the "browning" of beige fat cells (cells that could either become white fat *or* brown fat), and drinking coffee appears to nudge them into the fat-burning brown fat side. Plus, the researchers used thermal imaging and found that drinking coffee lights up brown fat–dominant locations on the body, indicating increased thermogenesis.

When I decided to suspend my "coffee tastes good" disbelief, I'd already been blending healthy fats into my teas for about a decade, thanks to some insights from my friend, nutrition expert Daniel Vitalis. Coconut oil, ghee, or grass-fed butter were some of my daily options. And as my wife's unpaid barista, she liked me to blend her coffee with grass-fed butter and a few drops of English toffee stevia. The sip I had from my grandfather's cup all those years ago most definitely didn't have those things in it. So, I decided to give my wife's favorite coffee recipe a shot.

First sip: Hmmm, this isn't so bad. I'm still prepared to chuck it down the sink, though.
Second sip: Wow... I might actually like this.
Third sip: I've seen the light!

All of the benefits seemed amazing, but I was never willing to get involved because of an experience from my childhood. Thankfully, I had the audacity to give it another chance. After further investigating the domain of coffee (which is currently one of the top five most traded commodities in the world), I found out that the disparity in coffee benefits and downsides is largely related to the quality of the coffee itself (pesticide-laden, moldy, lower in nutrients due to poor growing methods) as well as the low quality ingredients that are commonly added to peoples' cup of joe. These include highly processed sugar, coffee "creamers" made of vegetable oil and artificial flavorings, and/ or milk or cream from grain-fed cows that's lower in nutrients and higher in inflammatory omega-6 fatty acids (according to data from Washington State University). Coffee can be a healthful addition to your fat-loss nutrition plan. But the quality definitely matters! I've got my absolute favorite coffee recipe for you on page 389. It's formulated to enhance your metabolism, support your cognitive function, and make your taste buds do the Cha Cha Slide.

Green Tea and Black Tea

Although green tea has been utilized for thousands of years in other parts of the world, it hit the scene here in the U.S. a couple decades ago and spread faster than your favorite social media memes. And for good reason... the benefits of green tea seem to border on the miraculous.

When it comes to fat loss, the caffeine found in green tea works in similar ways to coffee (with a slight twist we'll talk about in Section Two), but it's not just the caffeine that supports your metabolism. A study published in the *Journal of Health Sciences* uncovered that antioxidants in green tea called *catechins* are able to increase the rate at which body fat gets burned for fuel. The eight-week study split participants into two groups, with one group receiving a beverage with the tea catechins and the other group receiving a control beverage without the tea catechins. All of the test subjects were also instructed to do cardio for 30 minutes three times per week. Here's what they found...

The test subjects consuming beverages with the tea catechins lost significantly more fat during exercise *and* during sedentary time (when they were not working out). So, whether you're exercising or not, sipping some green tea helps to stimulate fat burning. But this leads to an important point that I don't want you to miss. Caffeine and other unique micronutrients found in tea and coffee do work synergistically with exercise. These compounds help to *mobilize* the fatty acids to be used for fuel. And adding some exercise helps to ensure that mobilized fat actually gets *burned* (and not reabsorbed somewhere down the line). Again, there's a difference between fat cells releasing fat and the fat actually getting burned for fuel by your mitochondria. Green tea catechins help both to take place, but exercising a bit (even just taking a brisk walk) maximizes the benefits.

A study reported in *The American Journal of Clinical Nutrition* found that study participants who had a green tea extract before exercise burned 17 percent more fat than those who didn't. The researchers noted a greater improvement in insulin sensitivity as well. This highlights, once more, that green tea and exercise can go hand-in-hand. Though, just to reiterate, exercise is recommended but not required to see some impressive benefits. Another study published in *Physiology & Behavior* sought to find out what effect green tea would have on obese volunteers. At the end of the 12-week study, participants having green tea each day lost an average of 7.3 more pounds and burned 183 more calories per day than those who didn't have green tea. And here's what's most impressive about the study, all of the test subjects received three meals a day from the hospital facilitating the trial. Every test subject received meals that were calorically equal, yet those who included green tea lost more weight! Two to four cups a day seems to be the sweet spot for optimal benefits. But there's a green tea counterpart that I want to make sure isn't left out.

Black tea and green tea actually come from the same place, the leaves of the *camellia sinensis* plant. And like green tea, black tea has been prized for thousands of years in cultures throughout the world. What makes the two teas different in their appearance and benefits has to do with fermentation. To make black tea, the leaves are first rolled and then exposed to air to trigger the fermentation process. This reaction causes the leaves to turn dark brown and allows the flavors to heighten and intensify...plus a change in the micronutrient profile occurs as well!

A group of polyphenols found in higher concentration in black tea called *theaflavins* appear to have some phenomenal benefits on metabolism. Research cited in the *Journal of Functional Foods* revealed that black tea theaflavins have the ability to literally shift human gene expression to a profile that favors lipolysis and beta oxidation (burning fat for fuel)! To highlight this, scientists at the University of Oslo in Norway conducted a double-blind, placebo-controlled study that gave participants either three cups of black tea each day or three cups of a caffeine-matched control beverage. At the end of three months, the participants drinking black tea lost significantly more weight and had a greater reduction in waist circumference.

Another fascinating thing about black tea is that, even though it has caffeine that temporarily stimulates catecholamines (stress-related hormones), overall black tea has been found to actually *reduce* stress levels. A study published in the peer-reviewed journal *Psychopharmacology* found that drinking four cups of black tea each day for six weeks directly lowered cortisol levels in test subjects versus those drinking a placebo beverage. In the study, volunteers who drank black tea had 20 percent lower blood levels of cortisol after a stressful event compared with the control group.

As you've learned, elevated cortisol can be unfriendly to fat loss in the long-term. So, clearly, black tea is not to be overlooked when it comes to healthy metabolism for a multitude of reasons. So, whether it's black, green, or something in between, incorporating a couple cups of tea to your daily regimen can definitely be supportive of your metabolism. No matter which beverage you choose, just be sure to incorporate something that feels good and something you enjoy. And give yourself permission to switch it up if you want to. There are so many great options to discover and explore!

Veg Out

When it comes to micronutrients, the category of vegetables really does play in a league of its own. But there are a couple subsets of vegetables that are especially formidable when teeing off against body fat.

Greens

A study published in the journal *Appetite* uncovered that compounds found in green leafy vegetables like spinach and kale were able to significantly increase post-meal levels of the satiety hormone GLP-1 in study participants. This corresponded with a greater reduction in weight, body fat, and waist circumference over the course of the 12-week study period. We've already noted the meta-analysis published in the journal *Nutrients* revealing that for every additional serving of vegetables consumed each day, study participants lost an additional 0.36 centimeter from their waist circumference. This is so important and powerful that it's really difficult to put it into words. Incorporating more green leafy vegetables into your meals gives you a gigantic advantage in supporting fat loss.

The more green veggies you can get in during the day, the better. A huge leverage point so many people miss out on is getting in green leafy veggies with the first meal of the day. By incorporating them into your breakfast, you are starting your day with a greater metabolic advantage. A typical fat-loss supportive first meal of the day would look something like this: two to three whole eggs (prepared any way you like), one small serving of pasture-raised sausage, two servings of sautéed green vegetables (like spinach or kale) cooked in olive oil or coconut oil, and one serving of sliced avocado. This breakfast features foods and nutrients that spark the release of adiponectin, GLP-1, and CCK—all fat-fighting hormones. Plus, these foods and nutrients have been proven to reduce ghrelin, improve insulin sensitivity, and increase your overall metabolic rate. You can mix and match different protein-dense foods and fats, but the green leafy vegetables provide the ultimate edge due to their micronutrient density and their fiber. A meta-analysis of 52 studies uncovered that by simply increasing fiber intake you can boost adiponectin levels by 60 to 115 percent!

There's such a wide variety of green leafy fat burners to choose from. Along with kale and spinach you also have swiss chard, collard greens, mustard greens, bok choy, romaine lettuce, green leaf lettuce, arugula, and more. Include two servings in your first meal and shoot for five to seven servings each day.

Cruciferous Vegetables

Leafy vegetables like collards, bok choy, cabbage, and kale have dual citizenship, as they are also members of the cruciferous vegetable family. This group also includes cauliflower, rutabagas, Brussel sprouts, and the crowned king of the cruciferous category, broccoli. The remarkable thing about cruciferous vegetables is that they are abundant in micronutrients that are natural aromatase inhibitors.

As you'll recall from Chapter Two, estrogen is critical to the metabolic health of both men and women. When estrogen levels are too low, it can trigger reduced fat burning, increased appetite, and a redistribution of more fat to the visceral belly fat area. But, on the other side, when estrogen levels are too high, this can spark the rapid creation of more subcutaneous fat. And this fat, ironically, will then create even more estrogen!

The term *estrogen dominance* is much more common today than estrogen deficiency. This is in large part due to an abundance of xeno-estrogens we're exposed to in our environment, as well as increased rates of aromatization (where anabolic hormones like testosterone get "stolen" to make more estrogen). As we discussed, aromatization is encouraged by the chronic appearance of insulin. Yes, getting our insulin levels in check is a huge key to minimizing aromatization, but the cruciferous category of vegetables can make an impressive assist, too.

Data published in the peer-reviewed journal *Anti-Cancer Agents in Medicinal Chemistry* divulged that compounds found in cruciferous vegetables like broccoli and cabbage are able to effectively block excess aromatization from taking place. You may be curious why this information is cited in a journal that's dedicated to cancer research, and the answer is that this category of foods is also a potent defense against estrogen–driven cancers.

Another study published in the journal *Nutrition and Cancer* uncovered that *indole-3-carbinol* (I3C), obtained from cruciferous vegetables, is able to positively alter endogenous estrogen metabolism by converting estrogen into safer forms and supporting proper estrogen elimination in the body. Researchers noted that this also supports the healthful action of free testosterone in the body.

Spice It Up

You've probably heard the statement "variety is the spice of life." But, have you ever thought why life needs "spice" in the first place? And why is it "the spice of life" and not something else like "the figure-4 leg lock of life"? Well, it's because spice is important! Spice makes everything better. Not to say a well-executed figure-4 isn't a thing of beauty if you're a fan of the WWE. But it's "the spice of life" because spice is what makes things come alive. And variety in spices is what enables us to have an endless adventure with our food experiences. Remember, food isn't just stuff we eat...food is a gift for our taste buds, our hearts, and our experience of eating. So, here are a couple of spices that can accent your metabolism very nicely.

Turmeric

This potent spice has been used in cooking, medicine, and rituals in various cultures for thousands of years. Turmeric is part of the ginger family, *zingiberaceae,* the roots of which are used for making the spice that has become increasingly popular today. Turmeric and one of its most renowned micronutrients, curcumin, have well-noted anti-inflammatory effects. But what isn't commonly known is its surprising anti-obesity effects.

A study published in the *European Journal of Nutrition* uncovered that, in addition to downregulating inflammatory cytokines, curcumin also *up*regulates the activity of adiponectin and other satiety-related hormones. Turmeric has been found to improve insulin sensitivity, reduce blood fats, and directly act upon fat cells. It's a highlight of many curry dishes, but it's also easy to add to scrambled eggs and omelets, soups, and many other dishes as well.

Ginger

As noted, turmeric is a member of the ginger family. But the matriarch of the category itself has some fat-burning benefits you need to know about. A micronutrient in ginger called *zingerone* is being heavily researched for its influence on body fat. Remember the enzyme *hormone sensitive lipase* (HSL) that's responsible for ushering fatty acids out of your fat cells? New research has shown that zingerone in ginger is able to stimulate the activity of HSL and increase the breakdown of stored fat (lipolysis). Researchers discovered that compounds in ginger are able to substantially improve the ratio of blood fats and provide protection against nonalcoholic fatty liver disease.

Data published in the journal *Metabolism* demonstrated that participants consuming a hot ginger beverage with breakfast were able to boost the thermic effect of their food (they burned more calories digesting their meal) and they had reduced feelings of hunger throughout the day. It was a strange ritual I started to see, when after eating, my mom-in-law would offer everyone some ginger tea. Even though some of their traditional Kenyan meals would feature a little more carbs and beans than what would appear to be *en vogue,* I noticed that their family stayed very fit and enjoyed healthy, robust digestion. Could ginger be part of their health equation? The study used half of a teaspoon of ginger powder mixed in hot water, but you can make it with fresh grated ginger (as my mom-in-law does), boiling it in hot water, then straining it out. Ginger is pretty strong, and you can drink it as is. But she would tell you that you can mix in a little almond milk (or another milk of choice) and a low glycemic sweetener to make a drink that's more enjoyable to sip on.

Salt

Throughout the development of human civilization, you'd be hard-pressed to find a foodstuff that's been more valuable than salt. In fact, the word *salt* is derived from the Latin word *salarium* which means "salary." Salt has literally been used as *money* because its value was understood. Today, salt's story is sketchy, at best. We've lost touch with its value, partially because it's ever present, and partially because the information on salt has been a bit skewed.

In our modern world, salt is the most common thing you'll find in the spice cabinet. It's the go-to for livening up just about any dish. It provides more body to the flavors, heightens the taste of other spices, and it even simmers down the bitter notes. We, as a people, have been loving salt since the richest human lived in a four-story cave and wore the finest designer wooly mammoth jeans.

Yet, when you think of salt nutritionally, right now, you might conjure up thoughts about high blood pressure and heart attacks. This is mainly due to the amount of sodium found in salt. Salt (being about 60 percent chloride and 40 percent sodium) is, by far, our biggest source of dietary sodium. Because of this, the two words *salt* and *sodium* are often used interchangeably (though they are technically two different things). Sodium is one of the most crucial nutrients for human health. It's needed to help conduct the impulses of your nervous system, it's required for muscle contractions, and it helps to maintain proper fluid balance within our tissues. Without sodium, our tissues couldn't hold on to water, and our cells would end up drier than most dad jokes. And, most notably in the popular health–salt conversation, sodium is required to help modulate blood pressure.

To put it in simple terms, blood pressure is the force that blood is placing on the walls of your blood vessels as it circulates throughout your body. And *high* blood pressure is when that force is elevated to a point that increases the risk of damage to the blood vessels (and the cardiovascular system overall, including the heart).

The loudest gripe against salt is that it increases blood pressure, which is true, to a degree. But the research that initially vilified salt many decades ago originated from animal studies that gave rats *massive* amounts of salt (about 50 times the average intake) and deduced that salt is a major concern for high blood pressure. Yet, a large-scale, multinational study was just published finding that salt intake *does not* increase health risks, even at levels that were once deemed to be unhealthy. So, what gives?

The researchers concluded that elevated blood pressure is a *symptom* and not a *cause* of cardiovascular disease and morbidity. And dietary salt is on a much lower rung of things that contribute to the problem (with bigger issues being elevated triglycerides, stress hormones, and inflammation). The study found that even up to around 2 teaspoons of salt per day is not problematic for most people (noting that there are genetic predispositions for some folks to have challenges managing salt). This might seem like a pretty sizable amount compared to the conventional RDA. But what's even more eye-opening is that a salt intake closer to and below the RDA of about 1 teaspoon per day actually *increases* the risk of heart disease and high blood pressure! A meta-analysis published in the *Cochrane Database of Systematic Reviews* uncovered that study participants placed on a low sodium diet did have slightly lower blood pressure in the short-term, but found that the restricted sodium also led to elevated triglycerides, elevated stress hormones, and (accordingly) elevated blood pressure. Some experts might be salty to hear that, but they'll be even more shocked to find out how much salt can influence metabolism.

A study conducted by researchers at Harvard Medical School and published in the journal *Metabolism* found that a low salt intake directly increases insulin resistance in healthy test subjects. Salt supports cellular communication and improves the function of many of your major hormones. Additionally, research cited in *Scientific Reports* revealed that a low-salt diet could increase levels of the hunger hormone ghrelin.

Now, just to be clear, reducing salt intake can have a positive effect on weight loss. But (and it's a big but) this is primarily due to a reduction in water weight (since salt aids in fluid retention). A brand-new study set out to uncover if a reduced-calorie + reduced-salt diet would fare better than a reduced-calorie diet (without reducing salt) for fat loss. The study participants were provided three meals a day, and at the end of the two-month study period, those who were provided calorie-restricted low-salt meals lost more weight (noted to be specifically from extracellular water and total body water). However, people on the low-salt diet didn't lose any more actual *body fat* or *visceral fat* than the folks who got to incorporate more salt. They suffered through less tasty meals without any additional fat loss to show for it.

Again, an optimal amount of salt can actually be supportive of fat loss.

As you'll recall, the pancreatic hormone glucagon promotes lipolysis by opening up cellular doors to release stored fat to use for fuel. Recent data affirms that sodium aids in the performance of glucagon. Salt also influences the action of leptin, adrenaline, and thyroid hormone.

Now, this information is not an encouragement to install a feng shui salt lick in your home somewhere. This is a call to arms to be more adamant about providing your body the right amount of salt that it needs. There's no need to overdo it, but lacking in the right forms of salt can put you at a metabolic disadvantage.

Salt can be a pretty vague term because there are so many types, but just keep in mind that higher quality salts don't just provide sodium and chloride, they also provide a plethora of other micronutrients in the form of trace minerals. Celtic salt, pink Himalayan salt, black Hawaiian salt, sea salt, and Redmond Real Salt are all viable options to add flavor to your food and electrolytes to your water. Just to be clear, these are *not* the types of salt used in the vast majority of restaurants and processed foods. A study cited in the *Journal of the American College of Nutrition* estimates that at least 77 percent of the salt intake in the American diet comes from processed foods and not what you're adding from your salt shaker. This is primarily from low-quality, heavily refined salt that typically contains additives like anti-caking agents. It's devoid of other naturally occurring micronutrients and doesn't have the long history of use that these natural salts have.

By cutting down on processed, packaged food intake (and looking for products that use natural salt when you do purchase packaged foods) you'll find a simple way to cut back on the salt you don't want and open up space to add more of the salt that you do want. Salt is absolutely essential and valuable. If you're not in the small fraction of the population who has a true genetic defect that warrants a hyper-cautious salt reduction, you will probably find great value in fortifying your intake of high-quality salts. Use a variety of salts if possible in cooking and occasionally add some to your water. And from now on, if you ever hear Lil Jon say, "Shake it like a salt shaker," you know that you can humbly oblige.

Get Your Oil Changed

There are few things that can affect your health (and your fat loss) more than upgrading the fats and oils that you're consuming. As you know from previous chapters, dietary fats are absolutely critical to metabolic wellness. Let's take a look at some specific oils that provide premium fat-burning fuel for your metabolic engine.

Olive Oil

As you'll hopefully recall, we've already established that olive oil is supportive of beneficial gut bacteria, it's proven to beat the breaks off of conventional "vegetable oil" when it comes to fat loss, and it's jam-packed with potent antioxidants. But all of that is just an appetizer when it comes to this historically celebrated oil.

In a recent study published in *The American Journal of Clinical Nutrition,* it was revealed that consuming olive oil (a little more than a table-spoon) triggered the release of, not one, but *three* of the major satiety hormones associated with enhanced fat loss. Healthy test subjects instructed to include olive oil with their meal had significant increases in GLP-1 (enhances satiety and reduces visceral fat), CCK (reduces overall appetite), and PYY (decreases the likelihood of body fat stor-age). Olive oil appears to slide into your metabolic DMs and make your hormones work better.

Not only that, a new study cited in the *Journal of Translational Medi-cine* found that olive oil can potentially downregulate the expression of the FTO gene associated with excess body fat and obesity. Scientists found that a four-week diet intervention that included high amounts of olive oil appears to have epigenetic influences that result in improved body composition.

All of this is beyond impressive. But remember, quality matters a lot when it comes to olive oil! Refer back to the discussion on mono-unsaturated fats in Chapter Four for a refresher on choosing olive oil if you ever need to. And target 1 to 3 tablespoons of extra virgin olive oil each day to get the most hollers for your metabolic dollars.

MCT Oil

In our discussion of long chain, medium chain, and short chain fatty acids, the medium chain fatty acids (aka *medium chain triglycerides* or MCTs) hold a special place of prominence in the domain of fat metabolism. A randomized double-blind study published in the *International Journal of Obesity and Related Metabolic Disorders* placed participants on a reduced-calorie diet that included either supplemental MCTs or supplemental *long chain triglycerides* (LCTs). After the data was compiled it was revealed that the group who included MCT oil lost more weight, eliminated more body fat, and experienced higher levels of satiety.

What was particularly interesting about this study was that the people consuming MCTs were able to retain more of their muscle mass during the weight-loss process. As you know, muscle is an invaluable part of our overall metabolism. Many calorie-restricted diets sacrifice too much of our muscle tissue, which then reduces our metabolic rate in the long-term. MCT oil seems to have a muscle-sparing effect that could be supportive during any reduced-calorie diet program.

Something else unique about MCTs is that (because of the size of their bonds) they're able to bypass the typical digestive process and be used more quickly for energy in the body. When MCTs are absorbed they are driven straight to the liver. From there, they can be burned for fuel or converted into ketones for use as an alternative energy source. MCT oil can be added to many things, ranging from coffee and tea (especially emulsified MCT oil) to salad dressings and smoothies. Look for MCT oil that is derived from 100 percent coconut oil if possible. It's generally going to be better for you and better for the planet.

Most folks assimilate MCT oil just fine, but because it's metabolized differently in the body, if you come out of the gate getting too hot and heavy with MCTs, it can cause some people to have a little nausea or other digestive distress. If you haven't used MCT oil before, it's a good idea to start with a teaspoon and then work your way up to a max of 1 to 2 tablespoons per day. MCTs are a very simple addition to boost your body's energy expenditure and help regulate your appetite. And from now on, when we think about getting oiled up, we're not just going to think about *Baywatch*. We're going to think about providing high-quality, metabolism-supporting oils to our cells each day!

This marks the completion of Section One, Eating for Fat Loss! We've explored a tremendous amount of game-changing information so far. We've covered everything from optimizing your hunger and satiety hormones, to the microbiome–body fat connection, to uncovering some of the very best foods that are *proven* to support fat metabolism. All of the most pertinent tips, tools, and strategies are put together for you in the Eat Smarter 30-Day Program.

Next up, it's time to take a deep dive into the world of nutrition and cognitive health. You're about to learn how to improve your memory, enhance your focus and productivity, and a whole lot more. It's time for a major brain health level-up, so I'll see you in Section Two!

EATING FOR MENTAL PERFORMANCE, BETTER RELATIONSHIPS, AND BETTER SLEEP

CHAPTER SIX

Brain Games

Preserve and treat food as you would your body, remembering that in time food will be your body.

~*B.W. Richardson*

Theoretical physicist Dr. Michio Kaku said that the human brain is "the most complicated object in the known universe." Inordinately complex and powerful beyond measure, the human brain is the most valuable entity on planet earth. And the cool thing is that *you* own one of them. Now, the question is: *What are you going to do with it?*

You may have heard statements that we're only using 2 percent, or 10 percent, or 20 percent of our brains. But that's simply not the case. Neuroscientists will affirm that we actually use upward of 100 percent of our brain at various times throughout the day (a large portion of your brain is even active while you're sleeping!). The myth that we're only using a small percentage of our brain came from personal development literature and not from actual science. But, there is one thing we can all agree on . . .

Even though the vast majority of our brains are in active use each day, this does *not* mean that they are being used very well. In fact, if you are reading this right now, there is a high probability that you have the capacity to think faster, be more creative, problem solve more effectively, and become more laser-focused than you are right now. Though you may be using 100 percent of your brain, the capacity of your brain to improve in function is arguably limitless.

Since your brain controls your experience of life, it would not be a stretch to say that creating a better life would start with creating a better brain. You can play brain games, read books, and learn techniques to make your brain work better. But what's most overlooked is that **all of the changes you're able to make in your brain are dependent upon the food that you eat.** From the axons to the dendrites, from the neurons to the glial cells, from the white matter to the gray matter, and everything in between, your brain is made out of the things that you eat. A better brain starts with what you put in your belly. And this is why eating smarter can actually make you smarter.

ONCE UPON A TIME IN HOLLYWOOD

I really began to be interested in the health and functionality of the human brain when I was on the road over a decade ago. I was staying at a charming, vintage hotel in Hollywood, California (translation: a rundown dusty rust bucket in Hollywood, California) and there was an old TV that was supposed to "look like" it was from the '70s (and in fact it probably was). I was getting dressed while a PBS special was playing in the background, which was the only station that came in clearly, and I literally had to stop in my tracks and listen to what the speaker on the show was saying. The person speaking to a captivated studio audience was Dr. Daniel Amen. I was hanging onto every word as he was revealing some of the mysteries of this powerful organ sitting atop our shoulders.

Dr. Amen is a multi-time *New York Times*–bestselling author, double board-certified psychiatrist, and a pioneer in the field of brain imaging to monitor brain activity and blood flow using a technology called *SPECT imaging* (single photon emission computed tomography). During the special he said that in psychiatry, "We're the only field of medicine that doesn't look at the organ that we treat." Though psychiatrists are entrusted with supporting patients' mental health, it has largely been the same guesswork that's been utilized for hundreds of years. Conduct a brief conversation with the patient, quickly assess the symptoms based on what the patient says, form a diagnosis based on that communication, and then prescribe a medication or other treatment. He said, "Without a scan or another measure of brain function, it is like throwing medication-tipped darts in the dark at someone's brain." He wanted to find a better way to help his patients, so it lit a fire under him to utilize SPECT imaging to its greatest capacity. As a result, his clinics now serve over 4,000 patients each month and he has the world's largest database of functional brain scans relating to behavior, totaling over 160,000 scans on patients from 120 countries. Through this, he's been able to actually *see* the physical and behavioral changes that specific nutrients and lifestyle factors have on the brain. And several of these nutrients and foods that are proven to upgrade your brain are just a small slice of what you'll be learning about in this chapter.

The insights from someone with that type of knowledge base and experience is absolutely priceless, and I was over-the-moon excited when I learned that he and I would be speaking at the same event just a couple years after seeing him on that oldfangled television set. In our conversations since then, one of the most fascinating things I've learned is how fragile our powerful brains actually are. It's really paradox at its finest: The most complicated object in the known universe is about as delicate as my emotions after watching *Toy Story 3*.

You might be shocked to learn that your all-powerful brain is actually about the same consistency as soft butter. You might be even more shocked to learn that your brain is mostly made of water! In fact, the human brain is almost 80 percent water. After your lungs, this makes your brain (pound-for-pound) the second most water-dominant organ in your body.

Now, even though your brain itself is considerably fragile, evolution didn't show up to the party without a gift. Your mighty brain is the only organ that's fully enclosed in protective bone. You've got a homegrown helmet in the form of a cranium that keeps your brain protected from external intrusions. Even more remarkable, your brain has developed protection from internal intrusions, as well.

Furthering my research, I had a conversation with neuroscientist Dr. Lisa Mosconi. She shared with me that the brain is the only organ that's been granted its own state-of-the-art security system. It's a network of blood vessels called the *blood-brain barrier* (BBB). Since the brain is so complex and susceptible to injury, she told me, "Many substances typically circulating in our bloodstream could potentially cause great harm to the brain." Nature's solution to this was to develop the BBB, which is made of a wall of flattened cells linked so tightly that it's essentially impermeable (with the exception of very specific nutrients that are deemed safe to enter this VIP section of your body). With the BBB, your brain has 24/7 security detail that protects itself from harmful pathogens, toxins, and other dangerous compounds. In reality, many of the nutrients we consume, good or not, don't actually make it into your brain. Your brain has its own diet that's different from the rest of your body. It's an exclusive diet that Dr. Mosconi refers to as *neuro-nutrition.*

As we discussed in the introduction to this book, even though our brain only accounts for about 2 percent of our body's overall weight, it actually consumes 20 to 25 percent of our caloric intake! It's an energy and nutrient-hungry organ, but we need to provide it with "the right stuff," like that New Kids on the Block song. So, what makes the cut and what doesn't? And what is the rest of the brain actually made of? That's what we're going to dive into next.

WATER WORKS

The BBB stretches throughout your brain and uses the equivalent of retinal scans and white-glove pat downs to see who can pass through. Since water is so crucial to the form and function of the brain, it always has celebrity status to flow right through and liven up the neuro-atmosphere.

Another part of nature's protection for the brain is the colorless liquid called *cerebrospinal fluid* that keeps the brain afloat and provides cushioning from shock that may be caused by sudden head movements or trauma. This fluid is also critical for clearing out metabolic wastes from your brain to keep itself clean and functional. Trust me, your brain doesn't like having crumbs on the floor, and without adequate water, your cerebrospinal fluid is hampered in being able to do its job.

In addition to the air you breathe, water is also an assistive force in delivering oxygen to your brain. As you've learned, water isn't just an inert substance, it's a powerful solvent that's a carrier of nutrients. And many of these nutrients get to come along with water into your brain, strolling past security like, "I'm with him!"

This is why it's important to be mindful of the type of water you drink, as detailed in Chapter Four. Just like elsewhere in the body, there is a delicate balance that needs to be maintained with water and electrolytes to keep everything upstairs in tip-top shape. Electrolytes are minerals that carry an electric charge. And the brain is critically dependent upon these nutrients to help send electrical signals throughout all of your brain cells.

Take sodium, for example. Not only does this electrolyte help to maintain proper water balance, a study conducted by researchers at McGill University found that sodium functions as an on/off switch in the brain for specific neurotransmitters that support optimal function and protect the brain against numerous diseases (like epilepsy and neuropathic pain). Yet another reason that water and a little salt go together like Starsky and Hutch, Thelma and Louise, John Mayer and, well, everybody.

When talking about electrolytes and the brain, we definitely don't want to overlook our old friend, magnesium. A fascinating new study published in the journal *Neuron* found that magnesium is able to restore critical brain plasticity and improve cognitive function. Bestselling author and neuroscientist Dr. Wendy Suzuki shared with me that neuroplasticity is the ability of the brain to change and adapt. There was a time in neuroscience when the brain was believed to be "fixed" and minimally changeable, at best, once you surpassed brain maturity in your 20s. Generally speaking, what you've got is what you've got... and all you had to look forward to was a slow decline from there. But Dr. Suzuki's research revealed that an enriched environment and healthy lifestyle factors can increase brain plasticity early in life *and* later in life. Now we know that your brain can become better, whether you're a senior in high school or a senior citizen. And a big part of the equation is what you give your brain to eat and drink.

A double-blind, placebo-controlled study published in the *Journal of Alzheimer's Disease* found that improving magnesium levels in adult test subjects (age 50 to 70) could potentially reverse brain aging by over nine years! A younger brain also accompanies better performance. And the loss of plasticity that comes with unhealthy brain aging has been proven to coincide with dramatically reduced cognitive function. Clearly, electrolytes and minerals like magnesium matter, and this leads us back to its primary transporter, water, to hammer home how important hydration is for your brain.

A recent study cited in *Medicine & Science in Sports & Exercise* found that just a 2 percent drop in your body's baseline hydration level can lead to impairment in tasks requiring attention, motor coordination, and executive function (which includes things like map recognition, grammatical reasoning, proofreading, and mental math). Calculating a tip can be hard enough, but if your brain is thirsty, it makes even the simplest tasks that much more difficult.

Even though it might seem like Captain Obvious after learning how important water is to brain function, many people don't realize that insufficient hydration is the #1 nutritive trigger of daytime fatigue. Brand-new data published in the *International Journal of Environmental Research and Public Health* revealed that mild dehydration had a significant negative impact on fatigue, mood, reading speed, and mental work capacity in collegiate test subjects. And within a short amount of time, getting them properly hydrated alleviated fatigue, improved total mood disturbance, boosted short-term memory, and enhanced their focus and reaction times. The best supplements in the world can't outmatch the power of your brain's primary nutrient need, *aqua*. As we learned in Section One, water is invaluable for your metabolism, but it's also invaluable for your mental performance. Follow the hydration recommendations at the end of Chapter Four for the sake of your body fat and also that fat brain of yours.

FAT HEAD

When I was a kid, being called a fat head was a pretty universal diss. Today, it can be considered an ultimate compliment. After water, your brain's next major constituent is *fat*. Coming in at approximately 11 percent fat, 8 percent protein, 3 percent minerals, and a sprinkle of carbs and other compounds, your miraculous brain is a fatty organ that knows how to throw its weight around.

Since the "dry weight" of the brain (which excludes water) is mostly fat, you'd automatically assume that eating dietary fat would directly translate to the fat in your brain. But, just like eating fat doesn't directly end up as fat on your body, eating fat doesn't directly end up as fat in your brain either.

In our discussion of the different types of body fat in Chapter One, there's yet another type of fat to add to the mix. Body fat (visceral fat and subcutaneous fat) is in the category of something called *storage fats*. This is a type of fat that operates in the business of storing and releasing fat to be used for fuel. The fat found in the human brain is in a category called *structural fats*. It's a type of fat that works to provide cellular structure and acts as a form of "technical support" for your system.

Your brain cells (neurons) are wrapped in a form of structural fat, for example. The fatty membrane around each cell helps to provide external protection, but it also assists in allowing signals and nutrients to flow in and out of the cell. The brain's structural fats act as your internal *Geek Squad,* helping to put your hardware together and providing the tech support when it's needed.

While eating a surplus of dietary fat can translate to increased levels of storage fat, this doesn't affect storage fat levels in the brain at all — because there aren't any! Theoretically speaking, if the fat that makes up your brain was made of burnable storage fat, in a situation of food shortage your brain might start eating itself like homemade zombie food. Thankfully, it's not designed that way, but it begs for clarification on which foods help our brains to maintain its curvy, fat appearance.

Omegas

Only certain types of fat are able to finesse their way across the BBB. The most important and abundant structural fat in the brain is the omega-3 fatty acid DHA. For your brain, it's the fat king, and you need to make sure to deliver it into your crown every single day. Research published in *The American Journal of Clinical Nutrition* discovered that an increase of dietary levels of DHA was able to improve both memory and reaction time in healthy test subjects. DHA is such a critical part of memory formation that you can forget about making memories without it. Excellent sources of DHA include wild-caught salmon, herring, and sardines. Dr. Lisa Mosconi asserts that the best natural food source of DHA is going to be found in black caviar and salmon roe (both are types of fish eggs that have upward of three times more DHA per gram than the best fish sources!). Caviar might have you thinking of *Lifestyles of the Rich and Famous,* but it might be a new food that can provide nutritional wealth to your brain.

As we discussed in Chapter Four, the plant forms of omega-3s are viable options, but they're in the form of ALA, not DHA. Your body can convert a small amount of ALA into the brain-supportive DHA that you need, but approximately 75 percent of the plant-based omega-3s get lost in the conversion process. This calls on the need to supplement if you are taking a vegetarian or vegan nutritional approach. Getting yourself a high-quality marine algae oil would be a good idea. DHA is *essential* for healthy brain function, and you don't want your brain to struggle to find it.

Now, let's not forget about the other brain VIP omega-3, *eicosapentaenoic acid* (EPA). EPA and DHA typically come as a tandem. They're so important for the structural integrity of the brain that a study published in the journal *Neurology* using MRIs revealed that people consuming the lowest amount of EPA and DHA in their diets had accelerated brain shrinkage! This isn't the type of shrinkage that happens because it's cold outside, this is more like the permanent kind that can lead to significant long-term problems. The researchers noted that the lack of EPA and DHA in the diet was particularly harmful to the memory center of the brain called the hippocampus, which lost neurons at a rate equivalent to two additional years of abnormal aging. They stated that people who ate less than 4 grams of DHA per day showed the highest rates of brain shrinkage, while those who ate 6 grams or more had the healthiest, shrink-proofed brains.

One of the most common sources of EPA and DHA today is in the form of fish oil supplements. A randomized placebo-controlled study cited in the *Nutrition Journal* found that healthy test subjects taking 3 grams of fish oil per day for five weeks significantly improved cognitive performance compared to participants taking a placebo. Fish oil is an easy way to meet your omega-3 needs, but be sure that you're mindful of the source and quality. As new innovations continue, I'll be sure to keep you updated on the best food and supplement resources in the Eat Smarter Bonus Resources Guide at eatsmarterbook.com/bonus.

Outside of that, how much fish should you target if you're going the whole food way? Two to three servings per week appears to be ideal, but as noted in a study conducted by researchers at Rush University Medical Center, adults who eat at least one seafood meal per week do, in fact, perform better on cognitive skills tests than people who eat less than one seafood meal per week. So, have at least one serving of fatty fish per week to hit that minimum effective dose. Plus, add in a little fish oil or algae oil to hit the target of over 4 grams of DHA per day, and you'll have a pretty effective strategy to help round things out.

Additionally, grass-fed beef, pastured egg yolks, and other types of fish like mackerel and trout are all viable sources of brain-healthy omega-3s. Again, these are some of the very few fats that can actually cross the BBB and support your cognition.

Now, let's take a look at the next type of fat that makes the list.

Phospholipids

This category of fats is present throughout your entire body, but much more so inside your brain. Another type of invaluable structural fat, *phospholipids* help give all of your brain cells shape, strength, and elasticity.

Phospholipids are made almost entirely out of omega-3s, echoing how important omega-3s are dietarily, but you can also derive phospholipids from certain foods. Fish, crabmeat, salmon roe, krill, soybeans, milk, oats, and sunflower seeds are all good sources. But egg yolks, cracking into the top of the list in yet another category, pack a big nutritional punch with over 10,000 milligrams of phospholipids per 100 grams of product.

One of the most interesting things about phospholipids is their contribution to cellular communication. Not only are they involved in signal transductions (allowing your brain cells to communicate with each other), research cited in *Advances in Biological Regulation* revealed that phospholipids play a crucial role in regulating receptor sites for our all-important thyroid hormones that help to regulate metabolism *and* cognition. You may not have heard much about the connection between thyroid hormone and mental performance before, but it's yet another amazing connection in the body reaffirming that doing good things for one area (metabolism) is probably going to be good for something else (brain health). Data published in the journal *Hormones and Behavior* asserted that thyroid hormone influences the brain's processing speed, efficiency in executive functions, and overall learning behavior. But, keep in mind, as important as thyroid hormone is, it can't do its job properly without phospholipids.

Another compelling feature of phospholipids is their ability to potentially support mental performance under stress. A recent double-blind, placebo-controlled trial found that the consumption of phospholipids helped to enhance attention and improve reaction time when test subjects were placed under acute stress. The study participants also reported reduced participation anxiety and a heightened sense of mental energy.

Phospholipids can be further broken down into their four most common subcategories. These are phosphatidylserine, phosphatidylethanolamine, phosphatidylcholine, and phosphatidylinositol, which each have a substantial impact on the performance of your brain. Take phosphatidylserine, for example. A study highlighted in the journal *Lipids in Health and Disease* investigated the influence that phosphatidylserine could have on short-term memory function (name/face acquisition and remembering phone numbers) in test subjects with reported cognitive decline. After just three weeks of increased phosphatidylserine, they observed a substantial improvement in their short-term memory. In comparison to the control group, patients with improved levels of phosphatidylserine were reported to have "rolled back the clock" of their cognitive age by several years! Ample food sources of phosphatidylserine include Atlantic mackerel, tuna, chicken liver, chicken heart, turkey, beef, white beans, and soy lecithin.

Phosphatidylserine is one of the top two phospholipids used by the human brain, while the other one that we need to make a virtual sticky note about is phosphatidylcholine. A fascinating study published in *Clinical Neuropharmacology* found increasing the amount of dietary phosphatidylcholine in healthy study participants led to a significant improvement in explicit memory versus a placebo. Explicit memory (also referred to as declarative memory) is one of the two main types of long-term human memory. Explicit memory involves conscious recollection of information. Meaning, when you want to proactively grab a piece of data from your mental rolodex, you're able to easily scroll through and find it.

What's even more compelling about phosphatidylcholine is that it acts as a precursor for one of the most important compounds in brain development and the creation of memories. Your body uses phosphatidylcholine to make a brain chemical called *acetylcholine*. Acetylcholine works to support and improve a form of your memory called *working memory*. This is a crucial part of your memory that allows your brain to briefly hold new information while it's needed in the short-term. In essence, your working memory enables your brain to capture a short video and play it back. This is used for things like remembering instructions, recognizing patterns (helpful in solving math problems, for example), and remembering what you should be focused on! With that last one, this asserts that acetylcholine is also vital for focus and attention. Clearly, supporting your body's intake and production of acetylcholine can be a game-changer.

Acetylcholine is one of your brain's main neurotransmitters, having marquee roles in both memory and learning. Phospholipids are one part of the connective tissue for acetylcholine, while another part is a B vitamin, choline. This nutrient might just be one of the most important things for developing your lifelong memory capabilities. Research conducted by scientists at the University of North Carolina postulates that your memory characteristics are heavily impacted by how much choline your mother ate during pregnancy and lactation. Choline appears to influence the development of the memory center in the brain (i.e., your hippocampus). This is a new affirmation for new and pregnant moms to ensure they're eating an ample amount of choline-rich foods, and for all of us to optimize our levels, regardless. Because even if you didn't start off with a great game of Hungry Hungry Hippocampus gobbling up choline early in life, you still have a tremendous opportunity to step your neuro-nutrition game up and win!

About 10 percent of the choline circulating in your system is produced by your liver. And the rest of your brain and body needs must come from your nutrition. The highest source of dietary choline you're going to find is from beef liver, followed by chicken liver, cod, shrimp, eggs (again), and plant sources like broccoli, Brussels sprouts, and cauliflower. There is an incredible interaction between our structural brain fats and other key nutrients to make the magic happen.

Up next is another powerhouse dietary fat that can dance its way into the VIP section and get the party jumping in your brain.

MCTs

In Chapter Four we worked to clear up the confusion surrounding saturated fatty acids. To recap, saying that saturated fats are "bad" is a dangerous oversimplification we need to be cautious about. Not only have natural food-based saturated fats been vindicated in the scientific literature as a causative agent behind heart disease, but saturated fat is actually one of the main fats that make up your brain cells! But before you go bobbing for apples in a bucket of coconut oil, listen to this . . .

Though the brain is made of some saturated fats, hardly any of the saturated fats a person eats actually makes it into the brain once you reach adulthood. The security check at the BBB doesn't allow it. According to Dr. Mosconi, the brain consumes a sizeable amount of saturated fat in early development, but doesn't consume much after adolescence. Restated: *Saturated fat is critical to brain development early in life.* In fact, nature's first food, breast milk, can be upward of 50 percent saturated fat. From there, various food sources of saturated fats are assimilated into young brains, but in adulthood that assimilation is all but turned off. And if your brain needs any more saturated fat, it can actually manufacture it on its own. There's essentially no need to restock it from your diet for your brain's sake. Plus, the latest research indicates that consuming too much might be problematic.

Once the brain reaches maturity, consuming high amounts of saturated fat has mixed results in clinical trials. A meta-analysis published in the journal *Neurobiology of Aging* found some studies reported increased cognitive decline with high saturated fat consumption, while other studies found that higher saturated fat intake improved cognition. Again, the studies typically don't account for the source nor type of saturated fat. I just want to make sure you have the data to make an informed decision on your food choices. Clearly, the source of the saturated fat matters (whole food–based versus processed food–based). But there is also a type of saturated fat that the brain really seems to have a crush on.

Medium chain triglycerides (MCTs) are still up on a poster in your brain's bedroom, even long into adulthood. Researchers at Yale University published data purporting that MCTs can readily cross the BBB and be utilized by brain cells. Getting access into the VIP section should be enough proof as to their importance, but there's more. A remarkable study published in the *Annals of the New York Academy of Sciences* sought to find out if MCTs could have an impact on improving the condition of patients with Alzheimer's disease. It is now well-noted that Alzheimer's disease is consistently accompanied by an impairment of glucose uptake into the brain cells. There is a form of insulin resistance taking place in the brain that accelerates the degradation of neurological function. The scientists in the study discovered that, since MCTs are quickly metabolized by the liver, prompting the production of ketones, those ketones are then able to easily cross the BBB and provide an alternative fuel source to the glucose-impaired brain cells of Alzheimer's patients. The scientist found that the consumption of MCTs directly led to improved cognitive function in mild-to-moderate forms of Alzheimer's disease and cognitive impairment. The research here is still in its infancy, but it is very promising.

Not many people realize that Alzheimer's disease has been inching itself into the top five causes of death in the United States. Alzheimer's isn't just about losing memories, people with this devastating condition are subject to neuronal damage and death that can eventually impair their ability to perform essential actions, such as walking and swallowing. It's a heartbreaking process that far too many families are subject to today.

The rates of Alzheimer's have skyrocketed in recent years, and many experts affirm that it doesn't "just happen." There are genetic factors, yes, but the huge epigenetic influences of diet, exercise, and environment clearly play a major role. Part of having optimal brain performance is working toward prevention of chronic illnesses like Alzheimer's and other forms of dementia. With where we are currently in science, once these conditions take hold of the brain, it's very difficult to see improvement. It's beyond impressive to see that these types of fats can warrant a positive benefit, but let's work to create preventative brain-healthy practices within our families and communities at large. In addition to brain-healthy nutrition, a recent study analyzing participants with inherited Alzheimer's disease genes revealed that 30 minutes of exercise five days a week could dramatically lower their risk of Alzheimer's expression. Plus, researchers at Washington University School of Medicine in St. Louis found that getting adequate amounts of sleep (which we'll talk about soon!) can lower your risk even further.

To summarize, MCTs may provide both a direct and an indirect brain fuel source (via their ability to cross the BBB and their ability to generate ketones). Whole food sources of MCTs include coconut oil and dairy products (from cow's milk, goat's milk, and other sources). Concentrated MCT oils can also be purchased and added to things like coffee, tea, salads, smoothies, and more.

EVOO

With healthy brain performance, we not only want to provide key nutrients that can cross the brain's security system (the BBB), we also want to provide support for the security system, itself! Through things like neuroinflammation (inflammation in the brain), exposure to toxins, and nutritional deficiencies, the BBB can become dysfunctional over time. By not allowing the right things in, or keeping the wrong things out, a damaged BBB can further exacerbate poor mental performance and cognitive decline.

Groundbreaking new research published in *ACS Chemical Neuroscience* asserts that oleocanthal-rich extra virgin olive oil (EVOO) is able to restore the function of the BBB! What's most impressive is that EVOO appears to have multiple means of action by which it improves the health of the BBB. The Auburn University scientists conducting the study found that EVOO effectively supports the reduction of neuroinflammation, increases the activity of a potent metabolic protein called AMPK, and improves the process of autophagy in the brain. Let's take a moment and touch on each of these benefits further.

You're already aware of the devastating impact of excessive inflammation, thanks to our discussion in earlier chapters. But inflammation in the brain is especially troublesome. Acute inflammation in the brain can cause everything from disorientation, to nausea, to loss of consciousness. Chronic inflammation in the brain is heavily tied to memory loss, vision loss, and the provocation of conditions like Alzheimer's and dementia. Foods and nutrients that support the reduction of inflammation in the brain are truly invaluable.

The metabolic protein *AMP-activated protein kinase* (AMPK) has numerous beneficial impacts on the brain. One of the consistencies we've noted in reduced cognitive function is a reduction in glucose reaching the brain cells. According to researchers at the University of Massachusetts Medical School, AMPK is one of the rare compounds that's able to improve glucose transport across the BBB and enhance delivery to the neurons. And if that doesn't get you amped enough, AMPK is also supportive of autophagy.

Autophagy is part of the brain's self-cleaning process. It's the body's way of cleaning out damaged cells in order to "make room" and regenerate newer, healthier cells. In the brain, impaired autophagy is another ingredient seen in neurodegenerative diseases. As part of normal metabolism, brain cells produce wastes that need to be removed (sort of like taking out the trash). A major waste product that can accumulate in the brain is a harmful form of amyloid beta peptide, a toxic protein that's linked to Alzheimer's disease. The clearance of the resulting amyloid "plaque" out of the brain appears to be enhanced by the oleocanthal (antioxidant and anti-inflammatory phenol) contained in olive oil. Supporting autophagy is serious business, as a new study published in *Current Biology* states that autophagy is actually *required* for new memory formation. So, the bottom line is, having a sharp memory isn't just about getting the good stuff in, it's also about getting the not-so-good stuff out.

Other research cited in *The Scientific World Journal* reaffirms olive oil's ability to reduce BBB hyperpermeability. But another interesting thing is that sufficient intake of monounsaturated fatty acids found in EVOO is found to help prevent the age-related deletion of mitochondrial DNA in the brain, according to data cited in *Frontiers in Cellular Neuroscience*.

EVOO is rich in fats that support the brain in a multitude of ways. So, how much should you target? Researchers at the Rush Institute for Healthy Aging found that people who consumed at least 24 grams of these fats per day had an 80 percent reduced risk of Alzheimer's compared to those who consumed 15 grams or less. It only takes 2 to 3 tablespoons of EVOO to hit your daily dose of high-quality brain-protective monounsaturated fats. Plus, there are plenty of other brain-boosting foods you can add to the mix to hit that target and provide some other unforgettable benefits, as well.

BRAIN HYGIENE

In our society, when we talk about hygiene, we're generally talking about practices of cleanliness to maintain health, to prevent disease, and to just generally not stank. If you consistently smell like you rubbed a stick of onion-scented deodorant under your arms, people would likely say that you have poor body hygiene. If your teeth are so yellow that when you smile traffic slows down around you, then people would likely say you have poor dental hygiene. Even though we've all been stinky or had some weird stuff on our teeth at some point or another, it's how we address these things on a consistent basis that tells the tale of our hygienic prowess.

Within our culture, we generally use the look and smell of things to establish their cleanliness. Your brain requires a level of hygiene too, but (unless you have brain imaging tech handy) you generally can't see your brain, and you definitely can't give it a sniff test. To ensure your brain stays sparkling clean and clear of obstructions, here are some foods proven to support brain hygiene and boost your mental performance.

Turmeric

Noted for its exceptional antioxidant capacity, turmeric has also been found to enhance brain hygiene by giving your brain a virtual spa treatment. Scientists from the Department of Neurology at USC found that the active ingredient in turmeric (curcumin) is able to help eliminate amyloid plaque, slow down the aging of neurons, excavate heavy metals, and reduce inflammation in the brain.

Something really noteworthy about curcumin is that it's also been revealed to improve the function of resident macrophage cells that operate as the frontline of the brain's immune system. In the instance that an unwelcome invader is able to finesse its way past the BBB, these cells are there to pull up on them and open a can of whoop ass in order to protect your brain at all costs. Known as *microglia,* they participate in overall brain maintenance and are constantly scavenging your brain and the rest of the central nervous system for plaques, damaged or unnecessary neurons and synapses, and, as noted, any infectious agents that sneak their way through. Because of these incredible features, turmeric has been noted in multiple studies to improve memory function. And to put a hygienic final touch on it, research published in the journal *PLOS ONE* revealed that curcumin is capable of improving neuroplasticity and stimulating the creation of new brain cells.

Walnuts

Compounds found in walnuts have been shown to help scrub your brain clear of the harmful amyloid beta peptide that leads to bona fide amyloid plaque buildup. The data highlighted in the journal *Neurochemical Research* demonstrated that walnuts have the potential to reduce oxidative stress, reduce inflammation, and protect your brain cells from an early demise.

Walnuts are packed with brain-healthy vitamins, minerals, and fats. And recent research from UCLA suggests that eating a handful of walnuts per day may help boost memory, concentration, and the speed at which your brain processes information.

Cinnamon

Scientists at the University of California–Santa Barbara discovered that phytonutrients in cinnamon can help comb out tangles of tau proteins in the brain. These neurofibrillary tangles are actually one of the primary biomarkers of Alzheimer's disease. Not only does cinnamon inhibit these tangles from happening in the first place, it also reduces oxidative stress and improves the overall health of neurons.

Another study cited in the *Journal of Neuroimmune Pharmacology* discovered that cinnamon has the potential to improve the learning speed of folks with learning challenges by stimulating hippocampal plasticity. It's easy to add cinnamon to things like smoothies, coffee, oatmeal, savory-sweet chicken and pork dishes, sweet potatoes, and more. A little goes a long way, so shoot for at least ¼ teaspoon per day!

BRAIN, BRAIN GO AWAY

A big part of improving our mental performance is avoiding the things that bring harm to our brains. This might seem obvious on the surface, but many of us are unaware that some of the foods we eat can give our brains an express pass to catastrophe.

You already know that your powerful brain is your most energy-demanding organ. Scooping up at least 20 percent of the calories you consume, your brain is like a competitive eater scarfing down as much fuel as possible to power the 100 billion neurons that make it up.

Since glucose is your brain's primary fuel source, there are custom sugar gates in the BBB to allow glucose to pass through in droves. As far as your brain is concerned, it's expensive to keep the lights on upstairs, and Harvard researchers affirmed that the brain will gladly confiscate half of the sugar energy in your body.

Since sugar is always funneling into and throughout the brain, insulin activity in the central nervous system has become a huge topic of discussion in science the last few years. Research published in the journal *Frontiers in Endocrinology* states, "Insulin in the brain contributes to the control of nutrient homeostasis, reproduction, cognition, and memory, as well as to neurotrophic, neuromodulatory, and neuroprotective effects." The report goes on to affirm that there's a delicate balance of glucose needs and glucose overburden through high sugar intake. The researchers noted that excessive glucose can directly lead to insulin resistance extending to the central nervous system, higher incidence of type 2 diabetes, and a dramatically increased risk of Alzheimer's disease. In fact, they declared that "a close association between type 2 diabetes and Alzheimer's disease has been reported, to the extent that Alzheimer's disease is *twice* more frequent in diabetic patients, and some authors have proposed the name 'type 3 diabetes' for this association."

This is critical to understand! To reiterate their findings: Excessive sugar intake and insulin resistance is so connected to Alzheimer's disease that scientists are now referring to it as type 3 diabetes. The overconsumption of sugar is devastating for your brain. And our society doesn't just have a sweet tooth, it has an iced-out grill full of sweet teeth.

Estimates are difficult to calculate due to the variance of natural sugars, added sugars, and concentrated forms of natural sugars (like those found in fruit juice). But it's clear that we're far surpassing the recommended dietary guidelines of about 30 grams of added sugars per day. Even though we're down from our peak sugar consumption of more than 100 grams of sugar per day in 1999, some estimates show that the average American is still eating over 90 grams of added sugar per day. This equates to about 77 pounds of added sugar per year! Again, this is only calculating the *added* sugars/caloric sweeteners, and it's not taking into consideration the natural sugars contained in various foods and beverages.

Though most people know that we, as a society, have a problem with sugar, it's so deeply ingrained in our culture that we often struggle to make the changes necessary. I mean, how can you villainize something that's so connected to love and significance in our lives? It's the cake with icing we give our child on their very first birthday. It's what we give our sweetheart on Valentine's Day to signify our love. It's what we give our kids after their game to celebrate a victory or to console a tough loss. It's what we tie into celebration on nearly every holiday…from Halloween candy to Christmas cookies to cold sodas on the 4th of July. And on Easter there's apparently a bunny out there laying eggs full of candy. That one's just weird. And don't get me started on those marshmallow Peeps.

When I was a kid, no matter where we moved in the city, we always had a neighborhood corner store. You see, a corner store isn't anything like a 7-Eleven or QT. Yes, you can get your usual chips, sodas, candy bars, and personal care items, but you can also get a meat order with fresh sliced bologna (an oxymoron), the attendant knew your name like Norm on *Cheers,* and they had my most favorite thing of all: penny candy.

Before folks were whole grazing the bulk food bins at Whole Foods, penny candy was pioneering candy purchases in 'hoods across America. If you've got 1 cent, you could buy one piece of candy. A Swedish Fish, a JuJu Coin, a Tootsie Frootie Roll, a Sour Fruit Chew, and the list goes on and on. You've got 10 cents, that's 10 pieces. And don't let me walk in with a dollar! I'm leaving there with a brown paper bag full of 100 pieces of those loose candies…and enough sugar to make me black out while playing video games and *still* keep my fingers moving to finish the level.

Candy wasn't just sweet and tasty, it was an adventure. And so many of our sugar-filled experiences hold a special place in our lives like that. To suddenly tell yourself to stay away from it is like when Ralph Fiennes found out that Jennifer Lopez wasn't who she said she was in that movie, *Maid in Manhattan*. We had such a good time together, and you really livened things up in my life, but now the media says you're bad for me. Even though sugar lied right to your face, the happy ending is you keep hooking up with sugar anyway, just like Ralph and J-Lo.

We don't want to break up with sugar. And there's a couple of reasons beyond the fact that it tastes good. I interviewed Dr. Robert Lustig, who's one of the world's leading authorities on sugar consumption and cognitive function. He stated, "We're biologically programmed to like sweets." In nature that sweet taste is an indicator of a dense source of nutrition. But food manufacturers have manipulated our biological programming and led it astray. Nowhere in our evolution were we ever able to access so much sugar, so quickly, and (usually) without the accompaniment of essential micronutrients. Drinking one bottle of typical soda, you can knock down 15 to 20 teaspoons of sugar which easily stresses your microbiome, overburdens your liver, and aggressively ransacks your brain. And, to top it all off, it's highly addictive.

Dr. Lustig shared that sugar lights up areas of the brain associated with pleasure and reward. And the amount of sugar many people consume in an average snack or meal makes it light up like a sea of glow sticks at a concert. The problem is that very quickly after the concert, the intense sugar glow sticks start to lose their spark and end up working pretty crappily. One of the main regions of the brain affected by excess sugar is the nucleus accumbens. Similar to drugs like cocaine, sugar actually spikes dopamine release in the nucleus accumbens. This is a hallmark reason behind the pleasure connected to gnawing on sweet things. Dr. Lustig stated that, as we consume copious amounts of sugar over time, the dopamine signal attenuates and gets weaker, "So you have to consume more to get the same effect...and if you pull back (on the sugar), you go into withdrawal."

Due to legalities that surround creating addiction in human test subjects, many clinical trials currently available are using animal models. One of the most eye-opening was conducted by researchers at Princeton University who discovered that rats who were fed excessive amounts of sugar and then forced to go through "withdrawal" experienced physical symptoms like teeth chattering, head shakes, and tremors. The researchers reported that repeated sugar consumption will cause a demonstration of all three criteria of addiction: increased intake, withdrawal, and cravings that lead to relapse. In the slightly altered words of Rick James, "Sugar is a helluva drug."

Home Alone

In the classic holiday movie *Home Alone,* Kevin McCallister (played by Macaulay Culkin) went up against a couple of burglars who dubbed themselves the "wet bandits." The movie orchestrated multiple scenarios to show that these two burglars were not the sharpest tools in the shed. An 8-year-old kid beat the pants off of them with homemade booby traps and the wet bandits seemed to get more and more foolish by the minute. Even after all of the abuse and getting caught, they went through it all over again in *Home Alone 2* (another holiday classic and [clears throat] we'll just pretend that part 3 didn't happen). No matter how hard they tried, things just kept getting worse. And, believe it or not, certain foods cause your brain cells to turn into the wet bandits (or sticky bandits if we're talking about part 2). You start making poor decisions, you don't remember what you need to remember, and you end up getting hurt, over and over again.

Sugar parlays itself into this domain as well. Harvard researchers recently cited a study that linked excess sugar intake to an obstruction in cognitive abilities such as memory and learning. While another study published in the journal *Neuron* found that overeating sugar creates dysfunction in a neuropeptide that regulates arousal, wakefulness, and appetite. The abnormal impact to this neuropeptide, *orexin,* results in increased mental fatigue and drowsiness. On the other hand, it's important to note that the researchers also acknowledged that protein consumption helped to normalize orexin and *boost* mental alertness. If you're going to outsmart life's booby traps, you've got to be alert and ready. Too much sugar tosses virtual Micro Machines on the floor in front of us to slip on. We have to beat sugar at its own game, which we'll talk about in the next section. For now, just be proactive about reducing your intake of added sugars. And remember, all sugar is not "bad," but going over your carbohydrate tipping point we talked about in Chapter Four can spell big trouble for your brain and a sequel for your waistline.

Artificial sweeteners are another category that's home alone in the nutritional domain. They give the appearance that the house is empty (there's no calories in sight and seemingly nothing to worry about). But little did we know there were some *Angels with Filthy Souls* stowing away that can send your brain cells running for their lives.

Artificial sweeteners hit the scene as a guilt-free way to enjoy your favorite sodas, snacks, and treats. I can still hear the slogan in my mind, "Just for the taste of it, Diet Coke!" It wasn't a caloric sweetener like cane sugar or high fructose corn syrup, and it still tasted good. I literally saw family members order a quarter pounder with cheese, an order of fries, and a Diet Coke because they were trying to watch their figures. Go figure.

The marketing for artificial sweeteners was fantastic. Sure, it was made in a lab. Sure, it wasn't made from anything natural. Sure, there wasn't any long-term research done on it. But it was safe to consume, right? Well, our society thought so...until studies began coming out warning of the increased rates of cancer seen in laboratory animals consuming artificial sweeteners (saccharine) and damage to the microbiome (sucralose). And they even appeared to have some negative impacts on your brain.

A recent study conducted by researchers at the Boston University School of Medicine and published in the peer-reviewed journal *Stroke* discovered a surprising link between drinking diet soda and two debilitating health issues. The study found that people who drink diet soda daily are almost *three times more likely* to have a stroke and develop dementia. Now, just to be clear, this is a strong correlation, not causation. The researchers did an excellent job taking into account adjustments for age, sex, education (for analysis of dementia), caloric intake, diet quality, physical activity, and smoking. But other factors like family history of dementia can be accounted for and additional studies can be completed, of course, to try and repeat the results. Artificial sweeteners being linked to neurodegenerative diseases is a big deal that needs further testing to be sure. But, as with everything in eating smarter, I want you to possess the latest information we have so that you can make smart decisions for your own body and brain.

An additional study I want to make mention of was conducted by scientists at the University of Bordeaux and published in the peer-reviewed journal *PLOS ONE*. In the study, the researchers set out to find how an artificial sweetener (saccharine) stacks up in addictive behavior against a strong narcotic like cocaine. They gave rats (with no prior experience with refined sugar or artificial sweeteners) the ability to choose eight times per day between two mutually exclusive levers—one that gave them a dose of cocaine and one that gave them a dose of saccharin-sweetened water. The results showed that a shocking 94 percent of the time the critters became hooked on saccharine and not cocaine. And get this, even rats that were already addicted to cocaine quickly switched their preference to saccharine once it was offered as a choice.

The scientists in the study concluded: "Overall, research has revealed that sugar and sweet reward can not only be a substitute to addictive drugs like cocaine, but can even be *more* rewarding and attractive. At the neurobiological level, the neural substrates of sugar and sweet reward appear to be more robust than those of cocaine (i.e., more resistant to functional failures), possibly reflecting past selective evolutionary pressures for seeking and taking foods high in sugar and calories." The researchers also swapped in sugar in place of the artificial sweetener and saw the same results. The sobering truth is that the sweet taste drives us to consume more, and this offers us an explanation as to why so many people have difficulty controlling the consumption of highly sweetened, processed foods and beverages when continuously exposed to them. It's not simply a matter of willpower; it's a matter of biology. And awareness can start the healing process.

Why this matters to me on a purely logical level is that artificial sweeteners actually do their work by tricking your brain. The taste receptors send messages to your brain that you're consuming something sweet. It would usually mean that your brain should expect some calories to accompany the sweetness but (surprise!) that's not the case.

With the sweet taste coming in, and your body's primal programming to handle sweetness a certain way (through releasing insulin), I just don't think we can fool our bodies that easily. And a study from scientists at the Washington University School of Medicine confirms that. A recent clinical trial involving 17 obese test subjects (who did not regularly consume artificial sweeteners) found that the artificial sweetener sucralose elevated their blood sugar levels by 14 percent and insulin levels by 20 percent on average. Artificial sweeteners can pretend that they're home alone, but you can rest assured that they're laying out a trap or two that's applying a little pain to your brain and hormones.

Seriously, if you or anyone you know has seen success by reducing sugar intake and switching to artificial sweeteners, no one in the world can knock that. Your success in formulating what's best for your unique metabolic fingerprint is up to you! My job is just to ensure that you have the data to do it as healthfully as possible. There's a huge wave of *natural* calorie-free sweeteners coming to the forefront that have some potential upside, and some unanswered questions as well. Going back to our 80+ Rule, as long as your diet is built around a strong foundation of whole foods, adding some of these calorie-free sweeteners here or there can possibly support you in not drinking Pepsi late at night like Kevin's little cousin, Fuller. But you want to be careful to not wet the bed by going too far, whether it's a calorie-free sweetener or not.

One more thing that can have your brain operating like you're on team wet bandit is swinging too far in one direction with your BMI. Even though the structural fats of your brain are pretty stable, being malnourished and underweight can cause significant reductions in the size of the brain. Researchers at Yale and the University of Cambridge discovered that underweight individuals have significant deficits in their brain's gray matter volume. In analyzing various patients, they found that this lowered gray matter could lead to slower functioning, memory loss, and other learning difficulties. This is a call to arms to ensure that we are nourishing ourselves, not excessively dieting and/or exercising, and providing ourselves with the specific neuro-nutrition that we need every day.

On the other hand, being significantly overweight has a potential connection to our brain size, too. A brand-new study published in the journal *Neurology* found that as the size of our waist gets bigger, the size of our brain tends to get smaller. Specifically, the gray matter of our brains shrink considerably. The study authors noted that this area of our brain that shrinks is responsible for things like self-control, muscle function, and sensory perception. It's not clear if abnormalities in brain structure lead to obesity, or if obesity leads to these changes in the brain. But the two do go together like the wet/sticky bandits, Harry and Marv.

Now you know some of the real booby traps that can sabotage the form and function of your brain. Next up, it's time to dance into some of the specific foods and nutrients that can help you to think faster, be more focused and productive, and even improve your memory.

DANCE WITH THE ONE WHO BROUGHT YOU

One of the unique things about your brain cells is that they don't readily get replaced like the rest of the cells in your body. The vast majority of our brain cells are actually formed while we are in the womb. After our birth (hello, world!), certain parts of our brains continue to create new neural cells through infancy. But, after that, there's a hard stop in production.

For many years, it was concluded that the brain cells you have at birth (and shortly after) are the only brain cells you will have throughout your entire life. In recent decades, however, it's been affirmed that the brain has a limited capacity to regenerate itself and create new brain cells in *some* areas of the brain. The creation of new brain cells (*neurogenesis*) has been identified to primarily happen in the hippocampus (the memory center of the brain). But, outside of that, what you've got is what you've got. This is why caring for our brain cells is of the utmost importance and one of the most crucial things to do in our lives. When we're born, we're bringing a certain number of brain cells with us...and we've got to dance with the ones we came with.

Caring for your brain cells and practicing good brain hygiene can supercharge your cognitive function and enable new connections (via neuroplasticity) for a lifetime. Here are some foods and beverages that support the health of your brain cells and unlock mental dance moves that will help you perform better in every area of your life.

Spinach

Chicago's Rush University Medical Center found that people who ate one to two servings of leafy green vegetables like spinach each day experienced fewer memory problems and cognitive decline. Compared to people who rarely ate leafy greens, study participants who ate about two servings a day had brains that performed as if they were about 11 years younger!

The test subjects underwent a battery of annual tests to assess cognitive function in areas like episodic memory, working memory, visuospatial ability, and more. After accounting for other lifestyle factors, eating green leafy veggies stood out as a clear brain-booster. Target two servings per day of leafy greens like spinach, kale, and various types of lettuces. This is easy to get in a fresh salad or green smoothie, or you can sauté up some spinach with brain-healthy fats, high-quality salt, and some of our next brain-healthy food, garlic.

Garlic

The benefits of garlic have been cited in over one thousand scientific publications in the last decade alone. But its use dates all the way back to the ancient Egyptians who prized garlic for its utilization in both food and medicine. This little, bulbous plant has body-wide benefits that extend itself right up to your neurons.

A study published in the journal *Drug and Chemical Toxicology* revealed that garlic can help improve memory and learning speed, even when brain cells are damaged from toxin exposure. Another study found that garlic has neuroprotective effects that defend brain cells against amyloid plaque build-up, toxicity, and early cell death.

Finely chop or mince fresh garlic and add it to your guacamole, add generous amounts to cooked veggies, and many chicken and seafood recipes are easily livened up when garlic hits the dance floor.

Blackberries

The polyphenols in blackberries have the potential to slow and even reverse age-related declines in cognitive performance, according to research published in *Nutritional Neuroscience.* The vitamin C, vitamin K, and antioxidants packed into these little berries are all supportive of optimal mental performance. Toss a cup of blackberries into a smoothie, add them to your favorite yogurt, or simply enjoy them as a solo act.

Chocolate

Very few foods can make your brain move and groove like chocolate can. Fascinating data cited in *Neuroscience & Biobehavioral Reviews* revealed that the flavonoids in dark chocolate can actually be observed penetrating and accumulating in the brain regions involved in learning and memory, especially the hippocampus.

As we discussed previously in the book, the quality of the chocolate we eat matters a lot. And, according to a recent study featured in *The Journal of Nutrition,* eating as little as ⅓ of an ounce of high-quality chocolate each day can help protect your brain against age-related memory loss. That's a square or two of a typical organic dark chocolate bar, or about a tablespoon of cacao nibs added to your yogurt, oatmeal, or smoothie. And one more thing to note about chocolate: It's also been well-documented to induce positive effects on mood (clearly), and one of the ways it does this is through improving blood flow to the brain and also through stimulating neurogenesis. Yes, chocolate is one of the handful of foods that are proven to spark the creation of new brain cells!

Green Tea

One of the most brain-healthy beverages that Dr. Daniel Amen recommended all those years ago to improve mental focus was green tea. The caffeine contained in green tea has been found to improve reaction time, increase attentiveness, and reduce mental fatigue. But in some ways the caffeine, alone, has a limited amount of dance moves. And that's what makes green tea so special. It has an array of other powerful nutrients that are also supportive of improved mental performance.

In addition to being an excellent source of antioxidants, green tea contains a unique amino acid called *L-theanine*. As one of the rare nutrients that can gracefully waltz its way across the BBB, L-theanine is able to increase the activity of the neurotransmitter GABA, which helps reduce anxiety and makes you feel more centered and relaxed. This is definitely helpful when you want to be more productive!

Even folks who are sensitive to caffeine find that green tea works with their system thanks to the balancing effects of L-theanine. Another way that L-theanine works to improve focus is noted in the peer-reviewed journal *Brain Topography*. The researchers observed that L-theanine intake increases the frequency of alpha brain waves, indicating reduced stress, enhanced focus, and even increased creativity. Sipping on two to four cups per day was noted to carry the greatest brain benefits.

Spirulina

The data surrounding spirulina and brain health is really impressive. A recent study published in *PLOS ONE* revealed that spirulina has the potential to 1) improve neurogenesis in the brain, and 2) reduce neuroinflammation. These are two very remarkable attributes. Not to mention, it's loaded with antioxidants and other nutrient precursors to help make vital neurotransmitters. A teaspoon of spirulina a day is plenty to provide your brain with some added insurance. As long as you're prepared to turn your snack into a color cascade that resembles the *Swamp Thing,* spirulina is an easy addition to smoothies, fresh-made juices, and even guacamole.

Mushrooms

A six-year study found that the inclusion of culinary mushrooms can improve your memory and reduce the risk of age-related cognitive impairment by upward of 50 percent. Mushrooms like golden, oyster, white button, and shiitake were all noted to be beneficial in the study. Many of these mushrooms are an excellent source of nutrients like potassium, copper, and B vitamins that are known to be supportive of cognitive function. Add two to four servings of mushrooms per week and you'll dramatically reduce your risk of tangoing with memory problems.

Lion's Mane

In addition to culinary mushrooms, there's an entire class of *medicinal mushrooms* with their documented benefits tracing back thousands of years. One of those long-renowned medicinal mushrooms is called *lion's mane* (thanks to its resemblance of a flowing hairdo you might see on Simba). Today researchers are analyzing lion's mane for its profound impact on brain health.

Scientists at the University of Malaya discovered that compounds in lion's mane are able to significantly improve the activity of *nerve growth factor* (NGF) in the brain. NGF is essential in the regulation of growth, maintenance, proliferation, and survival of various brain cells. This medicinal mushroom reminds us of the incredible amount of foods and nutrients we have access to that many people have yet to discover! Lion's mane mushroom is generally utilized via an alcohol extraction or a hot water decoction like a tea. As always, I'll have the best resources available for you as new products and innovations are made through the bonus resource guide at eatsmarterbook.com/bonus. There's even a favorite lion's mane coffee that combines two of the most potent brain-boosters in one!

Coffee

Many of us are well aware that coffee can improve mental performance. But few people know that regularly drinking coffee has been shown to help prevent cognitive decline and reduce the risk of developing Alzheimer's and Parkinson's disease. This attribute, referenced in the journal *Practical Neurology,* is yet another reason why smart coffee consumption makes the list of neuro-nutritious beverages.

Another study featured in the journal *Psychopharmacology* uncovered that drinking one large coffee in a day (200 milligrams caffeine) or four smaller cups (65 milligrams caffeine each) had some remarkable benefits on mental performance. The researchers found that both methods of coffee intake led to equal improvements in alertness and improved reaction times, as well as enhanced performance on cognitive vigilance tasks, activities involving multitasking, and tasks involving deep concentration. As you'll recall from our earlier discussions, coffee is also one of the biggest sources of dietary antioxidants (providing many additional benefits on their own). If you are doing the cha-cha with the java, remember that the sweet spot appears to be between 50 and 250 milligrams of caffeine per day. This creates a nice choreography opportunity to enjoy a cup of coffee or two, or a combination of a cup of coffee and a few cups of green tea.

Broccoli

If it wasn't for broccoli, I don't know if I would be here right now. It was the one and only green vegetable that I ate as a kid, and thankfully each bite was providing some much needed nutrition for my brain.

One of the most valuable things about broccoli is that it's a rich source of fat-soluble vitamin K. This fat-soluble vitamin has been found to be a critical component in the synthesis of another form of structural brain fats called *sphingolipids*. According to data cited in the journal *Nutrition Reviews,* the interaction between vitamin K and sphingolipids plays a major role in our cognitive function.

On top of that, adequate consumption of vitamin K has been found to improve episodic memory. Episodic memory is a form of explicit memory (involving conscious recollection of information). Your episodic memory is essentially recording autobiographical events (times, places, associated emotions, and other contextual who, what, when, where, why knowledge) that you can proactively refer back to when you want to. In addition, broccoli is also an excellent source of nutrients called *isothiocyanates.* These powerful compounds have been found to help reduce brain inflammation and provide protection against neurodegenerative diseases.

We've covered an incredible array of foods, spices, beverages, and more that are proven to support your brain health and help you to *eat smarter.* Up next, you're going to access one of the most powerful portions of this book. In the next chapter we'll explore the deeper ways that food relates to our mental health, our emotional health, and how we relate to each other.

CHAPTER SEVEN

Food Love Languages

Food is the ingredient that binds us together.

~*Unknown*

A huge part of eating smarter stretches beyond your plate and into your environment. The food you eat doesn't just affect you, it also affects the world around you. And, as you'll discover in this chapter, the world around you also affects what you eat.

Working with countless organizations and individuals over the years, I was always shocked by how much a person's environment affected their food choices (and how they often didn't realize it). Our environment shapes our tastes, food preferences, food accessibility, mental and emotional relationships with food, and overall eating behaviors long before we become aware of it.

Knowing this, addressing our eating behaviors solely at the point of personal choice is a huge mistake that's led to widespread struggles with dieting, higher rates of disease, and a continued socioeconomic burden that threatens the livelihood of our entire society. Recent estimates show that diet-related chronic diseases cost the U.S. economy a staggering $1 trillion each year. A study published by the American Heart Association shows that the cost of cardiovascular disease, alone, will exceed $1.1 trillion within the next few years if left unchecked, placing a crushing economic and health burden on the nation's financial and health care systems. A problem like this doesn't change just by telling people to eat healthier. It's changed by delivering real world solutions that treat the problem at every level. Food can be a powerful tool for happiness and healing, and it can also be a powerful weapon for degradation and disease. It starts at home, but it ends on the global stage. Let's take a look at how we can effect lasting change within our own bodies, within our families, and within our communities at large.

HOME FOR DINNER

We might be under the illusion that we are making choices about what we eat on our own free will. But the research clearly indicates that what you eat is heavily influenced by *how* you eat and, more interestingly, with *whom* you're eating.

Study after study has demonstrated how much the simple act of eating as a family can influence the outcomes of our food choices. For instance, researchers at Harvard University recently uncovered that people who consistently eat dinner with their families frequently consume more fruits and vegetables and less soda and processed foods. Their data analysis also showed that increased frequency of family dinner was also associated with higher intakes of several nutrients that support health and defend the body against diseases. Specifically, eating together as a family increased consumption of fiber, calcium, folate, iron, B-vitamins, vitamin C, and vitamin E; lowered glycemic load; and lowered the intake of trans fats. What in the entire world?! Who knew that the conditions in which we eat could have such a profound impact on *what* we eat? Again, if we're constantly trying to target the food choices themselves, without addressing the environment and the family culture around eating, we are really missing the point. Having a family ritual of eating meals together makes it *easier* to eat better things.

Growing up in a family with a strong history of obesity, I can literally count on my hand the number of times we actually sat down for a family meal together. We often ate at the same time, but it was more like a free-for-all. Everybody would grab something and eat wherever we could sit, often in front of the television, and often with processed foods.

When I lived with my grandmother earlier in my childhood, I did have more structure and sat down to eat with them more often than not (usually for breakfast). Interestingly enough, even though I'd have my fair share of processed foods there, I also ate more fruits and vegetables during that time (which is also echoed in the research). A study cited in the *Journal of Nutrition Education and Behavior* found that children who ate breakfast with their families at least four times a week were more likely to consume ample fruits and vegetables. The structure, intentional meal planning, and elimination of distractions are just some of the reasons this can have such a huge impact. The study went on to report that children whose TV was never or rarely on during family meals were significantly less likely to consume soda and chips. And children who consumed breakfast, lunch, *or* dinner with their family at least four days per week ate at least five servings (each week) of fruits and vegetables over 80 percent of the time.

What's specifically interesting about this study is that it was incorporating data from minority children who'd generally live within the construct of low-income communities. This shines a subtle, but hopeful, light that even if we don't yet have access to the best food options, creating and sustaining a new family ritual of eating together more often can dramatically improve the health outcomes of the family, including the parents. But, before I talk about the adults, I want to share one more advocation for our kids.

Children and adolescents are at vulnerable life stages for the development of environment-fostered obesity, according to data published in *JAMA Network* and the journal *Pediatrics*. Children and young adults who share family meals three or more times per week are more likely to be in a healthy weight range and have a healthier diet and eating patterns than those who share fewer than three family meals together. Additionally, and incredibly important, these children were far less likely to engage in disordered eating. Three meals per week is the minimum bar to set to provide an additional layer of real health insurance.

Of course, this isn't the only social factor. Some folks are already doing this activity at varying degrees, but may be missing out on some of the other critical insights (which we'll be targeting soon).

With these pieces of data, it becomes easier to place blame on our caregivers for our personal habits. But that's not what this is about. I simply can't blame my parents for my eating behavior. It was a cultural phenomenon. It's common in a low-income household for at least one parent to not be around for meals due to work obligations (just to afford the substandard food we were eating). This meant there was rarely an opportunity for all of us to eat together. Some of my best memories were when my mother would let me stay up late on Friday or Saturday night after my little brother and sister went to sleep. We all shared the same bedroom, so I still had to go to bed with them until they fell asleep. I can't tell you how upset I was when I would accidently fall asleep sometimes and miss out on my late night television opportunities! And I also missed out on an opportunity to eat.

After my siblings were officially passed out, I'd head into the living room with my mom and watch TV. My father would stroll in from work around midnight, and (since he got paid on the weekend) he'd usually get some food, like my favorite St. Louis–style thin crust pizza from Imo's or Elicia's pizza. I literally still remember the phone number to this day! It was an adventurous feeling for me as a kid. Staying up late, eating pizza, and even playing video games with my dad from time to time. From the third grade on, this was a consistent routine for me, until the environment and pandemic poor food access broke my family down.

We'll talk about the overwhelming access to poor food in a moment. But not eating together very often was a choice that we could've adjusted, had we known that it mattered. Even the times when only one parent was available to sit down and eat together, it might've wielded better health outcomes for all of us, according to the data. A study cited in the *Family and Consumer Sciences Research Journal* disclosed that sitting down to a family meal helped working parents reduce the tension and strain from long hours at the office. The researchers found that, even if test subjects had major stress at work, if they could make it home in time to eat dinner with their family, their employee morale stayed high. However, as work increasingly inter-fered with the ability to eat dinner with their family, levels of dissatis-faction at work began to creep up. As we've covered numerous times in this book, stress is a major contributing factor to a wide range of health issues. Eating dinner with people you care for is a surprising buffer against that stress that more people need to know about.

The cultural construct of one or both parents or caregivers not being home is more frequent, but not exclusive, to low-income house-holds. According to the Center for American Progress, we might have seen a slight drop in the number of hours worked per year today versus the work-centric paradigms of generations past, but there was still typ-ically at least one parent at home in these households. And making it "home for dinner" was a cultural norm. For example, in 1960, only 20 percent of mothers worked. Today, 70 percent of U.S. children live in households where all adults are employed. The researchers made clear that it doesn't matter which parent is home from work to cook and care for the kids, but when all adults are working (single or with a partner), that's a huge hit to the physical and emotional health of the family.

To stretch this out even further, the International Labor Organiza-tion reported that Americans often work hundreds more hours per year than the majority of industrialized nations. We might say, "Well, that's just good ol'-fashioned American gumption!" First of all, why are we saying "gumption"? And second of all, coupled with our much higher rate of work hours, we also have much higher rates of anxiety, depression, and chronic diseases than practically anywhere else in the Western world. Now, I'm in no way advising you to work less hours if you genuinely love what you do or it's out of dire necessity to support your family. I've been there a time or 20. What I'm saying is that we know that there's a clear connection between stress, lack of sleep, mal-nutrition, and excessive work hours. If work is costing you your health and the opportunity to create healthy family structures around food, it's about time to reassess your priorities and (at least) put a couple of simple practices in place to bring more well-being to you and your family. A powerful first step is scheduling a couple of meals together each week. Whether it's breakfast, lunch, or dinner, this one action can have transformative effects.

And let's not forget when we and the ones we love get a little older. A recent study revealed that eating together promotes healthy eating for seniors. The research found that seniors who regularly eat alone are often at higher risk for a variety of health issues, especially malnutrition. This is partly because we naturally tend to eat more around others and make better food choices. Often, seniors feel that cooking a larger, healthy meal for just one person is unnecessary and turn to pre-packaged foods instead. Plus, an overwhelming majority of the seniors in the study (around 85 percent) said that having someone to share their meals with makes mealtimes more satisfying. I feel that.

So, for our little ones, elder ones, and everyone in between, part of healing our health struggles is being more intentional about eating together more often. The dinner table can act as a unifier. Sharing a meal is the perfect opportunity to catch up, talk, and connect with those who matter most. It's cool that we have our hustle muscles flexing big time in our world today (we've got some work to do!), but it's also absolutely critical to decompress. And doing that along with good food can transform our reality.

YOU DON'T KNOW WHAT YOU DON'T KNOW

How on earth can I choose to eat healthier foods if I don't even know they exist? Today, millions of people are born into communities in the U.S. that have been inundated with substandard food, processed food, fast food, and eating practices that have proven to be flat-out deadly.

When I lived with my parents in some of the most impoverished neighborhoods in the inner city, all I saw around me was fast food and processed food. I literally had no idea there was any difference between real food and junk food. I just wanted to eat stuff that tasted good.

No one around me knew the difference between organic and conventional, grass-fed or factory-farmed, artificial flavors or natural flavors. We didn't know and barely cared, because sometimes food was scarce and we went hungry. I remember days of eating sugar sand-wiches while my mother hustled up a few bucks to help us make it to the next pay day. If she could beg, borrow, or steal to get $20 to feed our family for a couple of days, she's not going to spend it on an expensive organic chicken, potatoes, fresh greens, and seasonings. That would easily cost more than that $20 to feed all of us for just one meal! So, instead, we'd take that money to McDonald's and give everyone a burger and fries for under $10. We'd get a full belly of tasty food, with money to spare. It wasn't always about personal choice, it was about making ends meet in a community that didn't know of a better way. We didn't have CSAs to get fresh produce at affordable prices, we rarely had a parent available to cook a fresh meal, and most of the people in our community were already suffering from health issues related to their diet that depressed their energy and drive to make fresh food even when they had the chance. My mother was a great cook, but one of the things I heard her say repeatedly as I was growing up was, "I'm tired, Shawn, I'm just tired."

No matter how good your intentions might be, or how good of a person you might want to be, it's incredibly difficult to make better choices when you're just trying to survive. And it isn't just about the diet. Living in conditions with higher rates of crime (due to others' reduced capacity for empathy and ethics because they, too, are often struggling with their mental and physical health and trying to survive) can make it life-threatening just to walk down the street. As a result, there's less time spent outdoors in the fresh air and sunlight, there's less physical activity, and there's higher levels of stress from the dangers of the environment. It's a tremendous snowball effect that's often over-looked by those on the outside. This, in no way, takes away from personal responsibility. We all have choices to make that determine our destiny. But, when your options are limited and your environment is not conducive to basic personal health and safety, your ability to make changes is suffocated by the structure itself.

My mother had the best of intentions, but she lied, stole, and sold her blood many times to feed us. And someone might say, "Well, why didn't she just work hard?" She did. She worked her way up to being a manager at a convenience store, and on one of those days of hard work she was held up by an armed man with a knife and was stabbed several times. She fought back and fought for her life. After fending him off and making it to the hospital, the doctor later told her that her extra weight had saved her life. Not only did the dangers of the environment restrict her from taking healthy action in life psychologically, but also her weight became a defense from the world around her. And many other people have traumas that have become the catalyst for their unhealthy lifestyle choices. Again, many of us are born into conditions that foster the traumas. We have to address this as a sovereign community because it truly does affect us all. And each and every one of us has the power to do something about it.

IT'S A NUMBERS GAME

There are two things that don't lie. Hips don't lie (thanks, Shakira!) and numbers don't lie.

Today, there are disproportionately higher rates of chronic diseases in low-income areas in the United States. Hopefully, you're beginning to get a glimpse into how this snowball effect is taking place. There are a few more key insights to help make sense of it all and deliver some effective action. But first, let's take a look at the tale of the tape.

Currently in America:

- Approximately two out of three people are classified as being overweight.
- More than one in three people are clinically obese.
- Obesity is more prevalent in populations of minorities, with African-American and Hispanic citizens about one-and-a-half times more likely to become obese than white citizens.
- The U.S. Department of Health and Human Services Office of Minority Health (OMH) reports that African-American women have the highest rates of being overweight or obese compared with other racial or ethnic groups in the U.S.

- African-American women are 60 percent more likely to be obese than white American women.
- There are significantly higher rates of childhood obesity in minority communities.
- Type 2 diabetes and other diet-related illnesses are substantially higher in minority communities.
- Minorities are approximately two to four times more likely to die from complications related to diabetes.

These aren't just minority issues. These are people issues. As a society, we've had skyrocketing rates of obesity and chronic disease in recent decades. And our brothers and sisters, regardless of ethnicity, have felt the painful brunt of it.

The exciting news is that now, more than ever, people all over the country have been stepping up to do something about it. There is more education, better access to healthy food, and more litigation to protect our kids from detrimental food marketing. But, these improvements have not become pervasive in many of the communities that need them most. If I drive through my old neighborhood that I lived in during college, I still see the same layout of liquor stores and fast food restaurants nearly stacked on top of each other.

If I ever got tired of the McDonald's by my house that I was frequenting every week, I could simply cross the street and hit Jack in the Box for a slightly different tasting burger and menu items. I'm still surprised at myself because I'd go there all the time, even though the name of the place was *Jack in the Box*. A jack-in-the-box is a toy used to scare the crap out of someone. Which, appropriately, if you've ever eaten their Jumbo Jack and 2-for-99-cent tacos, digestively speaking, it will scare the crap out of you, too.

If that didn't suit me for the moment, just a few feet away was a Burger King, an Arby's, Lee's Chicken, and if I wanted a geometry lesson while eating a burger, I could go to Wendy's for a burger patty shaped into a square for no good reason at all. Keep in mind, these were all in walking distance from one another. Not to mention the

Taco Bell, pizza franchises, and convenience stores loaded to the hilt with candy, chips, and soda. My environment was shaping my choices, whether I knew it or not. There weren't any "health food stores." There wasn't an organic section of our local grocery store. And there wasn't a gym for miles and miles in either direction. I never saw one.

Living in this community is where my health ultimately collapsed. My dangerous and deficient diet led to the degeneration of my bones and the intervertebral discs in my spine. I crumbled under the weight of the environment as the food oppression around me rose higher and higher.

It took several years, but I was one of the very few that crawled, clawed, and scratched my way out of it. It wasn't because I was special. It was because I had exposure to another reality. Very early in life, I saw my grandmother make home-cooked meals. If only for a few years, I lived in an area that didn't have a liquor store and fast food restaurants on every corner. I saw what healthy relationships looked like. I saw the importance of education. I saw that, despite the fact that I was different from most of the other kids in that community, I mattered. That's all I needed. And that's what we all need.

Despite the most trying circumstances, human beings are able to rise above them and achieve the extraordinary. When I made that decision to turn my health around while living in an environment that was severely unhealthy, I turned to the internet, I turned to books, and (most important) I turned to people who could help. It was a friend from a chance encounter who first took me out of my environment and brought me to a health food store many miles away in another part of town. Again, *exposure*! It was one thing reading about this stuff on the internet. It was something even bigger to physically be around it.

Even though I was gaining access to new and better options, I still needed the money to take part in them. This is another troubling dimension of our current food system. It tends to only favor those who can afford it.

For many Americans, it doesn't matter if you want to improve your health and make better choices. Our socioeconomic structure is set up in such a way that poor quality, processed foods are made more affordable, while healthier foods are often priced at a premium. Even though heavily processed fast foods appear to be more costly to make, they're usually priced lower than most natural foods. For example, an organic avocado can easily cost you $3.00 in many grocery stores. But you can get *three* cheeseburgers for that same price at a McDonald's right now. So much goes into making that burger, from the procurement of the ingredients, to the labor, to the marketing. While an avocado literally falls off a tree. WTF?

Now, if you're like me, you might be thinking, "How in the world is that even possible?" Even though the cost to produce and sell their food is substantial, fast food companies are able to make their food so cheap and accessible that it's easy to say "Yes." If you're wondering how they're able to stay in business, let alone pull in a profit, it goes back to an economic principle called *elasticity of demand*. Basically, by making their food so cheap, fast food companies are able to elevate their demand and keep you buying more. Plus (and this is a big one), they make a lot of their money by cajoling you into buying accessory items. When's the last time you ordered just *one* item at a fast food place? When's the last time you bought a single burger without the fries? Buying a burger without the fries is like deleting the scene from *Jerry Maguire* when he says, "You complete me."

According to researchers at NYU, fast food economics relies on volume to work. They stated that a company "can increase its total revenue by lowering price if demand for the product is elastic (i.e., sensitive to price). For example, if the [company] lowers price 5 percent and quantity sold rises by 10 percent, then demand is elastic and total revenue will rise." Dealing in fast food is a numbers game. And they've got the numbers. But that's not the only way they win while communities suffer.

In an effort to show you the money (shout out to Jerry Maguire, again), we have to take a look at the amount of government assistance for these companies that's going on behind the scenes. From 1995 to 2010 alone, the U.S. government handed out $170 *billion* in agricultural subsidies to support the production of major commodity crops and farm foods that largely show up through the drive-thru window. And talk is cheap (like their "Value Menu"), so I prefer to show some real results of this activity. A recent study published in the peer-reviewed journal *JAMA Internal Medicine* set out to find if higher consumption of foods derived from government subsidized food commodities is associated with adverse risks to U.S. adults. The results were pretty shocking.

After adjusting for age, sex, socioeconomic factors, and other variables, the researchers found that those who had the highest consumption of subsidized foods had a *37 percent greater risk of being obese.* They were also significantly more likely to have excess belly fat, higher levels of blood sugar, and higher levels of inflammation (measured by elevated CRP). The government assistance programs for farmers may have started off with good intentions to feed U.S. citizens, but as the years have gone by, the funds doled out to farmers growing wheat, corn (used to make sweeteners and for cattle feed), and factory-farmed beef has dwarfed the amount of money going to farmers who grow fruits and vegetables. The results: Fruits and vegetables cost a helluva lot more, but you can ball out 'til you fall out on a fast food dollar menu.

Researchers at the Yale University School of Medicine chimed in on the disparaging circumstances many low-income communities face when it comes to finances and health. In a study cited in the journal *Diabetes Care,* the researchers asserted that fast food and processed food is widely available at low costs, enabling it to comprise a greater proportion of the diet of lower-income individuals. Their analysis revealed that being born into a low-income environment dramatically increased the risk of obesity which, in turn, increased the risk of staying in poverty.

So many people are trapped in this system. And it simply doesn't need to be this way. We have to stop blaming the victims who are born into this broken socioeconomic structure and create change as a society from the bottom up and from the top down.

For me to get out of the overwhelming financial and environmental pressure to eat poor-quality food, in many ways, I had to risk it all. I took chances on being able to hustle up the money to pay my electricity bill in order to buy higher quality food. In my personal situation, I became so enamored with the way that food could affect my body and mind that I went all in and bet on myself. Ultimately, by regaining my health and improving the epigenetic influences that we've talked about, I was able to have more energy, think more clearly, and feel good enough to pay it all forward by helping others. There were definitely some rough patches along the way, but shifting my priorities and investing in my health paid off mightily in the long run.

A risk like the one I took is one that most families simply can't take. But, from the bottom up, with information like what's in this book, each of us can be empowered to make some small improvements in our food choices, no matter where we are financially. When we know better, we do better. More people just need access to knowing how powerful they are to improve their health and the health of their families.

That being said, one of the biggest action steps in this book is to increase your level of exposure. And this goes in two directions:

1. No matter where you are right now, there are always people who are a little further behind that you can help. Help by giving other people exposure to healthier conditions. It could be a kid like me who simply needed to see what was possible to change their whole outlook on life. Participate in programs that provide field trips for inner city kids, community gardens, and healthier school lunch programs (better food is one of the most powerful forms of exposure because it changes you from the inside out!). Make it a mandate to share your time, talents, and/or resources to help uplift our communities. It's not going to be some nameless, faceless entity that solves this issue for us. *We* are the names and faces that will come together and make it happen. We're in this together, and we are powerful. If you need some help finding organizations and projects you can participate in, I have some options for you in the Eat Smarter Bonus Resource Guide at eatsmarterbook.com/bonus.

2. We're not just a product of our environment, we're also creators
    of our environment. Working to improve your own health and
    well-being is instantly up-leveled when you proactively get
    yourself around healthier people. Healthy habits are infectious,
    too. Your odds of making healthy decisions rise exponentially
    when you're around others who are making healthy decisions.

    If you're in an environment that creates constant conflict
    with making positive choices, it becomes exceedingly difficult
    to maintain a health-affirming lifestyle. This is just simple logic.
    But it plays out in the everyday lives of so many people. In my
    clinic, the #1 obstacle people complained about in improving
    their health was the people around them who seemed to make it
    more difficult. It was the people at the office...their friends...
    their parents...their kids...their significant other, etc. Here are
    some of the specific things I've heard people say:

    a. "My wife is always bringing unhealthy food into the house."
    b. "My husband isn't going to eat healthier foods, and I'm not
        going to make two meals, so I just eat what he eats."
    c. "My parents are set in their ways and aren't going to buy
        healthy food for us."
    d. "My kids won't eat it. So, I buy the easy foods they like
        (mac and cheese, chicken nuggets, hot dogs) and I just end
        up eating it along with them."
    e. They'd finish it off by saying something to the effect of, "I
        wish they'd change."

    Though all of the complaints about their social pressures
    are valid, many of us still have the opportunity to improve our
    social structures to promote health if we're truly driven to. In a
    conversation I had with bestselling author and multi-time fit-
    ness world champion Lori Harder, she shared how she dealt
    with the social pressures to eat unhealthy foods growing up.
    She, like me, came from a family struggling with obesity. She
    found that she had to remove herself more often to eat foods
    that were more health-affirming and avoid the fast food and

processed food free-for-alls that she was accustomed to. It was not easy to do so. She stressed how much she loved her family. But she also knew that if she was going to make long-term changes, she needed to change her environment.

For some of us, that might mean joining a gym and making friends and associates who are more into fitness. Have meals more often with friends or family members who live a healthy lifestyle (chances are, you're not going to plan a candlelight dinner together at KFC). Attend health- and fitness-inspired events (expos, workshops, and epic group workouts like the ones put on by my friend Shaun T). Join online health- and wellness-based groups to learn, be inspired, and engage in enlivening conversations about health and fitness (there's a great one at eatsmarter book.com/community). The most important aspect about participating in these things is that it builds more connective tissue that link you with a healthier lifestyle. And I'm not talking metaphorically, I'm talking about literal changes to your brain.

That exposure to healthier environments and activities literally changes the synaptic connections in your brain. And when you consistently place yourself in healthful circumstances, it lays down more myelin in your brain, making those healthy connections fire even stronger and more automatically.

As you change how your mind and body are working, you're better able to bring that influence and energy back with you to the environments that may need some attention. You become better equipped to effect change in your household. You become better equipped to deal with unhealthy social pressures (whether it's at work, with friends, or anywhere else). You're no longer carrying a you vs. them mentality. You don't need to convince anyone to help you make healthy decisions because you've gone from "doing" a healthy thing to "becoming" a healthy thing. It becomes who you are. And nothing can separate you from it, no matter where you go.

By getting yourself around more healthy people and conversations (in whatever ways you can!), you'll develop the
character traits that are needed to transform your personal
environment, whether it's developing more patience, more
self-awareness, more empathy and compassion, better communication skills, better planning and preparation skills (for
things like meal prep and buying/making tasty meals), more
perseverance, more fun, more objectivity, and even the ability
to detach yourself, if necessary. These are all traits that we have
the capacity to strengthen. Sometimes you may need to let go
of unhealthy environments and place yourself in new ones.
But the ultimate change is becoming a representation of a
healthy environment *yourself* and bringing it with you wherever you go.

Again, from the bottom up we can take personal responsibility and
proactively change our exposure. From the top down there are a number of changes we can help enforce by speaking up. You know who pays
for the government subsidies funding farming practices that contribute
to our processed food/fast food culture? You do. This is taxpayer money
being used to create oppression through food inequality. While it may
not have been the intention, it has become the outcome. It's our money,
and we can do something about it. These are conversations that need to
be had with your local and state representatives.

We need less bashing of each other, and more support for the health
of our communities. What comes out of politicians' mouths comes
from the issues that we demand attention to. Whenever you have the
opportunity, ask your representatives about policies to support healthy
eating, reduced processed food marketing to children, and food equality.

I don't want to just skip over this point about the aggressive processed food marketing to kids. Many countries have stronger regula-
tions on that behavior, while we still have a lot of progress to make
here at home. Research cited in the *Archives of Pediatrics and Adolescent
Medicine* affirmed that children who watch more television eat more of
the foods it advertises. The paper found that "each hour increase in

television viewing was associated with an additional 167 calories per day." And, not surprisingly, most of these extra calories were from heavily processed foods. The study also reported that the increased exposure to television advertisements led to a decrease in consumption of fruits and vegetables. The bottom line is that our relationship with television influences our diet more than we know. Let's get ourselves and our kids unglued from the TV more often. Play board games, talk, listen to music, podcasts, and audiobooks, work out together, cook together, read together, and create more real world memories. I'm not saying the Netflix and chill is out of order. We just need a little bit more chill time without the Netflix (whatever that may mean for you).

DOLLA DOLLA BILL Y'ALL

Another big way to support socioeconomic change is to support businesses that are doing the right things. You've probably heard the sentiment to vote with your dollar, but I want to take this to another level.

Public awareness of food quality has already been shifting the balance of power in major ways. For example, consumer awareness and demand for higher quality food has triggered consistent growth in accessibility of organic foods. In a food market that is relatively flat, sales for organic foods continue to outpace previous years. In fact, they now account for more than $21 billion in sales and are up nearly 9 percent in dollars and 8 percent in units sold. This is huge!

Clearly, our demand for better food is changing the way the market is moving and increasing the accessibility for so many of us. You may have noticed over the last few years how conventional grocery stores have expanded or created an organic section, and more restaurants are providing additional health-conscious offerings that include such labels as organic, free-range, local, and farm-to-table. They wouldn't do this (or be able to do this) if the demand wasn't high enough and they weren't making a profit. It's the way the markets work. The demand drives the accessibility.

Wherever it fits your budget, purchase foods that adhere to better standards. This might not always be possible, but when it is, casting that vote with your buck is adding another checkmark to the side that increases demand and lowers the price of real food.

Transforming our food system isn't going to happen overnight, but it will happen faster if we work with the food system instead of fighting against it. For instance, whether I like it or not, on any given day in the United States, an estimated 36.6 percent or approximately 84.8 million adults consume fast food, according to a recent report from the CDC. Whatever the reason to eat fast food might be — ease of access, low cost, busy and on-the-go, tastes good, etc. — changing the buying behavior of 85 million people daily to not go to their convenient fast food restaurant and instead travel (often further) to get wholesome food, spend more money, start doing food prep and pack their own lunch, or any other big change in behavior is a huge stretch. Instead, it might be a better idea to bring the improvements to them *where they are* to give more people accessibility to better choices.

I used to be against fast food restaurants adding healthier items to their menus. I felt like it was sort of like going to a drug dealer for a multivitamin. It's like, "What are you doing with this in your product line?"

Today, I see things a lot differently. With the deeply ingrained buying behavior of our society, and the expense associated with eating healthy, I feel that fast food can be a potential leverage point if used appropriately. The truth is, fast food restaurants speak with some of the loudest voices in our food culture today. If they start speaking the language of healthier options, higher-quality ingredients, and the elimination of dangerous additives, people who never have exposure to those ideas and options will now be able to see them. There are millions of people in challenging financial situations who want to be healthier, who want to lose weight, and who want to get out of pain. If they can, at least, get access to "Healthy Choice" menu items at the same low price when they go to their local fast food restaurants to feed themselves and their families, this radically increases the likelihood that they will, at minimum, give those foods a try. And if they taste good, that can seal the deal.

I used to believe that we shouldn't even patronize any fast food restaurants. Boycott them with our dollars by not showing up, and they'll eventually go out of business. It's simply not enough. For nearly 20 years, I've never stepped foot inside a fast food restaurant (except a few times when I had to pee really bad) and I vowed to inspire other people to do the same. But recently, a handful of thought-leading companies have stepped up to make more wholesome food, fast. They might not meet every standard that a militant health enthusiast might have, but several companies (making everything from burritos to burgers) have taken the initiative to improve the sourcing of their ingredients to include more fresh ingredients, organic ingredients, natural ingredients (largely omitting artificial flavors and sweeteners), local ingredients, pastured and grass-fed ingredients, and more. It's not about being perfect, it's about making progress.

I'm in no way, shape, or form recommending any of us to go to conventional fast food restaurants to buy healthier menu options if you have emancipated yourself from the fast food system. I'm recommending we work together through a comprehensive approach to improve the system (that 85 million people take part in every single day in the U.S.) to offer better options and eliminate ingredients that are blatantly doing the most harm. Fast food isn't going anywhere anytime soon. We just need to take measures to make the food they're selling better. Litigation to ban dangerous ingredients, food warning labels incorporating the updated science we have, improved transparency on nutrition facts, and (most important) folks spending money on healthier meal options at fast food restaurants will drive faster change. Passionate, vocal citizens have already circulated huge petitions and sparked legislation that's moved many of the most prominent fast food companies to eliminate some of the detrimental ingredients in their products. We've still got a ways to go, but it affirms that progress is possible. And progress is power!

Just to be clear, I'm not talking about when the market shift to eating low-fat foods inspired McDonald's to come out with the low-fat McLean burger back in the '90s. That was McNasty. And a poor attempt to pivot the buying behavior of their customers. There was less hamburger in the burger (I'll leave what they mixed into the ground beef as a filler up to your imagination) and it failed. I believe we don't want faker food. We want realer food. And it has to taste good.

These companies are fully capable of making something delicious using real food ingredients and eliminating synthetic chemicals. We just have to make our voices heard. As they lose business to companies that are making fast food more nutritious, and as we encourage our friends, family, coworkers, and ourselves to purchase the healthiest options available if we ever find ourselves in a conventional fast food pickle, that's how we effect change at yet another level.

A system-wide transformation takes time. But we're the ones endowed with the information, connectedness, and tenacity to do it.

Remember to proactively get yourself into health-affirming environments more often, help provide exposure for others in need of a healthy change, and vote intentionally with your dollars. These are all major keys to shifting the health of our communities and ourselves. But next up we're really catching fire by uncovering how food controls our ability to communicate and take action in the first place.

THE HUNGER GAMES

What we eat has a huge impact on how we feel, how we act, and how we relate to the world and people around us. Whether we're happy or in conflict, whether we're feeling united or struggling to connect, our nutrition is influencing how we show up in more ways than we realize.

Eating smarter isn't just about preventing illness and reducing body fat, it's also about getting in tune with our bodies so that we can be more in tune with each other. Nutrient deficiencies and abnormal fluctuations in your blood sugar can take you from being cool as a cucumber to hot as a habanero. And, oftentimes, we don't even know it's happening.

When our blood sugar is too low, the human body naturally responds by releasing the stress hormones cortisol and adrenaline to raise it back up. But the catch is that those hormones can also lead to strong irritability. A deficiency in our nutrition inherently leads to changes in our neurotransmitters, hormones, and profound changes in our brains. Put that together with a person or situation that might rub you the wrong way, and you've got a recipe for an overreaction omelet, an annoyed-as-hell aioli, or a double-decker shade sandwich that you're willing to throw at anyone.

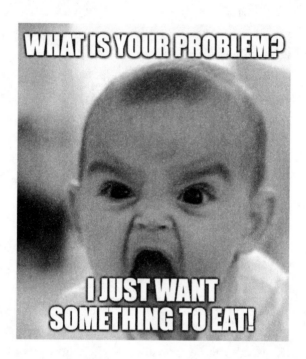

As noted in the introduction, a recent study from the Ohio State University on married couples found that the lower the participants' blood sugar level, the angrier and more aggressive they felt toward their partners. Even our perception of the people we love can be skewed when our bodies are not in balance. We often don't realize it, or can't seem to control it, because the more primitive parts of the brain can start to take over. The parts of your brain responsible for social control, for distinguishing between right and wrong, for perspective-taking (putting yourself in "someone else's shoes") and other executive functions can get hijacked by a part of your brain known as the *amygdala*.

The amygdala works to modulate all of our reactions to events that are deemed important for our survival. It's an absolutely critical structure because it aids in our ability to feel certain emotions. But the one emotion the amygdala is most keen on is *fear*. If you've ever been in a truly threatening situation where your senses are heightened, your heart is pounding, and you may need to fight or flee for your life, you can thank your amygdala for jumping in to take control. The amygdala is primarily concerned about survival of self, which is great when you actually need it. But in our basic day-to-day interactions, an amygdala hijack can take your relationships right to the chop shop.

Research published in the journal *Frontiers in Endocrinology* revealed that dramatic changes in blood sugar (shifting from a high blood sugar spike to an impending crash) can increase anxiety and trigger hyperactivity in the amygdala. An additional study reported that the increased activity in the amygdala reduced memory recall, lowered inhibitory control (the ability to delay or prevent acting on impulses), and increased psychological distress.

Nutrient deficiencies and abnormal blood sugar can put your brain on red alert. As crazy as it sounds, it's a fear for survival that can get projected out to the people and circumstances around you. Even if you love someone, it can seem like it's you versus them in a battle to see who will come out as the victor. But the reality is, Victor's Village can be a lonely place when you do and say things that you don't really mean. It really wasn't the best version of you who did and said those things. It was your *hangry* (hungry + angry) alter ego...and it can be a bit of a monster.

Knowing that food is a major controller of our mood, the wrong diet or poor management of our body's energy needs can lead to the appearance of your hangry representative. I believe we generally fall into one of these five categories on this all-star team of monsters.

What kind of hangry monster do you usually turn into?

Dracula—Creeping in the night...that's when your cravings start. You may be likely to say seductive things to others to get the food or drinks you want. You may also resort to biting if invoked.

Invisible Man/Woman—when you're hangry, you want to hide away and not be bothered with other people.

Werewolf—You're totally normal most of the time. But every-so-often when hanger strikes, you can run off the rails, snap, and even bark at people.

Frankenstein—when you're hangry, you find yourself mindlessly pulled to crappy food. You're not trying to hurt anybody, you just want to eat and be left alone by the townspeople. But you will step on someone if they get in the way.

Mummy—when you're hangry, you really get unraveled…you don't hold it together very well at all. You get a dusty attitude and you're not very fun to be around.

I'd have to say that my hangry personality would definitely fall under the werewolf category, while my wife is more of a Dracula-type. If you've ever seen any movies where vampires and werewolves share the screen, it usually isn't pretty. It took us years to home in on our hangry personalities and to learn how to keep ourselves from changing (and to lovingly support the other person during a metaphorical full moon or when the fangs come out). Being well-nourished intrinsically increases our capacity to have patience, positive rapport, impulse control, and the ability to see from the other person's point of view. These things are dramatically reduced when we're undernourished, and this can play out in acute situations or chronic problems that we need to become more educated about.

So, the next time you find yourself in conflict, grab your attention back from wanting to bite the other person for just a second, and do a quick internal check-in. Ask yourself, "Am I hungry?" "Am I dehydrated?" "Am I tired?" "Have I nourished myself today?" If you're lacking in any of these departments, it can pull the fire alarm in your amygdala and make your higher order brain functions run straight out of the building.

This is not easy to do when you're feeling irritated or attacked and the hangry monster is peeking its head out of its hole. But you are fully capable of doing it. It takes practice and a level of self-honesty, but over time, you'll be able to say, "I'm sorry, I'm just really tired" or "I love you, I just really need to eat something so I feel more like myself." You'll find that you spend a lot less time in conflict and more time enjoying your relationships. The bigger goal is to proactively ensure we're nourished using the information in this book, but everyone can get a little hangry from time to time. The bigger issue is when poor health and malnutrition becomes chronic. That's when the wheels can really fall off.

Nutritional Peacekeepers

Understanding that our nutrition affects our behavior, it should come as no surprise that violent behavior is also heavily linked to malnutrition. Yet, our society isn't talking about this enough. A study conducted by researchers at Oxford University set out to find if providing more essential nutrients to young, male prison inmates would have an effect on violent behavior and misconduct. They completed a double-blind, randomized trial that provided one group of inmates a multivitamin and essential fatty acid supplement, while another group only received a placebo. Here's what they found...

The average length of supplementation was approximately 4½ months and, during that time period, the disciplinary offenses enacted by the young men receiving additional nutritional support dropped by 35 percent! This was nearly a 30 percent lower drop in offenses than the placebo group. And what was especially eye-opening was that violent incidents in the inmates receiving nutritional support dropped by 37 percent. These are remarkable findings. And the results have been replicated in several other studies.

Another study published in the peer-reviewed journal *Aggressive Behavior* tested the cognitive, personality, and behavioral changes that providing additional vitamins, minerals, and essential fatty acids to prison inmates could have. Over 200 young men participated in the study, with some participants receiving additional nutritional support and some receiving a placebo. At the end of the study, the numbers of violent incidents in the group receiving nutritional support dropped by a startling 34 percent (substantially more than those receiving the placebo). But what was most interesting about the study was that there were no significant differences in any of the cognitive, personality, and behavioral testing measures used, just the actual incidents. On paper, it looked like the inmates were the same people, even though their behavior changed. Which means the cognitive measures aren't comprehensive enough, or the effect of better nutrition is just too subtle to understand right now.

The bottom line is, most people don't need to know what improved nutrition looks like on paper. What matters is the decreased number of incidents and the lives of the people who could be saved or improved by not being exposed to or participating in those violent events. Again, human behavior is very dynamic and influenced by many things. But we can no longer overlook the profound impact that food has on the way we feel, think, and act.

The lead scientist in the first study stated, "Having a bad diet is now a better predictor of future violence than past violent behavior. Likewise, a diagnosis of psychopathy, generally perceived as being a better predictor than a criminal past, is still miles behind what you can predict just from looking at what a person eats."

Food affects our minds and bodies more than we may realize. I know from firsthand experience in working with thousands of people (and seeing it play out in the data) that oftentimes, people don't do well because they don't feel well. It's very difficult to express compassion and understanding for another human being when we're physically unhealthy and suffering inside. As a society, it would benefit us all if we work to ensure that misconduct-prone citizens, along with those in a position to protect others and police the misconduct, are better taken care of.

I don't think most people recognize the amount of psychological stress citizens living in communities disposed to crime and citizens who participate in law enforcement are under. Swinging to the other side of the pendulum in the criminal justice system, a recent report conducted by researchers at the National Institute for Occupational Safety and Health uncovered that police officers have one of the poorest cardiovascular disease profiles of any occupation. They're nearly four times more likely to be sleep deprived than the general population, a higher percentage of officers are obese than in other occupations, and the percentage of officers with depression is nearly double that of other fields of employment.

Again, we're dealing with a systemic problem that overlooks the actual humans involved in it. According to award-winning psychiatrist and addiction specialist Dr. Indra Cidambi, "Police officers are often in the midst of other people's crises—fights, domestic violence, shootings, bloody crime scenes, and fatal car accidents, which, sometimes, puts their own lives at risk. (Officers) face high-stress situations several times a week, especially in urban areas. They are charged with making instant decisions in these immediate situations." She continued, "In addition, police officers' schedules can be grueling, often working rotating and overtime shifts. As a result, officers can often be fighting fatigue and lack of sleep, which can impair hand-eye coordination and reaction times. These untraditional work schedules can often deprive officers of time with their families."

High stress, lack of sleep, lack of family connection time, and challenging health issues have been breaking down another vital demographic of people in our society. As a result, there are strikingly high levels of substance abuse among officers today (at two to three times higher than the rest of the general population) and police officers rank near the top of all occupations in suicide (with more officers dying from suicide than from shootings and traffic accidents combined). Why are we not talking about this?

This is one of the fields of work that needs the most socioemotional training, the most rest and recovery, the most mental and physical health support, and the most support for stress management, yet the system has let them down. It's a literal badge of honor to work yourself into exhaustion and breakdown. And the acknowledgment doesn't come, often, until it's too late.

I'm advocating for more mental and physical health support across *all* occupations. Especially for occupations where the lives of so many others can be on the line, like medical care, firefighters, and law enforcement, we, as a nation, need to take better care of the people who are entrusted with supporting and caring for us.

Reports published in *The American Journal of Clinical Nutrition* and *Case Reports in Psychiatry* affirm that malnutrition and the consumption of high-glycemic foods are a noted risk factor for depression, anxiety, and abnormal mental and emotional states. When we have citizens who are malnourished, sleep deprived, and suspected of engaging in crime, interacting with law enforcement officers who are malnourished, sleep-deprived, and pressed with the responsibility of policing crime, do you think the likelihood of violence goes up or down? It's simple logic what the outcomes will tend toward, and the data affirms this. Yes, we have the ability to express coherence, understanding, problem-solving, and empathy for others when we're not in a good physical and mental state of health. It's just harder. And all of us together have the power to change this.

We have to make sure that we're well-nourished as a basic premise for how we interact with each other...especially if we're entrusted to protect and serve; especially if we work with others; especially if we're human, period. It doesn't matter if you're a good person, it doesn't matter if you have the best of intentions: When you're malnourished and sleep deprived, the best version of yourself is no longer present.

Reaping Better Results

Looking at things from the top down earlier in this chapter, we talked about how money talks when it comes to making change in our food culture, particularly when it comes to uplifting low-income communities. Money talks when it comes to supporting our public service employees as well. Unfortunately, even though chronic disease rates are higher in some domains of public service, while poor mental health and suicide rates are higher in others, unless the systems behind them all are making money, it can be very difficult to change them. Most people are shocked to hear that physicians also have one of the highest suicide rates of any profession. Often tasked with life-saving or life-altering responsibilities, the medical system has ill-prepared and even encouraged dysfunction among its own members. Research from the American Psychiatric Association purported that "doctors who die by suicide often have untreated or undertreated depression or other mental illnesses." And researchers at Columbia University and the Irving Medical Center attest that the data is "alarming" but not surprising, given the amount of stress that doctors face systemically.

It's like a rite of passage to have medical students subjected to rampant physical and mental distress for months or even years at a time. The stress starts in medical school and continues in residency with high demands, long hours, insufficient nutrition, and lack of sleep. With the changing landscape of education, many universities are finally incorporating more training in nutrition and stress management. That's a good thing. But we clearly need to see more training in self-care, personal management, and (though it might sound strange) we need more training in business in the field of medicine. One of the major reasons that physicians are so stressed is that many tend to be forced to work in volume (like fast food) in order to meet costs. Plus, even the physicians who decide to work in large health care systems still need to develop skills in leadership, teamwork, and data analytics. Lacking in these key areas adds to a tremendous amount of stress. Better education in business (whether it's through traditional school or resources like books and podcasts) can lead to more quality time and care for patients, healthier, more efficient systems for physicians, and less stress for everyone.

Knowing that big business systems are reluctant to change unless money's involved, some interesting research was done recently including police officers and firefighters in the city of Reno, Nevada. After doctors analyzed the troubling blood work of these public servants, a comprehensive plan was put together to become the basis of a small pilot study.

For two years, the officers and firefighters were supported in following a reduced-sugar, low-carbohydrate diet and received counseling on how to improve sleep and reduce stress. The improvements in their biomarkers were so pronounced, it was estimated that the pilot program alone saved the city of Reno $22 million in healthcare costs and associated expenses! Again, money talks. And if prevention can save municipalities, cities, and states this much money, it makes it much more attractive for organizational decision makers to put health-supportive programs into practice.

Simultaneously, there is also a wave of people in numerous professions who are taking it upon themselves to take control of their health and well-being. A friend of mine who has been a Chicago city police officer for several decades shared with me how he had to create his own success routines and frequently remove himself from social situations in order to take care of his health and well-being. As a result of him staying true to his goals and leading by example, he has inspired countless other police officers to up-level their health as well. After 22 years on the police force, Jemal King has recently retired to travel the country and speak on personal development and financial wellness for the folks that need it most.

No matter what field you or your loved ones work in, there's always an intersection between health and wellness and how it influences the work that we do. We need systemic change, but we can also be the change. And moving in both directions is how we become unstoppable.

THE LANGUAGE OF LOVE

Food is so much more than the stuff we eat. As you've seen, food is a major influence on the function of our metabolism, the health of our brain, our mental and emotional well-being, and the way we communicate. And, in some aspects, food is actually *how* we communicate.

In the preface to *Eat Smarter,* I noted a connection to the bestselling book from Dr. Gary Chapman called *The 5 Love Languages.* In the book, Dr. Chapman acknowledges that we all communicate and receive love through five basic methods: Acts of Service, Giving/Receiving Gifts, Quality Time, Words of Affirmation, and Physical Touch. Though our love languages might be different from person to person, understanding and effectively speaking your own love language, along with understanding the love languages of others, is a huge key to health and happiness that's enjoyed by millions of people practicing these principles.

Let's take a look at how food speaks a language of love that can bring us all closer together and make us healthier and happier, one bite at a time.

Acts of Service — The day after my wife gave birth to our youngest son, Braden, my mom-in-law prepared a bunch of delicious food and brought it over to our house. She wanted to make sure that my wife was getting plenty of nutrition to help feed the baby (hello, mama milk factory!), to help support her recovery, and to just ease her mind by having one less thing to do.

That food was an incredible act of service that communicated love and elevated our household. Think about any of your friends, family members, or coworkers who may be going through a challenging time, exceptionally busy, or could just use a night off. Send them a message and let them know that you've got the food covered. Purchase or prepare them a meal (or a day of meals) of tasty, health-giving food to let them know that they matter.

Giving/Receiving Gifts—Many times, after I return home from travel for speaking events, media, etc., my mom-in-law would pick me up at the airport and she'd have an incredible meal prepared, plus a little dish that was just for me. I've said it several times, but I don't think she knows how much of a gift that was to me. After being on the road, likely eating at several restaurants (usually really awesome ones), there's nothing like coming back to food made by someone who really loves you.

Make a short list of your closest friends and/or family members (two to four people is plenty) and schedule a time to send each one of them a gift of deliciousness this month. Maybe you can send your best friend a box of her favorite energy bars, or send your mom a gift certificate to her favorite restaurant, or send your health fanatic brother a supply of healthy meals from his favorite meal prep company. Keep in mind, you don't need a lot of moola to do this. Homemade meals and treats can be the perfect gift to make someone's day.

Quality Time—Food is a centerpiece of holidays, celebrations, meetings, dating, sporting events, quality family time, and so much more. We bond through food. Food literally brings people together.

One of my favorite things in life is to sit around the table with my family to eat, laugh, and (for some reason) experience a post-dinner dance battle (true story: it's happened at least 100 times). Another awesome experience has been going over to my mom-in-law's for the holidays to get our grub on and spend quality time together. It's been so special for me to have that in my life since my grandparents passed away. I really didn't even know how much I missed that experience of having that consistent holiday hub until I met my wife and got my bonus family.

Another aspect of speaking the love language of quality time through food is cooking together. Making food together takes us back to a time when we used to do more stuff together as a family. Like back when we all used to go to Blockbuster video and hunt for movies together. This wasn't social media scrolling, it was real-life scrolling! And it was a battle for video victory. Standing by the door at the return box, asking the annoyed clerk if they've got the movie you want...ah, the thrill of the hunt!

We need to take making food together, and (especially) teaching our kids how to cook, off of the endangered species list of things to do together. If we're not teaching our kids how to cook, we're putting them at a huge disadvantage as they get older. I know there have been many times when my kids have asked to help cook and (because I was in a hurry, tired, or didn't feel like being a kinder, gentler Gordon Ramsey) I'd say, "Not right now. Next time." Well, I realized that "next time" typically turns into more next times. So, now, whenever they ask I always say, "YES." In fact, I ask for help just to get them in the kitchen with me.

Cooking and eating together is a powerful expression of love. As we demonstrated in the research earlier in this chapter, it's an excellent idea to sit down with your family at least three times each week for a meal together. An additional mission is to schedule a meal with extended family or friends once a month as well. And, remember, quality can be a lot more meaningful than quantity. So, get your phones away from the table, shut the boob tube off, and be completely present with the ones you love.

Words of Affirmation—From my little brother, to my wife, to my mom-in-law, I've seen how they put love into their cooking...

and I've seen how much it means to them when you let them know how much you enjoyed the meal. Especially for those who put a lot of intention into their food and love to feed people, sharing words of affirmation with the cook can put them on cloud nine.

Let the cook know how much you appreciate them. Tell friends, family, and even the chef at the restaurant (if you have the chance) how much you enjoyed their cooking. Sprinkle on the gratitude abundantly and often. Food is love made edible, and affirmative words say "I love you, too."

Physical Touch—Nothing touches us more deeply than food does. Our food becomes the muscles and bones that enable us to have movement, it becomes the cells in our brains that allow us to have thought, and it becomes the hormones and neurotransmitters that support us in having feeling and emotion. The food we eat truly makes us who we are!

It's such an intimate experience if you really think about it. When we eat food, we are choosing to take something from the outside world, put it inside of our bodies, and make it a part of us. What we eat touches our taste buds, but it also reaches out and hugs our hearts (literally!). This is the reason food is really the international language of love. And we can utilize that love to heal ourselves and the people around us.

Many years ago, the food my mom-in-law cooked for me made me feel welcome. Eventually, my new experiences with healthy foods enabled me to broaden my horizons and cultivate new ideas. And, ultimately, the gift of food in my life enabled me to touch the lives of millions of people.

Speak the languages of love by sharing the gift of good food with yourself and others. And always remember the power that food has to transform our hearts and minds!

In fostering healthy communication, healthy families, and healthy communities, what we eat is a critical component that's been overlooked long enough. Hopefully, this chapter has sparked some ideas and actions to help you better connect with the ones you love. We can all do our part on an individual scale, but we can also shift the tide of health and wellness in our society by coming together as a collective. We can usher in more peace, more compassion, and more cooperation by encouraging some of the systemic changes that we've discussed.

Food affects every area of our lives, and next up you're going to discover how to eat to enhance your energy, increase your longevity, and radically improve your brain health by improving your sleep. It's time to snack for some better zzz's, so let's dive into the next chapter!

CHAPTER EIGHT

Edible Sleep

I want to be like a caterpillar. Eat a lot, sleep for a while, and then wake up beautiful.

~*Anonymous*

If you've ever seen the movie *The Matrix,* you know that the main character, Neo, is able to be plugged into the Matrix to tap into accelerated learning, increased immunity against outside attacks, and seemingly superhuman powers. Believe it or not, sleep is the closest thing we have to jacking ourselves into the Matrix in the real world. It can make you smarter, protect you from things that might try to take you down, and basically make you better at *everything*. Let me show you how.

Each and every day, during our waking moments, we are constantly taking in bits of data from the outside world. The information we take in is used to create what we refer to as "memories." These memories help to fortify a broad range of experiences in our lives, from building healthy connections with the ones we love, to learning what to do in order to avoid pain, to strategizing the right actions to take to be successful in school and in our careers. Memories are vital to our progress as humans. And your memories are critically dependent upon the quality of your sleep.

A recent study published in the journal *Psychological Reviews* explains that the waking brain is optimized for the collection and encoding of memories, but the sleeping brain is optimized for the actual consolidation of those memories. Both rapid eye movement (REM) sleep and deep sleep play essential roles in taking what you learn while you're awake and consolidating it into your short-term and long-term memories. Basically, sleep enables you to take what you want to learn and make it 1) easier to recall and 2) more capable of applying it to what you want.

Another study cited in *PLOS ONE* reported that sleep has been most clearly shown to enhance *procedural memory* (i.e., skills and procedures) and *declarative memory* (i.e., recall of facts). To identify the impact sleep has on declarative memory, for example, researchers split a group of test subjects into two groups: Group one was given a declarative memory task at 9 a.m. and then tested for recall at 9 p.m. (12 hours later without any sleep)—while group 2 was given the declarative memory task at 9 p.m. then allowed to get a full night's sleep and tested at 9 a.m. the next morning. Even though it was an equal 12-hour time interval between learning and testing, the group that was allowed to sleep had a 20.6 percent greater increase in declarative memory! Sleep enabled them to retain more information and recall it when they needed to. But sleep doesn't just improve the memory capacity for your brain cells, it improves the memory capacity of your immune system, too.

Immunological memory is the ability of the immune system to quickly and specifically recognize a pathogen that the body has previously encountered and initiate a corresponding immune response. You *do not* want your immune system to be slow to remember things. And sleep is a huge key to taking your immune system from *Finding Dory* to *Searching for Bobby Fischer*. Research published by *Cell Press* revealed that the ability of our immune system to "remember" an encounter with a bacteria or virus is influenced by our quality of sleep. Specifically, slow-wave, deep sleep appears to improve the memory of T cells, while there's additional evidence showing that hormones released during sleep improve the cross talk between the cells that recognize foreign invaders and the cells that are sent to take them out.

In addition to preventing infectious disease, sleep helps to fortify your body's defense against chronic diseases like heart disease, diabetes, and more. A 14-year study reported by the World Health Organization found that poor sleep quality can double the risk of a heart attack, while scientists at the University of Chicago reported that even short-term sleep deprivation can increase insulin resistance.

What's most exciting (and alarming at the same time) in regard to the major role that sleep plays on our health is echoed in research cited in the journal *Current Neurology and Neuroscience Reports.* The study affirms that your sleep quality is a major regulator in the function of your DNA. Your genetic expression (determining everything from the health of your skin, to your body composition, to your ability to prevent chronic disease) is heavily influenced by your sleep quality. Getting your sleep wrong can have catastrophic consequences, but getting your sleep right can positively transform every area of your life.

This is just a small sample platter of how sleep deeply impacts the function of your mind and body. There's a full buffet on this and more, as well as 21 clinically proven strategies to improve your sleep quality, in my bestselling book *Sleep Smarter* if you're hungry for more on the subject. For now, let's chow down on one of the *biggest* entrées that controls your sleep quality: YOUR FOOD.

SLEEP'S LITTLE HELPERS

To understand how what we eat has such a profound impact on how we sleep, we have to take a look at what's happening where the food is digested, assimilated, and eliminated. You've already learned some game-changing insights on how your microbiome influences your metabolism back in Section One. Your gut bacteria help determine the amount of calories you absorb from your food and how quickly and efficiently caloric fuel gets burned, as well as modulating other factors like inflammation and hormone function. But that's just a few of the presents they deliver.

Your tiny gut bacteria also play a titanic role in regulating your sleep cycles. A recent report published in the journal *Sleep Medicine* uncovered that negative changes to your microbiome can have substantial detrimental effects on the quality of your sleep. What's more, the researchers discovered that, concurrently, poor-quality sleep can also have detrimental effects on your microbiome. Their report demonstrated that as the microbiome is negatively altered, and sleep quality is reduced, there's a direct reduction in our ability to switch between different mental tasks (something called *cognitive flexibility*). Clearly, when it comes to sleep and supporting our cognitive function, taking care of microbiome is of the utmost importance.

One of the major reasons that our gut health has such a profound impact on our sleep is due to the sleep-related hormones and neurotransmitters that are produced and/or stored in the gut. Take serotonin, for example. Serotonin is well-noted to promote positive mental and emotional health, while low levels of serotonin are associated with anxiety and depression. On top of that, serotonin also plays a major part in sexual function, bone health, regulating the movement of your digestive system, and sleep quality.

A 2007 report found that low levels of serotonin can contribute to insomnia. Serotonin is a potent neurotransmitter with many jobs, and even though it's often associated with things happening in our brains, the vast majority of serotonin is actually located in our gut!

Approximately *90 percent* of the human body's total serotonin is located in the gastrointestinal tract. And scientists at the California Institute of Technology (Caltech) reported that there are specific bacteria that interact with the cells in the gut that produce and secrete serotonin for us. These cells (called *enterochromaffin cells*) are interacting with your bacteria cells all of the time, and if the north pole of your microbiome goes south, the only thing coming down your chimney will be a big box of sleep problems.

Not only does serotonin improve sleep on its own accord, one of the most important things your body does with serotonin is use it to make your #1 sleep-regulating hormone, melatonin. Yes, melatonin is glorified as a "sleep hormone," but it's really so much more than that. It's involved in regulating your body's circadian timing system (influencing when various hormones are released throughout the day and night, mental energy, digestive function, etc.), as well as regulating blood pressure, body temperature, cortisol levels, antioxidant defenses, and immune function. Saying melatonin is just a sleep hormone is like saying Michael Jordan is just good at putting a ball into a circle.

When I was in college, I was taught that melatonin is produced via the pineal gland in the brain, end of story. Today, we know that melatonin is also synthesized in other cells outside of the pineal cells, such as bone marrow cells, lymphocytes, and, most remarkably, cells in the gut. Scientists have uncovered that, although some pineal-derived melatonin has been seen in the gut, the primary source of melatonin is being produced by the enteroendocrine cells in the gastrointestinal tract mucosa. In fact, a study published in the *World Journal of Gastroenterology* revealed that the human digestive tract could contain more than 400 times more melatonin than the pineal gland at any given time! This may come as a surprise because, again, we often relate sleep to being a "head thing." But sleep is a powerful event orchestrated by your entire body, and if the bacteria in your gut decide to catch a Bobby Brown attitude and get out of sync with the rest of the system, getting good sleep at night will no longer be your prerogative.

A new study cited in *Frontiers in Psychiatry* purports that our microbiome helps regulate our sleep and mental state through the action of the microbiome-gut-brain axis. Your microbiome is at the very root of your sleep wellness, and, referring back to Section One again, the health of our microbiome is largely controlled by the food that we eat. We want to consistently provide the right fuel (prebiotics, resistant starch, polyphenols, etc.) that help keep our ratio of friendly flora robust and healthy. We all have a small percentage of what we would consider "unfriendly flora" or "opportunistic bacteria." But even they have important roles to play in things like digestion and immune system function. The real problems arise, however, when the ratio of friendly bacteria to unfriendly bacteria gets skewed and the bad bugs start taking over—i.e., gut dysbiosis.

In order to protect your microbiome to support your sleep, it's not just what you consume, but also what you avoid consuming. Here are a few things to be mindful to limit your exposure to, if at all possible.

Peer-reviewed studies have shown that each of these can have detrimental effects on your gut bacteria:

- Agricultural chemicals (pesticides, fungicides, herbicides, etc.)
- Processed foods (excessive sugars are shown to feed pathogenic bacteria)
- Artificial sweeteners
- Haphazard or repeated antibiotic use
- Lack of movement and exercise
- High levels of stress
- Chemical food additives and preservatives
- Chlorinated water (Chlorine is a known antibiotic—though it's an excellent cleaner, even in small amounts it can damage your bacteria cascade; it's best to get yourself a water filter that removes chlorine if your municipality uses it.)
- Sleep deprivation

Ironically, your microbiome helps regulate your sleep, but your sleep also helps regulate your microbiome. Research reported in the journal *Cell* tracked microbial changes of study participants after altering their sleep schedule via a ten-hour flight spanning multiple time zones. This simple, acute change in sleep schedule increased the test subjects' ratio of "fat bacteria" known to be more prevalent in people with obesity and diabetes. Then, once the travelers got back on a regular sleep cycle, their levels of these microbes dropped back to normal again.

Clearly, supporting your gut buddies is critically important to your sleep wellness. We want to incorporate prebiotic and probiotic-rich foods like we covered in-depth in Chapter Three, as well as do our best to avoid the things that blatantly damage our microbiome. These simple actions will help to keep your friendly flora in good health *and* prevent your unfriendly bacteria from krump dancing all over the place and messing up your sleep.

To take this one more edible step further, there are specific nutrients that act as precursors to sleep-related neurotransmitters, hormones, and processes that we want to be sure that we get plenty of in our diets. Next up, let's cover some of the most important good-sleep nutrients and some of the best foods to find them in.

GOOD SLEEP NUTRIENTS

Even if you've got the best nighttime routine in the world, a simple nutrient deficiency can seriously foul up your sleep game. Here are some of the most valuable and well-studied sleep-supportive nutrients to target every day.

Tryptophan

As one of the nine essential amino acids that we *must* obtain from our diet, tryptophan stands out as a key building block for better sleep. A tryptophan deficiency has been found to create disruptions in REM sleep, while improving tryptophan levels has been shown to reduce wakefulness at night and increase mental alertness after waking up in the morning, according to research cited in the journal *Nutrients*.

As you'll recall, serotonin is a key building block of melatonin. Well, tryptophan is a key building block of serotonin! Your body needs tryptophan in copious amounts. Some of the best sources of tryptophan include chicken, turkey, lobster, eggs, cheese, tofu, chocolate, spinach, pumpkin seeds, peanuts, and spirulina.

Vitamin B6

Also known as *pyridoxine,* vitamin B6 is a critical cofactor in the tryptophan-serotonin pathway. Coming into the game in its short-shorts and unsuspecting demeanor, vitamin B6 plays the role of John Stockton making the big assist in the production of both serotonin and melatonin.

When your system is jazzed up, this essential vitamin helps to modulate your body's stress response and relax your nervous system. Some of the best sources of vitamin B6 are yogurt, salmon, tuna, eggs, chicken liver, chickpeas, spinach, sweet potato, and avocado.

Glycine

Another amino acid that's been found to be particularly supportive of sleep is glycine. A study reported in *Neuropsychopharmacology* revealed that glycine appears to improve deep sleep time and reduce wake after sleep onset (meaning you wake up less often). Excellent sources of glycine include beef, chicken, turkey, salmon, peanuts, quinoa, spirulina, and Brazil nuts; one of the most remarkable sources is bone broth. In addition, the collagen contained in bone broth has been found to help support thermoregulation to lower the body's core temperature at night and improve sleep cycles. Try sipping on a cup of hot bone broth about an hour before bed as part of your wind-down ritual.

Vitamin C

Data cited in the journals *Appetite* and *PLOS ONE* demonstrated that insufficient intake of vitamin C increases the likelihood of sleep disturbances and shortens the duration of overall sleep time. Moreover, a 2009 study showed that a combination of vitamin C (100 milligrams) and vitamin E (400 IU) taken twice daily, in addition to continuous positive airway pressure (CPAP) administration, significantly reduced episodes of apnea. The inclusion of vitamins C and E also improved sleep quality and decreased daytime sleepiness.

Excellent sources of vitamin C include "superfoods" like camu camu berries, amla berries, and acerola cherries, as well as more everyday foods like bell peppers, green leafy vegetables, broccoli, kiwifruit, strawberries, citrus fruits, and papaya.

Vitamin D

This fat-soluble vitamin has one of the most fascinating relationships with sleep. It's well documented that sunlight exposure helps to fortify our levels of vitamin D. And although it could be considered a "daytime" hormone, a recent study published in the *Journal of Biological*

Rhythms determined that vitamin D is able to modulate the expression of and synchronize genes involved in our circadian rhythm.

We've already established that the circadian timing system helps to regulate the release of hormones during the day *and* night. Our circadian clock determines which hormones get released, how much gets released, and at what time they get released. Vitamin D appears to be a major part of the nutrient team ensuring that body clock keeps time accurately, which enables you to get good sleep at night and have great energy during the day.

An additional study in the *Journal of Clinical Sleep Medicine* found that getting your vitamin D levels up can help to reduce daytime sleepiness. Salmon, sardines, cod liver oil, oysters, shrimp, egg yolks, and culinary mushrooms are all great sources of food-based vitamin D. But, remember, an important way to make sure your vitamin D levels stay up to par is getting an ample amount of safe sun exposure.

Potassium

A study cited in the journal *Sleep* found that potassium can help improve sleep efficiency (meaning you go through your sleep cycles correctly) and reduce wake after sleep onset. Bananas are often touted as the best source of potassium, but there are far better sources (especially if you want to avoid the excess sugar). Avocados, green leafy vegetables, sweet potatoes, sea veggies (especially dulse), coconut water, black beans, white beans, yogurt, mackerel, and salmon are all exceptional sources of potassium.

Calcium

Calcium and bone health are synonymous with each other, but if you're deficient in calcium, your sleep can get fractured, too. A peer-reviewed study in *Current Signal Transduction Therapy* demonstrated that a calcium deficiency can cause disruptions in your REM sleep, and deep sleep as well. You can find great sources of calcium in sesame seeds, chia seeds, almonds, yogurt, cheese, beans, lentils, sardines, collard greens, kale, and spinach.

> ## Under the Weather?
>
> Getting a good night of sleep is one of the most effective treatments for things like colds and flus. But, unfortunately, sometimes being under the weather can cause problems with getting good rest. If you need a little assistance to sleep better when you're dealing with symptoms like a grody cough, look no further than your favorite beekeeper. A randomized, double-blind, placebo controlled study revealed that honey was able to outperform a placebo and significantly reduce cough frequency and severity at night *and* improve sleep quality. Honey is also a remarkable source of antioxidants, and it's even been found to reduce blood fats when used as a replacement for sugar. Pretty sweet!
>
> But honey isn't the only superfood in the bee arena. Bee pollen, propolis, and royal jelly are some of the most nutrient-dense foods ever studied. Bee pollen, for example, is a complete protein, containing upward of 22 different amino acids in total. It's also a rich source of vitamins, minerals, and enzymes. Plus, numerous studies have found bee pollen to be protective of your all-important liver function. A couple of teaspoons a day is enough to keep your metabolism buzzing!

Magnesium

As we discussed in Chapter Five, magnesium is one of the most valuable nutrients for the human body. It's involved in over 600 cellular processes in the body that we're aware of (meaning, there's over 600 things your body can't do — or can't do efficiently — without magnesium being present). That's all Hakuna Matata until you find out that at least 56 percent of the U.S. population is deficient in magnesium. It's crucial to ensure you're getting in plenty of magnesium-rich foods or you might find that your sleep is getting scarred up.

A 2016 study reported that magnesium is able to reduce the activity of your sympathetic (fight-or-flight) nervous system and turn on the activity of your parasympathetic (rest-and-digest) nervous system. Another study published in *Pharmacological Reports* states that magnesium is able to interact with inhibitory GABA receptors and induce antianxiety effects. Sounds like Timon and Pumba would be super-into magnesium.

One other double-blind, placebo-controlled study published in 2012 found that improving magnesium levels appears to improve sleep efficiency, improve melatonin function, reduce cortisol, and reduce wake after sleep onset. Excellent dietary sources of magnesium include avocados, pumpkin seeds, almonds, dark chocolate, leafy greens, tofu, black beans, fatty fish, and spirulina.

Omega-3s

Scientists at the University of Oxford found that improving your intake of omega-3s can reduce sleep disturbances and help you get deeper, more restful sleep. An additional study cited in *Frontiers in Neurology* discovered that the anti-inflammatory action of omega-3s (specifically DHA omega-3s) is able to reduce the symptoms of sleep apnea. You'll find great sources of DHA omega-3s in salmon, mackerel, sardines, cod liver oil, caviar, salmon roe, oysters, and algae oil. Make sure to refer back to Chapter Four for the full breakdown on the conversion of plant-sourced omega-3s into DHA. The best sources in the plant-based omega category include chia seeds, flaxseeds, pumpkin seeds, hemp seeds, and walnuts.

RED LIGHT, GREEN LIGHT

Every single second, the human brain is processing billions of bits of information. We might not think about it often, but in the blink of an eye our amazing brains are directing the movement of blood through our veins, keeping our hearts beating, digesting our food, healing our damaged cells, defending our bodies from diseases, taking in data from all of our senses, processing our memories, regulating our temperature, plus a list that would go on longer than the amount of time customer service keeps people waiting on hold (at least pick some better hold music for crying out loud!). The bottom line is, your brain is constantly engaged in a lot of labor. And, as with anywhere a lot of work is taking place, the area can get a bit messy.

With all of the work the brain is doing, there is a tremendous amount of metabolic waste products that need to get excavated from the building. Unlike the rest of your body that has an extracellular waste management network in the form of your lymphatic system, your brain, as you'll recall, has tight security detail covering what gets into and out of the virtual vault that it's in.

It wasn't until a few years ago that researchers identified the clean-up crew that keeps your brain in tip-top shape. The crew was given the name *glymphatic system* as a little shout-out to the glial cells that help regulate it. Though the glymphatic team does some light work throughout the day, it's really a night-shift team that gives your brain a complete makeover while you're sleeping. In fact, it appears that the glymphatic system is ten times more active putting in work while you're asleep! A recent study published in *Science Advances* reported that during sleep (and especially deep sleep) your glymphatic system kicks into high gear, washing away wastes and toxic proteins. Anything that impairs sleep can disrupt the function of the glymphatic system and be a driver of disease and reduced cognitive function. So, if you want to green light your brain's waste removal and support overall brain health, here are a few things to yield on or even stop in relationship to your sleep schedule.

Sugar

Up to its old tricks again, added sugar has been found to cause major disruptions to sleep quality. A six-month study conducted by scientists at the University of Copenhagen found that the consumption of added sugar and sugar-sweetened beverages can lead to an objective loss of 1 hour's worth of sleep each night! With total calories remaining the same in the diet, a higher ratio of added sugar can steal some of the sweetness from your dreams.

At the intersection between your diet and metabolism, we've already put a hefty case together to leave added sugar sitting at a red light. Now we know that sugar can be disruptive to your brain health and sleep quality, too. Just to be clear, we're talking about *added* sugar and not carbohydrates overall. Another important factor in your metabolic fingerprint and carbohydrate tipping point is identifying how carb consumption affects your sleep.

We're all unique in how carbohydrates can influence our sleep quality. One study published in the journal *Nutritional Neuroscience* reported that a very low-carbohydrate diet significantly improves deep sleep but reduces the amount of REM sleep. While another study published in *The Lancet* found that a low-carb diet improved both deep sleep *and* REM sleep. The main thing to take away is that avoiding added sugar is clearly helpful for improving sleep, and while reducing carb intake can be helpful too, how carbs affect sleep is going to vary from one person to another. Obviously, targeting the high-quality carbs we talked about in Chapter Four is going to be ideal for your waistline, and driving to Dreamville as well.

Alcohol

As one of the Starting Five of our macronutrient team, alcohol can get quite a bit of playing time for some folks. Depending on the type of alcoholic beverage, the data shows that low to moderate alcohol consumption can have benefits ranging from improved heart health, to increased bone density, to protection against cognitive decline. However, crossing a razor-thin line into excess alcohol consumption is heavily linked to increased visceral fat, increased risk of cancer, and an increased mortality from all causes. Whether your alcohol consumption is on the low end or not, one thing that's clear across the board is that sipping close to bedtime can have your sleep cycles stumbling around like Captain Jack Sparrow.

A recent meta-analysis affirmed that drinking alcohol close to bedtime does, in fact, help some people fall asleep faster...but there's a catch bigger than OBJ reaching back and posterizing a defender. Cited in the peer-reviewed journal *JMIR Mental Health,* researchers found that even one drink close to bedtime can impair sleep quality. Moderate alcohol consumption was found to lower restorative sleep quality by 24 percent, with high alcohol intake damaging sleep by nearly 40 percent. A hangover isn't from the alcohol alone, it's from the detrimental impact that it has on your sleep cycles.

Specifically, alcohol is shown to cause what's known as a *REM rebound effect*. With alcohol in the system, even after the person is asleep, REM sleep is delayed and/or suppressed leading to insufficient recovery of crucial brain and bodily functions.

To jettison the effects that alcohol has on sleep, we can 1) not drink alcohol, or 2) employ a couple of important tactics if we ever plan on drinking.

It's ideal to give your body at least 2 to 3 hours from the time you finish your last alcoholic beverage to the time you go to bed. This gives your body a head start on metabolizing the alcohol before you hit the sack, and it also gives you a chance to utilize the next important tip, which is to drink more water. Upping your hydration can help nullify the effects of alcohol faster. Not only does this help flush out metabolic waste products, but alcohol is also a diuretic, meaning that it can increase your likelihood of dehydration. Dehydration is another one of the primary causes of hangovers and poor quality sleep. Having two 8-ounce glasses of water for every serving of beer or wine is a good rule of thumb to start with.

Coffee

We've discussed many of the remarkable benefits of coffee and other naturally caffeinated beverages like green tea and black tea throughout this book. But one thing that these drinks don't play nice with is your sleep.

A fascinating study looking at the effects of caffeine on sleep quality was published in the *Journal of Clinical Sleep Medicine*. Scientists at Wayne State University School of Medicine had test subjects consume caffeine at various intervals of either 6 hours before bed, 3 hours before bed, or immediately before bed and tested their objective and subjective sleep results. The researchers discovered that consuming caffeine even as much as 6 hours before bed was enough to have a measurable detrimental impact on their sleep quality!

Even though study participants may have subjectively reported that they got 7 hours of sleep, for example, the objective measurement of their sleep cycles demonstrated that caffeine consumption (even 6 hours before bed) led to a 1-hour loss of sleep. This means that, even though they may have been unconscious for 7 hours, their body only received the benefits of 6 hours.

The researchers noted that moderate to large doses of caffeine commonly found in increasingly popular energy drinks and coffees are the particular culprit. In the study, 400 milligrams of caffeine was used, which is just above the amount you'd currently find in a "grande" cup of coffee at Starbucks. Though many people wouldn't down a grande close to bedtime, even a smaller amount can be sketchy for some folks (depending on your unique metabolism of caffeine).

According to the American Academy of Sleep Medicine, caffeine has a half-life of approximately 5 hours. *Half-life* essentially means that after a specific amount of time (say, 5 hours), half of the substance is still active in your system. So, using the 5-hour half-life as an example, if you consumed 400 milligrams of caffeine, after 5 hours, you'd have half of it (or 200 milligrams) still active in your system; after another 5 hours, you'd have 100 milligrams; after another 5 hours, it would be 50 milligrams; and so on. This is why having caffeine even 6 hours out from bedtime still caused sleep disturbances in the study. If someone has a high caffeine metabolism, that half-life can be shorter, say 3 to 4 hours. If someone has a slow caffeine metabolism, the half-life can be substantially longer at 6 to 7+ hours.

Some people can have coffee a bit later in the day and sleep fine (objectively and subjectively), while others can hardly tolerate caffeine well at all and would be best to skip it (outside of a small amount much earlier in the day).

With that said, one of the best tips for enjoying coffee and caffeinated teas without interrupting your sleep is to create a caffeine curfew for yourself. I've found that most people do well hitting a yellow light with caffeine late in the morning and hitting a full red light stop in the early afternoon (by noon to 2 p.m. if they plan on getting to bed sometime between 10 p.m. and midnight). It depends on you, but it's a great tip to execute because, believe it or not, caffeine is definitely impacting your sleep quality.

Still, some people are like, "Nah, I can drink a pot of coffee before bed and sleep like a baby." First of all, babies' sleep patterns can be straight-up nuts, so, to that, you'd be correct. The incorrect thing is that the peaceful, low-stress sleep a baby *does* get, your caffeinated sleep just doesn't compare to. Research cited in the journal *Circulation* revealed that caffeine acutely stimulates the sympathetic (fight-or-flight) nervous system of even experienced coffee drinkers. A caffeine curfew is a good idea for everyone, even if you believe your blood is probably 20 percent java.

NUTRITIONAL SLEEP ACCESSORIES

Our sleep quality is critical to everything from cognitive performance, to disease prevention, to regulating our metabolism. For example, researchers at Stanford University found that insufficient sleep can reduce levels of the satiety hormone leptin, increase levels of the hunger hormone ghrelin, and directly increase your BMI. Clearly, getting plenty of good-sleep nutrients is crucial to optimizing our sleep. But there are some nutritional accessories that can support the look of your sleep, too.

One of our biggest tenets in *Eat Smarter* is to cover our nutritional needs through food first. Food is the main outfit that keeps you looking and feeling your best, while specific supplements can provide some fly accessories that give your outfit the finishing touch.

Now, if you go out wearing only your accessories (buck-naked with no outfit), it will have you looking and feeling like a crazy person (unless you're at Burning Man or something). That's the mistake most people make when they think they can lean heavily on supplements to support their health. Supplements are only meant to *supplement* a good diet and lifestyle. So, please, never mistake supplement/accessories for real food/outfits (the folks at Burning Man don't tell you how long it takes to get that sand out of their nether regions).

With all of that said, here are a few useful, sleep-supportive supplements that I want to make sure are fashionably on your radar.

- **Reishi**—Research published in the journal *Pharmacology Biochemistry and Behavior* found that the renowned medicinal mushroom reishi was able to significantly decrease sleep latency (meaning you fall asleep faster), increase overall sleep time, and increase non-REM, deep sleep time. I love having reishi tea 30 to 45 minutes before bed. Some of my favorite sources are listed in the Eat Smarter Bonus Resource Guide at eatsmarterbook.com/bonus.

- **Chamomile**—A randomized controlled trial cited in *Complementary Therapies in Medicine* demonstrated that chamomile extract was able to significantly improve sleep quality in test subjects versus a placebo. Chamomile is another excellent tea to have before bed, or it can be taken in capsules as well. As with anything, look for organic and no questionable fillers or binders in the capsules, if possible.

- **Valerian**—With centuries of documented use and efficacy, valerian has become one of the most popular sleep-supportive supplements in the U.S. Compared with a placebo, valerian extract resulted in a statistically significant improvement in sleep latency, sleep quality, and number of nighttime awakenings, according to a study published in *Pharmacology Biochemistry and Behavior*. Valerian root tea, dried valerian root capsules, and valerian root extract have all been shown to support sleep in clinical trials.

- **Magnesium**—Magnesium makes yet another list because 1) it has such a wide range of benefits in the body, and 2) it's used in so many processes it can easily get depleted. There are a wide variety of oral magnesium supplements on the market that can be utilized. I'm a big fan of topical sources of magnesium, too (i.e., they're absorbed through our skin). This can range from storied Epsom salt baths to sprayable supercritical extracts.

- **L-theanine**—Earlier in this section we noted the remarkable benefits L-theanine provides in reducing stress and anxiety. We also noted that L-theanine is able to increase the activity of the neurotransmitter GABA (another helpful sleep-supportive supplement for some people), which encourages a sense of calm and relaxation. L-theanine is most recognized for its ability to counteract stress, and it's one of the reasons that the caffeine in green tea doesn't tend to hyper-stimulate people (it's one of the best natural sources of L-theanine!). A double-blind, placebo-controlled study found that test subjects taking supplemental L-theanine improved their sleep duration and sleep efficiency. The research indicates that supplementing with between 250 and 400 milligrams a day appears to be most effective.

- **Melatonin**—Being that it's one of the most-used and well-researched sleep supplements, it should be no surprise that melatonin is on this list. What is surprising for most people is that melatonin is not actually a sedative, and it doesn't help you sleep like you'd assume. As mentioned previously, melatonin is one of our body's most powerful biological time regulators. Melatonin helps your body sync with your environment and regulates the release of other hormones. That being said, it's important to proceed with caution when using it.

  ○ Melatonin is a potent hormone, and just because you can pick it up over-the-counter at your local store, doesn't mean that it's appropriate to go commando with it. A study published in the *Journal of Biological Rhythms* discovered that faulty timing or large doses of melatonin can cause a desensitization of melatonin receptors. Essentially, haphazard use of melatonin can start shutting down your body's ability to use it effectively. Because of this, many people who've consistently taken melatonin notice that over time they've had to take more and more. We need to intelligently and respectfully use melatonin if it's part of our sleep wellness strategy. Staring into a blue light-emitting screen (from our computer, phone, or TV), which has been confirmed to suppress melatonin secretion and increase cortisol at night, and then downing some melatonin expecting to get better sleep is just counterproductive. We need to have healthy practices for our overall sleep hygiene. Many of those things have to do with our lifestyle, but adding melatonin in a thoughtful fashion can make it one of your valuable accessories.

○   According to a meta-analysis cited in the *Nutrition Journal,* one of melatonin's most efficacious uses appears to be in helping to prevent phase shifts from jet lag. If you're traveling and changing time zones, bringing along some melatonin can help you to quickly adjust. That's pretty awesome. Outside of that, melatonin has been found to improve sleep efficiency in some people, as well. Utilizing melatonin in spot cases to get your sleep back on track, or microdosing over longer stints, appears to be the most appropriate uses. There are capsules and sprayable forms of melatonin supplements on the market. Do your best to purchase from reputable companies using natural sources, if at all possible.

BRAIN GAINS

This section of the book has been packed with tips, tools, and insights to help make your brain as fit and healthy as possible. From improving your memory and focus, to better regulating your emotions and sleep quality, food has the power to influence every single aspect of your brain's performance.

Now that your brain has gotten a nice pump, it's time to press our way into the final section and access one of the most powerful aspects of eating smarter. What you're about to discover can make you stronger in every area of life, so let's flex those fingers and turn the page because it's time to take things to the next level!

THE SCIENCE OF MEAL TIMING AND THE EAT SMARTER 30-DAY PROGRAM

CHAPTER NINE

Food o'Clock

When people ask me what is more important, food or love, I don't answer because I'm eating.

~Unknown

Three square meals a day. That's the way we're "supposed" to eat according to the unwritten nutrition laws of our culture. If you're like me, you've tried to live by that food code...and have been led to believe that others around you are abiding by that law, too. But if you dig a little deeper, you'll discover that this law is more rickety than my first car. I got by with it for about a week, then it broke down on the side of the road and left me eating snacks at a random gas station.

A study published in the peer-reviewed journal *Cell Metabolism* tracked the eating habits of a group of adult test subjects to see how often the average person actually eats. The researchers discovered that, not only does the average person not eat three square meals a day, most people tend to eat sporadically throughout the day (more of what would be considered snacking) and many people eat some pretty random combinations of things when they snack. For example, one person ate a cream cheese–Cheeto sandwich, while another person had a Rice Krispies treat along with some spicy trail mix. The head researcher said that the people in the study were "very creative," which is science-talk for being pretty weird.

Now, I'm not judging as though I haven't put cheese and ketchup on my eggs or put red hot potato chips on my sandwich and smashed it down ever-so-slightly. Humans *are* weird. And that's what makes us amazing. And, as I stated in the introduction to this book, humans have tried to eat everything you can imagine at some point throughout our evolution. Our ancestors tried and tested foods to find out what's actually good for us. They discovered health-giving foods, foods that are a party for your palate, and foods that taste so bad people had to say a prayer after the meal instead of before it. They discovered foods that are medicines, foods that are poisons, and everything in between. A big difference for us, today, is that we no longer have to rely on mother nature to tell us what to eat. For many people, the food knowledge of our ancestors is no longer cherished. Humans have now invented *thousands* of new foods through chemistry, selective breeding, and even splicing and dicing up genes. Unnatural is now normal. And natural is out of fashion.

Another unusual aspect of our current food culture is something I call *the paradox of convenience*. Yes, having more food available year-round has helped civilization to grow. But, with 24/7 access to hundreds or even thousands of different food items, the pure accessibility of so much food has led to a much higher frequency of eating. The aforementioned study found that the average time between the first bite of breakfast and the last bite of dinner (or an evening snack, or drinks at the bar) was 14 hours and 45 minutes. That means the average person is eating something for a span of about 15 hours a day, which is nearly the entire time most people are awake. Throw in some sleep to round out that 24-hour clock, and that might not seem like a big deal. But, to your genes, it might be one of the biggest deals ever.

The scientists in the study decided to see what would happen if they simply shorten the window of eating for some of the test subjects. There was no other dietary advice given—no restriction on calories, macronutrient ratios, or anything else. They simply had study participants reduce their eating to a period of 10 to 12 hours a day, and here's what happened...

After 16 weeks, the study participants lost an average of over 7 pounds, and they subjectively reported that they were sleeping better and having a lot more energy. An analysis of their diets also uncovered that they'd naturally reduced their calorie intake by about 20 percent (even though there was no calorie restrictions placed on them). They were losing weight, eating foods they enjoyed, and experiencing a lot more energy. It might sound too good to be true on the surface, but there's a lot more going on behind the scenes. We're going to break down some of the things that happen with your metabolism when you shorten your eating window in a moment...and it's going to knock your metabolic socks off! This method of eating is generally called *intermittent fasting* and has been growing in popularity recently. There are many different ways to employ it. But, you may be wondering if it's just another newly invented fad that'll be here today, gone tomorrow. But, the truth is, intermittent fasting isn't a new invention—breakfast is.

THE FIRST BREAKFAST

Personally, I love the idea of breakfast foods. Pancakes, omelets, waffles...and don't even get me started on cereal. But these foods, and any other foods for that matter, don't have a time requirement on when they're supposed to be eaten. It's a cultural construct that cereal is eaten in the morning, sandwiches are eaten at lunch, and meat loaf is eaten at dinner. A lot of these cultural habits are based on convenience, marketing, and social programming.

There was a time before processed foods came along that food wasn't separated into teams of times when we are allowed to eat them. Many of us have found ourselves in a virtual *Groundhog Day* with our eating habits. But it's time to jump into the *Hot Tub Time Machine* and see how all of this got started.

For the vast majority of human history, there wasn't any concept of waking up and having a morning meal. Food historians have purported that breakfast is a recent invention made in a deliberate effort to get people to change their eating habits.

Before agriculture, humans were not mere laborers getting up and grinding at a 9 to 5. They thrived by engaging in shorter, strategic work...hunting, gathering, and spending a lot of time in leisure. The data suggests that most pre-agriculture humans didn't work very long hours at all. There was no need to stockpile on energy to start the day, expending a lot of energy doing manual labor was not very common, and they definitely weren't knocking down a big breakfast to hit a CrossFit workout that may have included deadlifting a boulder, burpees, and throwing a spear at a woolly mammoth.

Through the process of hunting and gathering, and a regular variance in food accessibility, humans evolved to have what scientists refer to as *thrifty genes* that are exceptionally good at managing energy. They're very good at storing fat when food is in abundance, and equally as good at burning fat when a meal isn't around.

It's important to note that the same genes are still alive and well within us today. Agriculture may have helped to create civilization as we know it, but it also threw a sharp, spiked monkey wrench right into our metabolism. Prior to our friends with benefits relationship with modern agriculture, humans developed the metabolic machinery to readily burn stored body fat for fuel. But after agriculture was embedded into society, that soon changed. If you were going to work a full day in the field, then you'd *better* chug down a big breakfast, because you were going to need it!

This was a time of much less cerebral work, and much more physical work. You did use your hungry brain, of course, but this was tied to a lot more manual labor than the average person is accustomed to today. Humans were forced to adapt. Eventually, a "high-energy breakfast" became the order of the day. But a study published in the *Journal of Applied Physiology* stated, "This lifestyle (of eating constantly throughout the day) collides with our genome, which was most likely selected in the late Paleolithic era (50,000 to 10,000 BC) by criteria that favored survival in an environment characterized by fluctuations between periods of feast and famine. The theory of thrifty genes states that these fluctuations are required for optimal metabolic function." Repeat: *optimal metabolic function*. We might be onto something here.

Even centuries after the Paleolithic era, when humans traded in their bison-skinned loincloths for breezy designer togas, breakfast still wasn't a regular part of the human diet. For example, the people of ancient Rome didn't really eat it, according to food historian Caroline

Yeldham. They believed it was healthier to eat their first meal at mid-day around noon. As you likely know, the Romans had a substantial influence on many other cultures around the world, and this way of eating impacted what people ate for a very long time.

Cut to the Middle Ages, when monastic life largely shaped when people ate. This is likely when the word *breakfast* initially hit the scene. People still weren't necessarily eating early in the day (unless it was a hard laborer, someone who was ill, or in their elderly years), as eating before morning mass was frowned upon. But, after mass, around 10:30 or 11 a.m., people would break their overnight fast (literally, *break fast*) and eat their first meal of the day.

Another historian, Ian Mortimer, suggests the Tudors invented the timing of breakfast (as we know it) in the 16th century as a side effect of popularizing the concept of employment. As people increasingly went to work for an employer, rather than working for themselves on their own land, they lost control of their time. A big breakfast allowed them to work the long, uninterrupted day, often without additional nourishment.

The well-to-do folks began to join in the breakfast charades as they were able to sleep in and play out their own version of the Bruno Mars "*Lazy Song.*" Breakfast in bed, yes, please! And there were now records of decadent morning feasts for the aristocratic circles to get together and chop it up about who's the most noble or who's rocking the best wig.

There was actually a statute established in the year 1515 insisting that craftsmen and laborers should start work at 5 a.m. and continue until 7 or 8 p.m. between mid-March and mid-September (when they had the most daylight). They would be allotted 30 minutes for break-fast and 90 minutes for lunch. The work hours were a little less when the days were shorter, but when you've only got a small amount of time to eat and rest, you'd better use it.

When the Industrial Revolution took place, along with the advent of the lightbulb and the ability to light up factories, this is when systemic, yearlong working hours came along. From the head honchos to the factory workers, it was not uncommon to see 100 hours of labor in a week. And this is when it became commonplace for all social classes to eat a meal before going to work.

With all of this understood, breakfast may be a new invention, but that doesn't mean that it's not a viable option. Breakfast wasn't a normal part of life, but neither was bathing. So, I'm definitely not saying that breakfast isn't an advancement that we can't healthfully participate in. But, unlike regularly washing your private property, not eating for a little bit larger portion of the day can yield some remarkable upgrades that we're going to talk about next. The *Eat Smarter* 30-Day Program has one version with a traditional breakfast time and one with the Smart Intermittent Fasting protocol (which we'll talk about soon!) built in. Both are incredibly effective, but let's talk about why *intermittent fasting* is so valuable.

INTERMITTENT FAST AND THE FURIOUS

There are many types of well-documented versions of intermittent fasting being utilized today. Some versions involve eating "normally" one day and then fasting the next day (eating little to no food—often noted to be 500 calories or less during fasting days). Some versions instruct folks to eat normally for five days and then fast for two days, rinse and repeat. Other versions generally recommend a 24-hour fast one or two times a week. While others simply promote skipping some random meals wherever you see fit and keep living your life one quarter mile at a time.

Over almost two decades in this field, I've seen a lot of stuff come and a lot of stuff go. One of the things I've seen the most people have success with is simply creating a daily fasting window of 12 to 16 hours (there's a lot of wiggle room here, which we'll get to!), with 16 hours of fasting and 8 hours of eating having the most evidence behind it. Although there's about as many personality types of intermittent fasting as there are personality types in *The Fast and the Furious* movie franchise, the research demonstrates pretty similar effects. That said, these benefits you're about to learn about can universally be applied to a variety of approaches. But, again, the most successful driver, and the vehicle used in the *Smart Intermittent Fasting* program, is based on a daily eating and fasting window.

Intermittent Fasting Improves Metabolic Function

As you've discovered in earlier sections of the book, your metabolism is largely governed by your hormone function. One of the most incredible things about intermittent fasting is that it initiates hormonal changes that make stored body fat more accessible. Data published in the peer-reviewed journal *Obesity* states that employing intermittent fasting is like flipping a "metabolic switch" that shifts the metabolism from fat creation and fat storage to mobilization of body fat in the form of free fatty acids and fatty acid–derived ketones to be used for fuel. Translation: Instead of storing more fat, intermittent fasting flips the switch to start using it.

In Chapter Two, when we went through the hormonal roles of our metabolic theater, we noted that insulin is a primary driver of fat storage, while its twin brother, glucagon, is a major driver of fat release and utilization. Intermittent fasting helps put glucagon into the driver's seat while simultaneously improving insulin sensitivity. Researchers at the University of Copenhagen found that intermittent fasting is able to quickly reduce insulin resistance and nullify the effects of insulin-created roadblocks that stop fat from being released from the cells. Their study also revealed that intermittent fasting has some significant effects on our vital satiety hormones.

Getting our hunger and satiety hormones back online is a huge key to long-term success with our health and fitness. Several studies indicate that one of the body's most important satiety hormones, adiponectin, is increased through intermittent fasting. As you'll recall, researchers discovered that optimal levels of adiponectin can support fat loss *without* increasing appetite. Adiponectin is also noted to help your body move fat away from the viscera (belly fat) region to the subcutaneous fat region, while low levels of adiponectin have been associated with obesity, higher levels of belly fat, and insulin resistance. Research published in the journal *Endocrinology* also reports that intermittent fasting can improve the function of other satiety-related hormones like neuropeptide Y, while supporting fat loss and retaining lean muscle mass.

This leads us to a very important point. Intermittent fasting is *not* conventional calorie restriction. Often times, by partitioning your calorie intake into your fasting window, you will not need to significantly restrict your calories to lose fat. Your metabolism will literally be working more efficiently and be more acclimated to burning fat for fuel. Plus, and this is a huge leverage point of the Smart Intermittent Fasting program, intermittent fasting is protective of your body's major "fat-burning machinery," which is your muscle tissue.

A startling percentage of people who lose weight through conventional calorie restriction regain their lost fat and find it exceedingly harder to lose weight over time. A huge player in this metabolic conundrum is a loss of their body's valuable muscle mass. Muscle is expensive for your body to carry around (calorically speaking). Generally, having more muscle on your frame enables you to burn more calories during activity *and* at rest. Too many people think that exercising is going to enable them to *Tokyo Drift* their way into having the body they want. But, in reality, there's only so much exercise you can do. **It's what your metabolism is doing when you're not exercising that makes all the difference in the world.** This is known as your *resting metabolic rate* (RMR) or *resting energy expenditure* (REE). A study cited in *The American Journal of Clinical Nutrition* concluded that a large drop in the resting metabolic rate from weight loss is due to the loss of muscle mass. And this is where intermittent fasting takes *The Fate of the Furious* who've struggled to keep the weight off and allows them to get a hit of nitro.

A new study featured in *Advances in Nutrition* asserts that over 35 percent of the weight lost through a standard calorie-reduced diet is from the loss of muscle mass in healthy individuals. Upward of 30 percent of the weight lost from someone who is overweight or obese is coming from the loss of their valuable muscle tissue. According to a report from the *International Association for the Study of Obesity,* intermittent fasting is remarkably more effective for retaining muscle mass than daily calorie restriction! It appears that the changes in gene expression and improved hormone function through intermittent fasting upregulate the retention of muscle tissue while boosting the rate of fat loss. Pretty cool. When talking about intermittent fasting and fat loss, I can't omit the fact that intermittent fasting has been shown to increase the conversion of beige fat cells to fat-burning brown fat cells, too.

In the aforementioned study cited in *Obesity,* the researchers stated that the metabolic switch typically occurs 12+ hours after cessation of food consumption. Simply finishing your last meal of the day by 8 p.m., hanging out for a bit and getting a good night's rest, then having your first food after 8 a.m. the next morning is an easy example of kickstarting these benefits. Add to this all of the powerhouse supportive nutrition from *Eat Smarter* that improves hormone health, enhances digestion, and fortifies liver function, and you have a baseline formula that helps your metabolism pump out sequels with bigger and better results.

Intermittent Fasting Improves Brain Health

Intermittent fasting can stimulate the production of new brain cells, according to data published in the *Journal of Molecular Neuroscience.* As you know from Section Two, new brain cells are hard to come by. And intermittent fasting is one of just a handful of ways to give your brain some new, active cells to drive around your brain and make memories with.

Not only does intermittent fasting stimulate the creation of new brain cells, it also makes the neurons you already have work better. Numerous studies have revealed that intermittent fasting increases our levels of something called *brain-derived neurotropic factor* (BDNF). BDNF is a powerful assistance in the healthy development and survival of our brain cells. It's been shown to improve neuroplasticity, enhance cognitive function, and protect our brains from a myriad of diseases.

Research featured in the journal *Psychiatry Investigation* illustrated that a deficiency of BDNF is linked to higher rates of depression, panic disorder, and other mood disorders. This is another phenomenal benefit that intermittent fasting brings to the table. In a study featured in the journal *Psychiatry Research,* clinicians found that short stints of fasting were able to improve symptoms of depression and improve anxiety scores in 80 percent of patients.

In a conversation with physician and *New York Times*–bestselling author Dr. David Perlmutter, he told me that BDNF is like Miracle-Gro for your brain cells. It's able to support and improve so many functions, and our diets have a huge impact on its production. What he shared with me was echoed in a study published in the journal *Neuroscience* finding that a diet high in refined sugar and damaged fats can reduce levels of BDNF in the brain. Sugar is able to strip your brain's land of BDNF production, while intermittent fasting is one of the rare things that can boost the production of this Miracle-Gro to help you harvest the best results possible.

In reference to the gut-brain-sleep connection that we discussed in Chapter Eight, a 2011 study revealed that intermittent fasting can potentially increase melatonin concentrations in the gut and brain! Melatonin is an absolutely crucial hormone that influences our circadian clock, which regulates our brain function *and* our metabolism.

There's clearly a plethora of ways that intermittent fasting improves brain function, but I've got one more to share with you because it just might be the most important. Intermittent fasting has been shown to directly improve *neuronal autophagy*. This is the process involved in the elimination and recycling of damaged brain cells. As noted in the previous section, efficient removal of brain waste is absolutely critical to the performance of your brain. So when your brain cells need a lift, intermittent fasting is there to have your back, like Dominic Toretto saying, "I don't have friends. I got family."

Intermittent Fasting Reduces Disease Risk and Slows Down the Aging Process

One of the most amazing benefits of intermittent fasting is the impact it has on inflammation. As we covered in the earlier sections of the book, excessive inflammation is a devastating force that can incinerate the health of your metabolism and brain. But there are some potent things that we can do to help put the fire out.

A study published in the journal *Annals of Nutrition and Metabolism* showed that a daily 12-hour intermittent fast was enough to significantly reduce levels of homocysteine and C-reactive protein, which are both major markers of heart disease and systemic inflammation.

An inability to effectively remove metabolic wastes is another one of the most overlooked causes of oxidative stress and inflammation. Researchers from the Department of Immunology and Microbiology at the Scripps Research Institute found that intermittent fasting has a profound effect on autophagy throughout our entire body (not just our brains). This cellular cleansing triggered by intermittent fasting accelerates the removal of metabolic waste products, enabling your cells, tissues, and organs to work more efficiently.

Massive research is now being done to examine the effects that intermittent fasting can have on chronic diseases like cancer. And the data so far is promising. An animal study published in *Mechanisms of Ageing and Development* looked at the effects of intermittent fasting on lymphoma (a cancer involving the lymph and immune systems). Intermittent fasting, which was initiated in middle-aged mice over a four-month period, reduced the incidence of lymphoma by 33 percent! The control group that did not employ intermittent fasting had a 0 percent reduction. Again, very promising, but more research involving human test subjects needs to be done.

The combination of disease prevention, reduced inflammation, and improved autophagy is a pretty good starting recipe for longevity. But to add a youthful cherry on top, intermittent fasting has been shown to consistently boost the production of human growth hormone (HGH). Intermittent fasting can increase blood levels of growth hormone by as much as five-fold, according to scientists at the University of Virginia Medical School. Often referred to as the *youth hormone,* HGH is well-noted for supporting muscular development, protecting against muscle loss, enhancing cellular repair, and improving overall energy and performance.

Creating your own strategic blocks of time when you're eating and not eating is one of the most powerful tools in your superhero utility belt.

But I want you to know up front that the windows you create are nothing you are required to live or die by. If you're particularly hungry a certain day during your fasting window, eat something. If you've got a family breakfast get-together or an important business dinner that conflicts with your eating window, eat something. Part of channeling what our ancestors were forced to do is rolling with the punches. No diet should hold dominion over your life and create more stress, including this one. As mentioned, I want to make sure you have the tools to make the best decisions for yourself...regardless of the different situations you may find yourself in. This book, and this program, is about *you,* and that's why it's so important to adjust things when needed and make the program your own.

I've met many people over the years who had struggled to lose weight in the past, and they frequently carried a subconscious belief that "if you're not hungry, then you're doing it wrong." And that's one of the most dangerous beliefs in the diet industry. Yes, we all can get hungry from time to time, but dealing with consistent hunger, and even aiming to experience more hunger, is like purchasing a first-class ticket for a cruise on the *Titanic.*

If we're seemingly eating healthy, yet we're experiencing constant hunger, that's more of a cue that something is hitting the skids rather than hitting a stride. Frequent hunger could be an indicator of several things, including nutrient deficiencies, hormone imbalances, and sugar withdrawals. It's not an accident that these are all things that we've targeted in *Eat Smarter.* We want to make sure that your nutritional bases are loaded so that you can knock your goals out of the park.

Obviously, intermittent fasting rides with some serious benefits, so now it's time to grab the wheel and drive right into the tips for the *Eat Smarter 30-Day Program!* But, unlike *The Fast and the Furious,* you don't have to hang out of the window of another high-speed diet program to get the results you really want. This program is about empowerment and catering your nutrition to fit your lifestyle. We're building and fueling your own unique vehicle to enjoy the rest of your life with, in a way that's fun, in a way that feels good, and in a way that transforms every area of your life.

CHAPTER TEN

Pre-Game: Smarter Tools for Lasting Success

Without strategy, execution is aimless. Without execution, strategy is useless.

~Morris Chang

It's been an incredible journey so far and I'm excited for you to take advantage of the powerful things you've learned. We've covered the remarkable ways that food influences your metabolism in Section One, including: how your fat-burning hormones and enzymes actually operate, clearing up the conventional calorie dogma once and for all, the Three Amigos that cause a virtual stampede over your metabolism, and a master class on the five starting players on your macronutrient team. Plus, we covered a plethora of the most effective, well-researched fat-loss-supporting foods that you'll be able to implement here in this program.

In Section Two, we shifted gears and took a deep dive into how food influences our cognitive abilities, our sleep quality (via the gut-brain-sleep connection), our mood, and our ability to connect with ourselves and others. Some of the most eye-opening data in *Eat Smarter* demonstrated how food deeply impacts the quality of our relationships. Not only that, we investigated how food can literally bring families and communities closer together. Surprising research revealed that the simple habit of sitting down for a meal with loved ones on a consistent basis can directly improve our food choices, reduce the negative effects of stress, and even improve our body composition. It's not just what we eat, but it's *how* we eat and *whom* we're eating with that can make all the difference in the world!

Section Three takes things to another level by examining the science of meal timing. We have examined the biological backlash of conventional calorie restriction that's been experienced by millions of people. Rampant muscle loss, increased hunger, and pervasive mood swings have become accepted as the normal price of admission when we sign up to haphazardly restrict our calories. This powerhouse section reveals how simply partitioning our caloric intake into "windows" of eating and fasting can help us to retain our valuable lean muscle tissue, improve the function of our most important metabolic hormones, and even enhance our cognitive abilities and stave off the signs of aging.

We've covered an incredible amount of information. And if you're ever feeling listless, curious, or just eager to learn more, you have full permission to go back and read any relevant chapters or sections to get a refresher. You're always guaranteed to find something new when you revisit something with fresh eyes!

This chapter is where the rubber meets the road, and all of the epic information you've learned in *Eat Smarter* gets put into action in your life in real time. But, you'd never go into any important endeavor without being prepared. We want to ensure that you have the tools and insights to guarantee that you are successful and, equally important, that you enjoy the process along the way. Here are some invaluable tips to support your *fast* transformation.

F.A.S.T. TRANSFORMATION TIPS

There are obviously massive benefits to incorporating some intermittent fasting into your regimen. But what makes *Smart Intermittent Fasting* so effective is that we strategically address the common pitfalls seen in conventional intermittent fasting and dieting in general. Utilizing the acronym *F.A.S.T.* you'll be able to accelerate your results and personalize things to keep you healthfully crushing your goals for many years to come.

F: Figure Out Your Ideal Eating and Fasting Windows

At the beginning of this section we highlighted a study cited in the peer-reviewed journal *Cell Metabolism*. The study revealed that simply having participants go from an unstructured eating window of about 15 hours a day to a more specific 10- to 12-hour window led to a significant increase in weight loss, improved sleep, and more energy throughout the day. Honing in on your ideal eating and fasting windows is the first step to maximizing the benefits of intermittent fasting.

A common error people make when shifting to intermittent fasting is making a big leap from eating "whenever" to creating a short window of eating for themselves that's too small, too soon. Prior to having a strategic eating and fasting window, eating is pretty breezy and unstructured for most of us. If we suddenly shut the eating window too quickly and cut off the breeze, it can get pretty stuffy, really fast. And many people will clamber to throw the window open again (and possibly jump out of it to run after a food truck). There's no need to instigate excessive hunger and a propensity to rebound binge. So, close the eating window just a bit at a time to allow your body and mind to get adjusted to the new routine.

Select a window of time each day that you will be fasting. Your fasting window can literally be anything you want. A 12-hour fast is a pretty simple place to start for most folks. The great news is that your time asleep is included in your fasting window, too!

You can begin with a 12-hour fasting window, then after a week or two, increase it to a 12½- or 13-hour fasting window and keep moving from there if it feels good to you. Remember, the data published in the journal *Obesity* found that after just 12 hours of fasting, a "metabolic switch" gets flipped that enhances the performance of many hormones and metabolism-regulating organ systems. A little smart fasting can go a long way.

A common place to begin a structured intermittent fast is to finish your last meal of the day by 8 p.m., and then simply wait until 8 a.m. (or later) the next day to have your first meal. Again, you will definitely initiate many of the benefits of intermittent fasting you've learned about. And to fortify your results, you can extend your fasting window out a bit more over time. If you finish your last meal by 8 p.m., for instance, extending your fasting window until 10 a.m., 11 a.m., or noon the following day is where even more impressive results take place for many people. A 16-hour window is the documented sweet spot for lots of folks (and pretty accessible thanks to the additional tips in this program). Anything from a 12- to 18-hour fasting window works best. Anything longer than that is just not necessary.

Paul B.

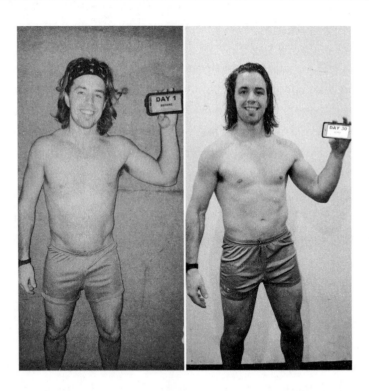

When I started the 30-day challenge I didn't have super-high expectations for myself. I never successfully stuck to a nutrition plan for more than two weeks and I haven't been to bed before 10 p.m. since grade

school. Between going to college full-time, working part-time, compet-
ing and coaching track and field, and being in a relationship, life would
always get in the way. I eat pretty healthy but I've never had a routine or
body I was proud of, that actually showed all the hours of hard work I
put into my workouts.

I made the decision to change my whole mindset. Instead of stress-
ing out about the details, trying to win the grand prize for the body of my
dreams, I dedicated myself to two things:

1. Feeding window: Commit to the intermittent fasting. Every day.
Wake up, hydrate, coffee. Eat around noon. Include quality proteins,
veggies, healthy fats, carbs from the earth. Eat slowly and don't force it.

2. Recovery: Wind down around 9:30 p.m. and ditch the screens.

I started at 207 pounds and now weigh in at 199 or 200. I set seven
personal bests in my squat and dead lift, and several sprint times faster
than when I was at 185 pounds. All this while training less hours, sleep-
ing more, and using the sauna three times a week.

My big takeaway is that committing to consistency allowed me to
make small wins and continue building on it emotionally and mentally. I
honestly forgot that this was a 30-day challenge because it felt like a
seamless transition into a new lifestyle. We're at the end of the month
and I'm down 7 pounds. I didn't have to starve myself to do it and my
performance improved. I feel like I did it the right way. Thank you Shawn
for a sustainable solution!

A: Adjust to Your Lifestyle

One of the other great things about Smart Intermittent Fasting is that
you can adjust it to your lifestyle. Whether your goal is improved cognitive function, increased fat loss, or enhanced protection against illnesses and early aging, Smart Intermittent Fasting can help you get
there with real momentum.

While writing this book, for example, my goal was to have
increased clarity, focus, and mental energy each day to deliver my very
best to the writing process. As a result, I structured things so that the
majority of my writing could be completed during my fasting window.

Not only has this enabled me to execute at a higher level mentally, it also eliminated a distraction that had hindered me while working on projects in the past.

Earlier in my career, though I was eating healthfully, I didn't realize that I'd conditioned myself to constantly be eating. My days revolved around when my next meal would be, and instead of creating, I'd be pulled away to find food or eat a meal and then deal with the post-meal cognitive deceleration. For me, Smart Intermittent Fasting actually took the stress away from procuring another meal at a time when I'd rather be enjoying my life. Plus, the enhanced brain capacity enabled me to get more done, more quickly, and free up more time in the day to hang out with my kids, exercise, work on other passion projects, and sit down to good meals with friends and family. I structured things to fit my lifestyle and the results that I wanted. And you'll be able to do the same thing, as well.

If you tend to be more of a night person, for instance, and generally don't get to bed until, say, midnight or 1 a.m., you can set your fasting window to be from 10 p.m. until noon the next day. That equates to a solid 14-hour fasting window, and you don't have to abide by the cookie-cutter fasting period that's often promoted in order to get some great results.

Another illustration of this point could be catering your fasting window to best fit your exercise schedule and training goals. The cool thing is that certain types of training can be even more effective if done during your fasting window (more on this in the meal plan bonus tips on page 361 if you want more information). But, let's say you're training in a team sport, and you want to implement some pre-training nutrition while still getting some of the benefits of intermittent fasting. Speaking strictly from a scheduling perspective, if you want to have some food or a protein shake at 7 a.m. for an 8 a.m. training session, you can set your fasting window to be from 6 or 7 p.m. the night before to reap the benefits of a daily 12- to 13-hour fast. Intentionally cater things to fit you and your goals. In just a bit, you'll be provided with a useful scheduling template that you can adjust to best fit your schedule.

Here are some other key points to pay attention to when adjusting things to fit your lifestyle:

- **Be consistent, but not neurotic.** Your brain and body are always looking for ways to automate things and groove into patterns of behavior. The more consistency you can have in your Smart Intermittent Fasting schedule, the more smooth and enjoyable things will tend to be. However, life happens! So, if you can't follow your normal routine to the T (maybe you're up late for work, or traveling and changing time zones, or there's a special brunch with family that doesn't happen very often), seriously, don't sweat it. Just adhere to the basic principles as best you can, and get back on the routine within the next day or so. An occasional disruption to the routine is to be expected. Just roll with the punches and continue to enjoy the benefits of your program.

- **Know the difference between hunger and habit.** A small percentage of people find that they are a little hungrier during their extended fasting window the first few days, but the body will quickly adjust. Because our bodies inherently look to automate behaviors, we can actually train ourselves to be hungry/eat at certain times if we do it long enough (even if we're not hungry). So, if you start making yourself eat each day at 6 a.m., for example, within a very short amount of time, your body will begin producing hormones, releasing neurotransmitters, and secreting digestive juices around 6 a.m. to prepare for food (whether you plan on eating or not!). It's programming. It's habit. And the good news is that it works the other way, too. As you build out your fasting window, your body will quickly become acclimated to eating at a different time. Most people who employ the Smart Intermittent Fasting protocol find that they're just not hungry as often as they used to be prior to the program. As long as you include plenty of the hormone-healthy foods that support your microbiome that you've learned about in *Eat Smarter*, rampant, frequent hunger should no longer be a part of your life.

Eliminating excessive hunger is part nourishment and part upgrading our routine. This program helps you to do both.

■ **Keep the basics in mind.** Many of us are incredibly talented at making things harder for ourselves. I know because I made myself president of the self-sabotage fan club. I finally gave up my position when I realized that a lot of the effort we put forth in "working hard" is due to the obstacles we unknowingly put in our way to begin with. As a model, let's use the goal of managing our hunger. Whether it's conventional calorie restriction, or the more effective Smart Intermittent Fasting, we make hunger a bigger obstacle in our lives when we don't cover the basic physiological need of getting adequate sleep, for example. As we discussed in the last section, scientists at Stanford University found that insufficient sleep can *decrease* levels of the satiety hormone leptin and *increase* levels of the hunger hormone ghrelin. That combination is a surefire equation that equals a lot more struggle with our food choices.

○ After utilizing Smart Intermittent Fasting for many years, the only time that I ever feel hungry in the morning is when I didn't get a great night of sleep. Not only that, I noticed that something with some extra sweetness sounds mighty seductive. It's like Betty Crocker is trying to slide into my mental DMs. Fortunately, I've been at this long enough to tune into those subtle messages my body is sending me. When that irregular hunger taps me on my shoulder, the *Minority Report* screen pops up and I go through my mental checklist: "Why am I hungry, right now? That's weird... Did I sleep well? Am I experiencing a lot of stress? Am I in need of some comfort and Betty Crocker is trying to spoon with me?" Of course, I check in to ensure that I'm well-nourished and properly hydrated, but I know that hunger can be driven by many other factors outside of what we consume. Learn from my mistakes and the mistakes of millions of dieters in the past. Make sure that you cover the basics to eliminate unnecessary challenges for yourself. Get the rest and recovery your body needs, be mindful of managing stress, and block Betty Crocker from your contacts. The most beautiful thing is that eating smarter helps you to improve your sleep, reduce stress, and keep supportive content on your metabolic timeline.

S: Safeguard Your Results with Supportive Nutrition

The biggest mistake people make with intermittent fasting is not so obvious. Because we have a specific eating window, there is a natural tendency for many people to eat less food over the course of the day. Not because they have to, but because they feel strong and satisfied.

Eating less food is not the issue. But not getting in the essential nutrients your body needs when you *do* eat is the issue. As we discussed earlier in the book, simple nutrient deficiencies can halt your fat loss, depress your cognitive function, and even disrupt your sleep cycles. During your eating window, it's absolutely critical to ensure you're getting in the nutrients your body needs to perform at a high level.

For instance, in Section One we noted data published in the peer-reviewed journal *Environmental Health Perspectives* affirming that micronutrients (like vitamins, minerals, and carotenoids) actually regulate our gene expression in a myriad of ways. The study stated, "Many of the micronutrients and bioreactive chemicals in foods are directly involved in metabolic reactions that determine everything from hormonal balances and immune competence to detoxification processes and the utilization of macronutrients for fuel and growth." One of the biggest driving forces of our hunger is to seek out and ingest key macro- and micronutrients that control the function of every cell in our bodies. Deficiencies lead to overeating and excessive hunger. This is a major reason many diets fail (including cookie-cutter intermittent fasting programs) and what sets Smart Intermittent Fasting apart.

During your eating window, our mission is to deliver your cells the macro- and micronutrients they need in the form of delicious foods that support fat loss, cognitive function, and balanced energy. These are the foods and nutrients we've been highlighting throughout *Eat Smarter* and have put together in tasty recipes you have access to in this book.

In addition to that, you're going to be able to include some nourishment *during* your fasting window, too! There are actually some specific foods and beverages that enhance the benefits of intermittent fasting. Nutrition researcher and bestselling author Ori Hofmekler shared with me that there is a class of "stress-mimicking nutrients" that yield many of the same benefits as dieting and exercise. These *fasting-mimicking compounds* in food support many of the processes seen with intermittent fasting, like improved autophagy, enhanced mental performance, and increased fat loss.

Let's take a look at a few sources of these fast-mimicking nutrients that you can include during your fasting window:

Coffee

Coffee has a plethora of nutrients that provide its fasting-mimicking properties. On a basic level, coffee has a negligible amount of calories (at about 2 calories per cup), so sipping some doesn't technically break your fast to begin with. In addition to that, coffee helps support satiety during your fasting window by increasing the release of the satiety hormone adiponectin. In addition, a study published in *The American Journal of Clinical Nutrition* revealed that coffee can also stimulate the release of another satiety hormone, CCK. Produced primarily by cells in the gut, CCK is a prolific hormone that plays a role in many aspects of fat metabolism.

Now, where it gets really interesting is that one of the nutrients found in coffee, called *chlorogenic acid,* has been found to increase the breakdown of stored fat *while* increasing the protection of muscle tissue. According to data published in the journal *Biochemical Pharmacology,* coffee is able to accomplish this feat through the action of AMPK (AMP-activated protein kinase). As you might remember from Section Two, AMPK has several awesome influences on our health, including improved glucose transport to our brain cells, regulation of inflammation, and enhancing autophagy to clear out cellular waste.

Anything that helps to maintain your valuable muscle tissue is especially significant. Coffee (without all of the problematic additives like sugar) can support and mimic the benefits of intermittent fasting thanks to its effects on AMPK and supporting your valuable muscles. But please understand, quality matters *a lot* when selecting coffee to provide these benefits. I share my recommendations (and updates as they come along) in the Eat Smarter Bonus Resource Guide at eatsmarter book.com/bonus. And your coffee will be tastier and accentuate your intermittent fasting benefits if you add some MCT oil to it.

MCT Oil

We've already revealed how MCT oil (a concentrate of medium chain triglycerides) has many phenomenal benefits for your brain and metabolism. On a technical level, introducing a small amount of MCTs during your fasting window *does* provide your body with some calories. Yet, there are several ways that MCTs can actually mimic and extend your intermittent fasting results.

One of the most coveted benefits of intermittent fasting is an uptick in the production of the illustrious ketone bodies. Yes, these ketones can provide fuel for your neurons, and, yes, these ketones can be used to support countless metabolic processes in your body. But one of the most valuable attributes of ketones is that they are incredibly protective of your muscle tissue. A report highlighted in the journal *Nutrition & Metabolism* affirmed that ketones defend against muscle protein breakdown *and* upregulate the absorption of amino acids into the muscle cells. Pretty amazing!

It's well noted that a very low-carb/high-fat diet can increase levels of ketones and fasting can increase levels of ketones, but consuming MCTs can also boost your levels of ketones (even if you're not fasting or eating a high-fat diet). Consuming MCTs during your fasting window mimics and supports the benefits of fasting in this way. Plus, according to data cited in the *International Journal of Obesity and Related*

Metabolic Disorders, MCTs have been found to boost the oxidation of stored fat while increasing satiety at the same time. The study also noted that MCTs enabled study participants to retain more of their muscle mass during the weight-loss process. That's what Smart Intermittent Fasting is all about…hitting the four targets of increased fat oxidation, improved cognitive function, enhanced protection of muscle tissue, while supporting satiety at the same time.

When it comes to MCT oil, we have to be mindful to not go after any hodge-podge product just because it says MCT on it. Getting a random MCT oil product can be like when I asked my mom for a new pair of Pumas and she ended up getting me a pair of Panthers instead (true story). It's not the same thing. And your body—just like the kids at my school—will know the difference.

Make sure to get an MCT oil that is 100 percent coconut-derived and has a higher ratio of caprylic acid (C8 on the carbon spectrum). During your fasting window, this can be added to coffee, tea, or even taken straight up like a shot at the healthiest saloon in town. There are basic MCT oils and emulsified MCT oils that look and blend like a nondairy creamer. Definitely lots of options to experiment with, but the most important thing is to feel good and enjoy the process.

Green Tea

Making an appearance on yet another list, green tea's benefits are as versatile as the career of Jamie Foxx. The massive antioxidant content in green tea is documented in living color in the medical research. Compounds in green tea like EGCG can sing to fat cells and make them applaud by burning their contents. The brain-boosting benefits of L-theanine in green tea have taken a starring role recently and are seen on the big screen of major media. But the truly funny thing about green tea that really makes it stand up are its benefits involved in supporting energy and metabolism while intermittent fasting.

A study published in the journal *Clinical Nutrition* revealed that study participants utilizing green tea had significantly lower levels of the hunger hormone ghrelin and higher levels of the satiety hormone adiponectin than those consuming a placebo. Another way that green tea supports *Smart Intermittent Fasting* is by supporting the process of autophagy that's up-leveled during fasting. New data cited in the peer-reviewed journal *Nutrients* indicated that the polyphenols in green tea induce autophagy to support the removal of cellular waste and "thereby revitalizing the overall health of the (person) consuming it."

As noted earlier in *Eat Smarter,* two to four cups of green tea per day appears to be ideal. Look for organic green tea whenever possible and you'll find that your body gets nominated for several awards that bring you more success and longevity.

Pu-erh Tea

Pronounced *poo-AIR,* this long-renowned tea has got to be one of the weirdest named food products, along with shitto spiced pepper sauce, wet bottom pie, and Nips butter rum candy (all real things!). But, unlike the rest of these strangely named foodstuffs, this legendary tea packs some serious nutritional benefits you need to know about.

Pu-erh is a fermented tea with a long history of use within regions in and around China. Today, pu-erh is well-respected for its profound benefits on metabolism and overall health. According to a study published in the journal *Phytotherapy Research,* pu-erh is one of the rare nutrient sources that has a direct, significant influence on the enzyme that unlocks fat from your fat cells, hormone-sensitive lipase (HSL), that we talked about in Section One.

Pu-erh is an effective adjunct to intermittent fasting because of its ability to support fat loss while protecting muscle mass, as documented in a recent study featured in *Clinical Interventions in Aging.* And to fan the flames of pu-erh even further, it's also proven to enhance our body's capacity to scavenge free radicals and eliminate cellular waste products.

On a scale of tasty to pu-erh, pu-erh is at a level of pu-erh. It's not very delicious in my opinion, but some folks seem to love it (and especially love its benefits). You can find convenient single-serving packets of pu-erh or purchase pu-erh in traditional tea "cakes" that you can prepare using a preferred tea infuser.

Rooibos Tea

Boasting upward of 50 percent more antioxidants than even green tea, rooibos (pronounced *ROY-boss*) is steeped in some surprising benefits that are a great complement to Smart Intermittent Fasting.

Native to southern Africa, rooibos has been utilized for centuries as a health-giving drink. And, unlike some other teas that sometimes can be an acquired taste, rooibos tea has a lightly sweet flavor with subtle hints of vanilla. Now, where rooibos really stands out is in its impact on metabolism. This caffeine-free fermented tea has been found to improve insulin sensitivity and even block the creation of new fat cells, as detailed in a recent study published in *Phytomedicine*.

Rooibos is also protective of your muscle tissue. Scientists at the Tokyo University of Agriculture and Technology discovered that a compound in rooibos called *aspalathin* stimulates glucose uptake into muscle cells and positively influences glucose homeostasis in the body. Rooibos can be found in the tea section of many grocery stores as a loose tea or in ready-to-use teabags. It's a great tea to drink during your fasting window or any other time during your day!

Other teas and herbal beverages (without added sugar) can be utilized during your fasting window. I've recommended several, but other notable options include matcha, yerba mate, gynostemma, reishi, and white tea. Keep in mind, these are just small implements that can provide additional benefits and make the process more effective. But the supportive nutrition you consume during your eating window will ensure that you receive the incredible benefits of intermittent fasting, plus a whole lot more.

T: Track Your Goals (of How You Look, Feel, and Perform)

You may have heard the statement, "You can't manage what you can't measure." In many ways, this is a fact of life. Tracking your physical metrics is *essential* to establishing a neural connection between your brain and body to affirm that the actions you're taking to improve your health are working. We *need* this feedback to thrive.

Physical metrics are objective measurements (hard data that can be measured by you or a third party). The physical metrics for you to monitor include waistline measurement, body weight, body fat percentage, and/or photos. The most valuable metrics for you to track before beginning your program are your waist measurement and your day 1 photo. You are going to be truly blown away at what you're able to accomplish in the next 30 days, but you need to take a quick moment to get the data on where you're starting from to know how far you've gone. I have some additional tracking tips for your physical metrics in the Eat Smarter Bonus Resource Guide at eatsmarterbook .com/bonus if you'd like more assistance on it. But there's another type of measurement that's equally important for you to know about.

Subjective Measurements

In research, subjective measurements often play second fiddle to objective measurements, and I get that. Objective measurements deal with the hard facts, while subjective measurements deal with your opinions and how you feel. Now, even though subjective measurements are not as prized in conventional data, tell me one thing that's more important than how you feel? I'll wait...

The reality is, our feelings are one of the most valuable gifts in our lives. It's an internal guidance system that is always directing our thoughts, actions, and outcomes in the world. It is our subjective feelings that often determine our objective results. So, this matters. And it matters a lot.

No one can tell you how you feel. This is something that you, alone, have the ability to monitor. In our excessively busy, hyper-distracted world, self-monitoring and paying attention to how you're feeling can easily be put on the back burner. And important feedback from your mind and body can be overlooked or flat-out ignored, and I feel it's at the root of many of our challenges today.

Minor, but frequent stomach problems, low mood, and low energy are all subjective symptoms that something is off. When these subtle alarms go off and we ignore them because we're "busy," eventually the alarm fades into the background. It's still going off, but we come to accept it as normal. If we're constantly ignoring our body's feedback, those minor stomach problems can evolve into an autoimmune issue, that low mood can evolve into depression, and that low energy can evolve into chronic fatigue. So often we don't address the small fires and then get surprised when our whole system gets set ablaze.

Part of eating smarter is getting reconnected to your internal feedback and paying attention to how you feel. Food is a major driver of how we look, feel, and perform, as you've learned throughout the book. Here are some subjective metrics to check in with to help usher in the health and vitality that you truly want.

1. **Track your hunger and cravings.** If you are well-nourished, cravings will be small and infrequent, and hunger will be underwhelming and subtle. If you experience stronger cravings or hunger at any point, take a moment and pay attention to them! Ask, "What is this hunger trying to tell me?" If you check in with yourself, you may realize that the hunger is indicating that you didn't eat enough protein at your last meal, you didn't get a great night of sleep, you may need to do a better job of getting in more micronutrients, or your stress is running too high. Aggressive hunger is not a sign that you're deficient in cupcakes and need an immediate transfusion. It's usually an indication that something is a little off with your nutrition, and it takes a little self-analysis to see what it is.

2. **Track your sleep quality.** There are a ton of objective sleep tracking devices on the market, but nothing is more valuable than your subjective experience. We've covered the intimate ways that your sleep quality affects your food choices and how your food choices affect your sleep quality in Chapter Eight. This is a valuable point of data to track because your sleep quality influences every other area of your life.

    Simply check in with yourself each day. Take note of how you feel when you wake up in the morning. If you found that you're sleeping a little better than usual, what have you been doing differently? That's good feedback! If you find that you didn't sleep as well or are more tired during the day, take note of that, too. It can provide valuable data that you can use to improve things moving forward. How do you feel when you wake up in the morning? How are your energy levels throughout the day? And how sleepy are you at night and ready for a good night's sleep? These are all subjective cues to pay attention to and utilize each day.

3. **Track your digestion.** How's that poop situation going? Are you as regular as the postman? Or are you as irregular as people who eat pizza with a fork? If you're eating every day, you should be pooping every day. This is not even close to being complex. How many times you poop each day is unique and can be debated. But the important thing is that you eliminate waste each day. If your poops are lackluster or irregular, this can give you feedback that you're not drinking enough water, you're not eating enough of the right types of fiber, or you're excessively stressed (stress can trigger constipation or even diarrhea in some people).

    Tracking your digestion is part subjective and part objective. Yes, you can objectively monitor the frequency of your poops and the "quality" of your poops (I'm pretty sure that quality and poop are not paired together very often). But, subjectively, when you eat certain foods or meals, it's important to monitor how your digestive process feels. Does your digestion feel natural, healthy, and robust? Or is your digestion uncomfortable, sluggish, or even painful? Digestive discomfort is abnormal, but, again, we can ignore the subtle feedback and begin to accept it as business as usual. When you do your business, it should be regular and the digestive process should be pain-free. If this is not the case, adjusting things to support your unique microbiome and following the advice in this book can radically improve your digestive wellness.

4. **Track your energy throughout the day.** Your personal experience of energy is one of the most subjective things in the universe, but it is very real! Our levels of energy are a conglomeration of so many measurable and immeasurable factors

that it would be impossible to calculate. From our discussions on adenosine triphosphate (ATP), we know that it's the "energy currency" of our cells. But that doesn't tell the full tale of the energy we experience in our daily lives. There are components of mental and emotional energy that reside well outside of the spectrum of ATP, for example. The important thing is to simply tune in to our energy levels and use it as a guidance system to make decisions that support our best selves.

We do know that what we eat has a tremendous effect on our mental and emotional state, thanks to the research we covered in Section Two. That said, it's a good idea to check in with yourself occasionally and notice if you feel a sharp decline in cognition after you eat certain things, or if you find yourself being hangry, or if something makes you feel especially balanced or lively. And what about your physical energy related to things like libido and performance in the gym? These are all things that offer up valuable data to help meet our body's needs. Remember, there are several factors that influence our energy (like sleep quality and stress), but what we eat each day is a major driving force of the energy we express.

Goal Measurements

Another huge component of tracking and leveraging your brain's reward system is utilizing the power of premeditated goals. The latest data clearly indicates that the way you set up your goals has a profound impact on what you're able to accomplish.

Whether we realize it or not, goals control our lives. No matter if it's a goal to get to work on time, a goal to hit the gym, or a goal to cozy up on the couch and watch TV, our goals and intentions drive all of our behavior.

Each broader goal is broken down into smaller goals in our psyche. Take the goal of getting to work on time. This includes a goal of getting up at a certain time, the goal of taking a shower, the goal of getting dressed, the goal of having coffee, the goal of walking to the car, the goal of driving safely, the goal of clocking in, and dozens of other micro-goals. These are not just things we do, these are goals we've set, and our goals (conscious or not) elicit corresponding actions.

We all are *always* living by our goals. But most of us are using our massive goal achievement power to accomplish minor, uninspiring things. The very best way to not accomplish big goals is to not have any big goals. A recent report in *Harvard Business Review* revealed that people who simply set specific, clear goals for their lives have radically higher rates of success. So many experts talk about the importance of setting goals, but I don't think it lands for most of us because it just doesn't make any sense. "Set a goal for anything I want, and I'm going to get it? Yeah, right! Unless I slipped and fell into the movie *Aladdin,* and unless there's a big, blue genie who never skips chest-day coming to take my order, there's no way I can ask for anything I want and get it."

And therein lies one of the core problems when it comes to setting, and achieving, goals. There is a very distinct difference between a goal and a wish. A goal follows a very clear set of steps backed by science. A wish follows a very clear set of steps backed by leprechauns, Santa Claus, and the Tooth Fairy on weekends. And although the science of goal achievement is very real, if you're missing any of the steps, you might as well go hunting for rainbows because your chances of getting lucky are about the same. You can absolutely accomplish some extraordinary goals, but my job is to make sure you know how this stuff actually works once and for all.

First things first, if you have big goals that are not written down, and, instead, choose to have them rattling around in your head like loose change, you are making a costly mistake. A study conducted by psychologist Dr. Gail Matthews looked at the rate of goal achievement for people who write down their goals versus those who don't. The study incorporated a diverse grouping of people in terms of age, ethnicity, and occupation. Participants were randomly assigned to either write their goals down or to just think about what they wanted to achieve, but not write it down. After the four-week study period, it was found that the mere act of writing goals down boosted goal achievement by 33 percent!

What in tarnation? How can simply writing a goal down increase your likelihood of achieving it? Well, writing it out tends to encourage a higher level of clarity and specificity that's often lacked in mentally speculating a goal. Writing the goal down also provides the opportunity to physically see the goal in the external world and refer back to it often. Plus, the small action of writing a goal down is actually a very *courageous* action. To write down a goal often forces you to get face-to-face with the negative voice in your head that immediately chimes in with all of the reasons you *can't* achieve the goal. But when you choose to write it down you are saying, "My self-doubt can politely go and sit in the corner. This is what I want, and I'm taking a stand on it!"

Instead of dwelling on the reasons you can't, writing down your goals provides an easy opportunity to write down the accompanying micro-goals that will help make it a reality. Just like when you are unconsciously setting the goal to get to work each day, those micro-goals (like getting up at a certain time and choosing which clothes to wear) are the actual steps that enable you to get there. The study also included a group that wrote down their goals plus wrote in some accompanying action steps that would bring the goal to fruition. This group significantly outperformed participants who didn't have written goals, as well. If the goal was to lose 5 pounds in thirty days, for example, three supporting micro-goals would look something like this:

GOAL	Three Things I Need to Accomplish This Goal	I Accomplish This Goal By
Lose 5 pounds	*Walk for 30 minutes each day *Implement Smart Intermittent Fasting *Avoid foods with added sugars	Date [30 days from today]

Your micro-goals are unique to you and your lifestyle. You know the things that need to be upgraded based on your strengths and struggle points. Your micro-goals make things more doable and transform a wish into real world action to get what you want. A great example of someone being blown away by the power of writing down their goals during my 30-day program is Mandy C.

Mandy C.

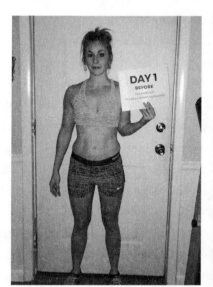 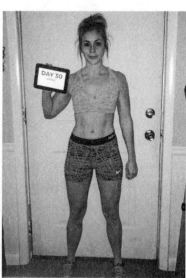

I'm still so proud of myself for the changes I can see. I went from a 27.5-inch waist to 25 inches, thighs 20 inches to 19 inches (my goal measurements), and I dropped ½ inch off my arms which I have NEVER accomplished before! I've dropped 8 pounds altogether. I feel amazing and I'm starting to like what I see when I look in the mirror.

In addition to my measurement goals, I've hit so many of my other goals too; I can't believe how much writing them down made a difference! I'm spending more time with my family, getting outside more, loving myself, and using positive thoughts to push myself instead of negativity. Thank you, Shawn, for helping me continue to change my life!!!

Writing down your major goals, plus writing the supporting micro-goals, is backed by science and the personal reports of countless people. But there's another piece that's often overlooked in goal achievement that you need to know about.

In the aforementioned study on having non-written goals versus writing your goals down, there was an increased rate of accomplishing the goal by 33 percent. But when test subjects had written goals *plus* social support and accountability, that success rate jumped up to an astounding 42 percent! In addition to writing down your goals, identifying who can help you get there might just be one of the most important steps in your success.

The best results in the goal-achievement study were seen by participants who sent their micro and major goals to a supportive friend and had weekly check-ins with them. Mandy also shared with me that she was conscientiously including positive, supportive people in her social circle. Supportive friends and/or family and groups like our online *Eat Smarter Community* are both excellent places to share goals and progress updates.

Another study conducted by the American Society of Training and Development on accountability found that you have a 65 percent chance of completing a goal if you commit to someone. The odds go even higher if you share a specific date that you'll achieve it by (this is important!). So, share with a supportive person in your life and/or with supportive folks in an online community. And one more *priceless* way that other people can help skyrocket your rate of success is by following in the footsteps of other folks who have already achieved what you want to achieve. This applies to every area of life! Ask yourself the question: *Who has achieved this before?* It could be a health and fitness goal, a financial goal, a relationship goal, or anything else. Consciously identify someone who's already done it and study them. Read their books, listen to their interviews, ask them questions if you have the opportunity. You don't have to know them personally, but find someone to model. Why on earth would you try to reinvent the wheel when you can simply realign it to fit your own life? If you want to be successful in something, make it a must to study successful people who've paved the way for you already. Success doesn't just leave clues, it leaves straight up GPS coordinates.

Julie G.

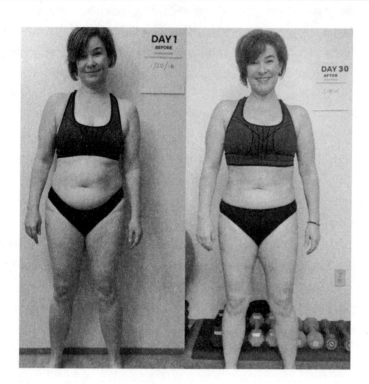

In my journal I wrote a quote from Shawn that I heard in one of The Model Health Show *podcasts, "Health is not something that you chase after. Health is something that you attract to you by the person you become." I am still one pound away from my 5-pound weight loss goal for the challenge, but I have gained a huge amount of strength and flexibility. I have lost 3 inches from my waist and 2 inches from my hips in the last 30 days. I have successfully established many exercise and nutrition habits. I've created the framework for health and fitness, and now the easy part is to just continue the work.*

I am thrilled with the physical results, but I am most proud of my extraordinary mental transformation and the active person I have become.

Even though people tend to have significantly better results by having a time stamp on their goals, some folks might wonder what to do if they don't hit their exact goal by the deadline. If you set a time constraint and don't achieve the exact goal, it's not the end of the world. But pressing toward your deadline and taking the necessary actions will land you far closer to the goal than if you just Mariah Carey lazy-danced your way through it and barely showed up for the performance. Julie G. is a great example. Her goal was a 5-pound weight loss, though she "only" lost four. But she also acknowledged that she gained a huge amount of strength and flexibility, lost 3 inches off her waist, 2 inches off her hips, and established new habits that will keep her healthy for many years to come. She didn't hit her exact goal, but managed to achieve a whole lot to be excited about. The most successful people simply recalibrate goals, set a new date, and keep moving forward until they hit them.

Tracking how you look, feel, and perform are essential parts of supporting your long-term transformation. It *starts* with establishing some clear goals. Just grab a journal and do this for yourself, or use the incredible goal achievement template I have for you at eatsmarterbook.com/bonus. Truly, the power is in your hands! You are the writer, producer, director, and leading actor in the story that is your life. You get to lead the charge as to where the story goes from here...and all you have to do is decide.

To help in that decision, and to give you even more insight into how to leverage the power of that amazing mind and body you have, I'm going to share with you five powerful tools to support long-lasting success.

THE FIVE INNER SECRETS TO S.M.A.R.T. EATING

The acronym *S.M.A.R.T.* outlines some of the most potent leverage points in our psyche that are often overlooked in diet-related programs. Even though we might see our results reflected in the outside world, all success is really an inside game. These five keys will not only enable you to achieve better results, they'll also enable you to have more confidence, happiness, and fulfillment along the way.

S: Solemnly Know Thy Dieting Self

Dieting is just as much America's pastime as baseball is. And, like baseball, dieting demonstrates a spectrum of personality types with different approaches to playing the game. Knowing your personality type when it comes to dieting will make you better equipped to avoid recurrent pitfalls and help leverage your strengths to achieve your higher potential.

The ancient aphorism to "know thyself" is an important tenet that can provide invaluable cautions and motivations to help you succeed on your journey. Here are four dieting personality types you can use to identify your tendencies. Once you can consciously identify how you approach things, you can start to play the game on *your* terms.

Type 1 — Swing for the Fences

This personality type comes out swinging and comes out swinging *hard* when they start a new diet or exercise program. Take it easy and start out slowly? Fuggetaboutit! This personality type is going in 1000 percent and it's their greatest strength and potential weakness.

Swinging for the fences can provide some epic results very fast. But, because this personality type tends to go so hard, they are more easily subjected to burnout and getting put out of the game prematurely. I recently had a conversation with someone who just seems to make things better wherever she goes. Sheri Salata is a phenomenal writer, producer, and storyteller. She served as the co-president of Harpo Studios and the Oprah Winfrey Network (OWN), as well as devoting about two decades to *The Oprah Winfrey Show* and serving as the show's executive producer. Her energy can light up a room, and her 1000-percent attitude served her mightily in helping to make her career endeavors an epic success. But, when it came to things like exercise, for example, going 1000 percent with an all-or-nothing-type vigor would come back to bite her on the benchwarmer.

She shared a story with me about dedicating herself to an intensive body makeover. She swung for the fences at the *hottest* workout facility, with the *hardest* classes, and the most *intense* agenda. And, though her swing could've knocked a few big hits, she ended up taking some big hits to her body. Nagging injuries forced her to miss several games and spend a lot more time on the sidelines. Before she knew it, the season was over. And her short (but passionate) stint on the field made her retire from the game altogether. Has this ever happened to you? Do you tend to swing for the fences? Have you ever gone 1000 percent into something causing you to get burned out and forced to retire before your time?

The great thing about folks who swing for the fences is that they are courageous enough to take big actions. But the potential drawback is that they tend to do too much, too soon. The very best power hitters who swing for the fences have also cultivated the trait of *patience*. More often than not, they don't just go swinging wildly and they don't go swinging unnecessarily outside of their zone. They get themselves prepared, they practice the fundamentals, and they strike fast when it's appropriate. They still swing hard, but their results are more consistent. They might not hit a home run every time, but their average rate of success is higher and, most important, they are far less prone to getting burned out.

Today, Sheri has put her passionate approach into smaller, consistent action, rather than going full tilt and trying to knock it out of the park on one swing. If you are someone who tends to swing for the fences, putting your 1000 percent attitude into consistent, yet smaller, actions will still land you some big home runs thanks to the power you carry. But, the difference is you'll be able to see a lot more long-term success.

In eating smarter, folks who tend to swing for the fences should consider a couple things:

- Focus on getting one to two meals a day that are dialed in instead of an entire overhaul of perfect meals every time.
- Pick one small action (keyword: small!) to consistently knock out of the park each day. It could be ensuring you drink the right amount of water, it could be making sure that you eat five servings of non-starchy vegetables, it could be getting in at least 3 grams of DHA omega-3s. Pick one thing to master for a few

weeks and lighten up a bit on trying to hammer everything else. (Lightening up can be a challenge for this personality type, but you can do it…especially if you know you are crushing that one targeted action!) Add more actions to point your mighty swing at over an extended time, rather than all at once, and you will end up with legendary success.

Type 2 — Easy Out

If you're not watching closely, this personality type can blow by faster than a 101 mph fastball. They're often here today, gone *today*. The easy-out personality type will easily jump into a new diet or exercise program, but they'll also easily jump out of one. If things don't go their way or don't feel comfortable, all you'll see is the back of their jersey as they trot on to the next thing.

The great thing about the easy-out personality is that they don't tend to hold onto their past mistakes and missteps. They cut ties and show up to the next thing with confidence as if nothing happened. As an aside in the game of baseball, it's great to have a short-term memory of past failures. In fact, the very best hitters fail about two out of three times. Having a .300 batting average (a little less than a one out of three success rate) virtually guarantees that you'll have an illustrious career, massive success, and end up in the hall of fame.

To have the presence to fail more than you succeed, and to still keep showing up ready to take your shot, is within the incredible potential of the easy-out personality type. The best version of the easy-out type knows that "failure" is only what's seen temporarily on the surface. Each failure contains a little bit of data that can help you with the next endeavor (if you should choose to use it!). The biggest curveball the easy-out type must learn to hit is deciding whether or not they're going to bring their optimistic approach back to the same game they originally committed to playing. To achieve great success they must learn not to move on to the next game, or team, or sport, so quickly.

If you tend to start things quickly and stop things just as fast, you can probably identify with the easy-out type. The easy-out type shows up to the new gym or new diet program all bright-eyed and bushy-tailed.

But, within a few days, weeks, or maybe even a few months, something throws them off their game, and they subconsciously say, "I'm out of here!" It could be an issue at work, an issue with the kids or significant other, an issue with finances, or a scheduling conflict. Something is bound to come up, but rather than making the adjustment, the easy-out type will leave the stadium and bring their easygoing attitude to the next thing once they get inspired again.

In eating smarter, folks who tend to be an easy out should consider these things:

- Plan on complications. Life is most definitely going to throw you some curveballs. But you, more than anyone, are equipped to hit them if you decide to. Use your lighthearted attitude toward the obstacles that come up, rather than being light-hearted about throwing in the towel and trying something else when the conditions are more ideal. If you keep starting and stopping things, you'll never be able to show your true talent. When things get challenging from time to time, just remember the mantra, "This is helping me to grow," and face the challenge with your special set of optimism to see the opportunity in it.

- If you fail, brush yourself off and get right back up for your next at-bat. If you are randomly busy with work all day and stressed, and don't follow your nutrition goals, so what! That doesn't mean your season has to be over. It simply means you had a tough at-bat or a tough game. Learn from your experience and use it to your opti-mistic advantage. For example, if you typically sit down for lunch at a healthful restaurant, but you know you've got a full day of meet-ings that won't allow for it, rather than picking up a McProblem with fries like you may have last time, this is your opportunity to bring your lunch from home this one day this week. The McProb-lem isn't the problem until it becomes the McStandard.

Type 3 — Caught Looking —

On the opposite end of the spectrum from those who swing for the fences you'll find those who tend to get caught looking. Rather than running up to the plate, guns-a-blazing, those who get caught looking can be exceedingly cautious. These are folks who often wait for everything to be perfect before they take their shot. They want to have every preparation box checked, every accessory on hand, and the perfect circumstances before they take their swing.

The admirable thing about those who tend to get caught looking is that they pay attention to details. They pride themselves on knowing what to do and they show up prepared—when they show up. The challenging aspect to this personality type, however, is that they can spend so much time getting prepared that they often delay (or even miss) their shot at big success. To use an exercise analogy, those who get caught looking decide, "I want to take my fitness to another level and do something fun and challenging. I'm going to start taking kickboxing classes!" Instead of simply googling "kickboxing classes in my area" and choosing a class to go try out that week, the caught-looking personality type will spend an excessive amount of time researching kickboxing classes and gyms (and maybe even tour a few without taking a class), go online and research the best kickboxing gloves, special kickboxing shoes, shin guards, mouthpieces, and kickboxing outfit. They finally show up to their first kickboxing class three weeks later looking like Jean-Claude Van Damme, while the rest of the class is in simple gym clothes and sneakers having fun and getting results already.

It's not that the caught-looking type doesn't kick butt like a universal soldier when they show up. It's that they tend to approach new things like it's a blood sport and overly prepare, instead of taking action and making the double impact they can make. With the excess time spent in preparation, it deeply increases the likelihood of being distracted, losing momentum, or simply giving up before you even get started.

Have you ever wanted to try a new diet or exercise program, but while trying to get everything perfect to get started, you got distracted and ended up not making it very far? There's a great line from Lemony Snicket: "If we wait until we're ready, we'll be waiting for the rest of our lives." If you can relate to the caught-looking personality type, it's important to know that waiting for things to be perfect has been the Achilles' heel of many people who have achieved far below their potential. You have such a gift in that you pay attention to details. Your eyes will catch the things that can make a major difference. But it doesn't matter much if you're not in the game!

Circumstances are rarely ever perfect, and there's practically never anything new that you can be fully prepared for. All real experience is on-the-field training. You've got to be in it to win it. So, instead of humdrumming over the details, your mission is to take action a little faster.

In eating smarter, folks who tend to get caught looking should consider these things:

- Use your attention to detail and desire for excellence *in the game* rather than on the sidelines. Rather than trying to be Van Damme Jr., you'd be better served to just select a class nearby, put on your shoes, and go! Your drive to perfect things and your attention to detail will help you know what you need to improve on in real time. You can get better, faster results than most if you're actually out there demonstrating that you have a lion-heart and not waiting around for everything to be perfect.

- Take an immediate action. Take on the mindset to "never leave the scene of a decision without taking an action." Yes, you can schedule meal-prep days. Yes, you can start a new grocery shopping list. But, today, I want you to select one new food or beverage you've learned about in *Eat Smarter,* buy it, and get it in your system. Again, on-the-field experience is more valuable than weeks and weeks of planning. Definitely use your planning skills to crush it long-term, but don't wait for momentum to pass you by because it can be a hard target to hit later.

Type 4 — All-Around Player

I was talking with Hall of Fame shortstop Ozzie Smith not too long ago and he shared with me how important it was to be an all-around player. Ozzie was well-known for his defensive prowess on the field. What he could do at the shortstop position seemed magical. And it rightfully earned him the nickname the *Wizard of Oz.* He told me that it wasn't just something that came naturally to him. He worked at it. Probably more than anyone else before his time. And the muscle memory he created in practice showed up magnificently in the game.

He was grateful for that. But what he wanted was to be known as an all-around player. He didn't want to be seen as great at one thing and then a liability at another. So, he worked to get stronger, lifting weights many years before it became *en vogue* for baseball players, he worked with a hitting coach, he worked on his base running, and he continued to work on his fielding and throwing. In addition to his 13 consecutive Gold Glove awards as the best defensive shortstop in baseball, Ozzie also racked up a Silver Slugger award as the best hitter at his position, 580 stolen bases, almost 2,500 total hits, and one of the most iconic home runs in baseball history. All-around player, indeed.

An all-around player personality type might not be great at any one thing, but they're pretty good at a lot of things. Or, in the case of someone like Ozzie, maybe they're excellent at one thing and then work to lift up the other dimensions of their game. All-around players, as a whole, can tend to do better at diet and exercise programs if they stay true to the fundamentals. They show up, they prepare, they demonstrate calculated confidence, and, most important, they take action. If you're an all-around player type, you're confident that you can jump in and make things happen. All you need is an opportunity. You can make just about any plan work, even a bad one. But with the right plan in your hands, you're tough to beat.

Practicing the fundamentals is important for *all* types, but that's especially true for all-around players. Because you're good at a lot of things, the all-around player can get caught up in what's working best right now. Maybe their five fundamental tools are 7 hours of high-quality sleep, 20 ounces of water to start the day, daily exercise, dinner with family five nights each week, and four to five servings of vegetables each day. But maybe they're seeing a lot of progress with their new exercise program and decide to extend it an additional 30 to 45 minutes. This, in turn, cuts into their sleep time. As a result, that fundamental tool starts bringing down the performance in the other areas. Their all-around confidence had them killing it in the gym at first, but then they saw a sharp decline in their results because they went with what was hot and not with what works long-term. Mike Dolce, multi-time UFC Trainer of the Year, comes to mind. He shared with me that he was absolutely dominating with his nutrition, hydration, and exercise, and the results showed, big time. But, it wasn't until he focused on getting adequate sleep that his results went from good to great. Mike is definitely an all-around player. When he put a little more attention on his fundamentals, he further cemented his outstanding performance.

In eating smarter, folks who tend to be all-around players should consider these points:

- Be cautious about overextending yourself in one area for too long. Yes, you can absolutely spend more time enjoying something new, fun, and exciting. Just remember not to venture too far past the foul line and end up falling into the dugout.
- Show up. When an all-around player shows up, their progress is virtually guaranteed. For long-term success, you just need to keep showing up. Now in his mid-sixties, I see Ozzie at the gym all of the time and he inspires me so much with his level of strength and well-being. He's demonstrating what's possible for us all, and that's what any all-around player has the opportunity to do!

Any personality type can work toward being another personality type. In reality, we all have a little of each within us. The most important thing is to identify your tendency so that you can utilize your strengths and no longer be surprised by your softer spots. In eating smarter, and in life, once one can "know thyself," the game gets a whole lot easier.

M: Mind Your Mind

Researchers at Yale University set out to uncover whether or not our beliefs about food could have an effect on our metabolism. To test the theory, they recruited test subjects and blended up a huge batch of milkshakes and poured them into cups. Now, before giving the milk-shakes to study participants, they slapped one of two labels on each cup. One label said it was a 140-calorie "sensible" shake while the other label said it was a 620-calorie "indulgent" shake. But, in reality, and unbeknownst to the participants, each milkshake was actually 380 calories.

The researchers monitored the blood levels of the hunger hormone ghrelin for each test subject to see how their beliefs about what they were drinking would affect their metabolism. As you'll recall, as ghrelin levels rise, it tends to increase our hunger and drive us to eat more. Once we eat, ghrelin levels decline, signaling the body that we've had enough and our biological systems for burning fuel can be ramped up. The response to our hunger and our metabolism depends on the nutrient-density of the food. In general, the more energy we consume, the more levels of ghrelin go down. After compiling all of the data, the study participants who believed they were drinking the more "indulgent" 620-calorie milkshake had their ghrelin levels drop as though they had consumed three times more calories than they actually had! Biologically, it would appear that their cells, hormones, and organ systems felt more satisfied with longer-lasting effects, simply because of what they believed.

These results shocked the researchers and have been eye-opening for the scientific community. This study uncovered a nutritional placebo effect that has far-reaching implications that can no longer be overlooked when it comes to diet and lifestyle choices. Our mind matters!

The lead researcher in the study, Dr. Alia Crum, said that placebos and our beliefs "create a whole host of neurobiological effects." Not only did believing that the milkshake was higher in calories and "indulgent" lead to a greater drop in ghrelin, believing that the milkshake was "sensible" and low in calories barely had an effect on ghrelin levels at all. In other words, if we believe that what we eat isn't very nutrient-dense (even if it is), ghrelin levels will stay higher and we won't be as satisfied. This has massive real-world implications for us. But, before we talk about some practical applications, we need to take a quick look at the placebo effect itself.

The placebo effect has been well-documented for many decades now. A *placebo* is essentially an inert substance or treatment that is designed to have no therapeutic value. This includes inert pills, inert injections, fake surgeries (where a patient is cut open and stitched back up without doing any actual therapeutic changes), and other procedures. Each and every type of medical placebo noted has been found to be effective in clinical trials. In fact, placebo treatments work so well that millions of dollars are lost each year in drug development and trials because the new drugs fail to significantly out-perform the placebos. According to research published by Harvard Medical School, placebos (fake drugs, surgeries, and other treatments) have proven to be effective in improving everything from migraines, to depression, to osteoarthritis, and more.

Blood pressure, infections, skin disorders, and even Parkinson's disease have all been documented to be improved by placebo treatments. In fact, a meta-analysis conducted by researchers at Rush University Medical Center in Chicago revealed that placebo-related improvements occur in *most* Parkinson's disease clinical trials. This is important. And it's about time that the public, at large, knows this information.

We also need to know that the placebo effect has an alter ego called the *nocebo effect* that is just as powerful. A placebo tends to be those things that invoke a positive, beneficial, or desirable expectation and response. While a *nocebo* is classified as a negative expectation given, resulting in a more negative effect than it otherwise would have been. This is when a physician or person of authority says, for example, a patient will experience negative side effects or unlikely improvements. A great demonstration of this was seen in another study conducted by Dr. Crum and her team where test subjects were given a histamine skin-prick test. The histamine causes an allergic reaction and a small rash to occur on the skin of the test subject where the prick took place. The size of the rash can be measured for changes over time. And here's where things get really interesting.

Six minutes after the skin prick test was administered, a physician applied a placebo skin cream instructing the various participants that

1) this is an antihistamine cream that will reduce the irritation and help make the rash go away, or 2) this is a histamine agonist that will increase the irritation and make your rash worse. Even though this was a totally inert cream with no therapeutic ingredients, the patients who were told that the cream would help make the rash go away had reductions in the size of their rash within 10 minutes. And the participants who were told that the cream would make the rash worse had their rash grow larger within those same 10 minutes! This, alone, affirms that the physiological responses to the treatment depended on the beliefs that the patient had about the cream. One set of patients received a placebo expectation from the physician that things would get better, and that's what happened. While the other set of patients received a nocebo injunction from the physician that things would get worse, and that's what they experienced.

The nocebo effect is so imminent that a study published in the peer-reviewed journal *Pharmacology Research & Perspectives* purports that the verbal and nonverbal communications of physicians can contain unintentional negative suggestions that may trigger a nocebo response. This raises the important mandate for physicians to be more intentional and conscientious with the words they choose and how they communicate with their patients. Dr. Crum's skin-prick study found that the more personable and competent the physician appeared to be to the patient, the stronger the effects of the placebo *and* nocebo.

But, more important, for our intents and purposes, it's essential to understand how powerful your mind is in driving the success of this program (or any other program) from here on out in your life. Your mind is your most valuable asset if you utilize it intelligently. This is another dimension of eating smarter that's often ignored in mainstream diet and exercise advice. For example, if you have a less-than-stellar track record on following through with your diet plans, you can be shooting yourself in the foot before you even get started. You can unknowingly place a nocebo effect on yourself based on your past experiences and not on your true capabilities or the quality of the program. If you've racked up enough L's, you can develop a state of learned helplessness that will lead you to approach a new diet with a subconscious belief like, "That sounds good and all, but nothing ever works for me long-term." It's like pumping the brakes on an already parked car. Feeling powerless to affect change invokes a nocebo effect that can literally change how your hormones and cells are operating. It's not that things can't work if you don't believe in them, it's that your belief in things can potentially make them work better or your lack of belief can slow down your progress.

On the surface we might say, "Yes! Here we go…I'm pumped to start this new program!" But, unconsciously, our programming can say, "Here we go again…I've made more attempts on diets than all the *Star Wars* movies they keep making. And with both, diets and *Star Wars,* I'm just confused now. Pass me that Cinnabon. It reminds me of Princess Leia's hairstyle."

We can nocebo ourselves to be less satisfied with our diet, more hungry, and more likely to self-sabotage. This, we know for certain. But, we can also Jedi-placebo ourselves if we choose to use our mind's true power. We can rave about how good a new diet makes us feel, how pleasurable it is, and how awesome our results are. Utilizing affirmative statements, we can literally placebo ourselves and change the way our body and brain responds to the changes we're undertaking. But if you think I'm just being a smart Wookiee, check out this recent study published in *Social Cognitive & Effective Neuroscience.*

In a collaborative effort by scientists at UCLA, the University of Pennsylvania, and the University of Michigan, they discovered that self-affirmation activates brain systems associated with self-confidence and reward and reinforces future behavior and beliefs. Essentially, the researchers discovered that self-affirmations can *literally* change your brain and the results you see in the real world. So, mind your mind. Practice changing the conversations in your head. View your healthy meals as delicious indulgences that you get to have. Speak to yourself in an affirmative, supportive manner. Speak highly of your results and progress, even if you haven't fully realized them in the outside world yet. It's not "fake it until you make it;" it's "be it until you see it." Placebo your mind because it is the ruler of your entire galaxy. And may the *Eat Smarter* force be with you.

A: Ask the Right Questions

You'd be hard-pressed to find a mental tool more practical for improving your results than improving the questions that you ask yourself. As we discussed in the preface of this book, there are specific regions of the human brain that are *controlled* by the questions you ask yourself. Questions trigger a mental reflex known as *instinctive elaboration.* When your brain is posed a question, it instantly kicks into gear to find an answer to it (whether you realize it consciously or not). Your brain *is driven* to find the answers to questions. And the quality of your questions will determine the quality of your results.

Being diagnosed with a so-called incurable bone and spine disease at just 20 years old did a real number on my psyche, as you would imagine. When I lost my health, I was also losing hope. And I would constantly ask myself questions like, "Why me?" "Why did this have to happen to me?" and "Why won't anybody help me?" Instinctive elaboration is a reflex. That means it's automatic. So, every time I asked these questions, my brain was scanning my internal and external environment to find answers to those questions. As a result, I felt more and more isolated as I continued to ask, "Why won't anybody help me?" I felt more and more like I was a bad or unworthy person as I continued to ask, "Why did this have to happen to me?" And I felt more and more like a victim as I continued to ask, "Why me?"

These questions were on repeat like that song we don't like that keeps playing on the radio until we eventually find ourselves singing along. My brain, accordingly, just kept feeding data back to me affirming *why me.* I felt like I deserved this terrible situation because I was different from the people around me, because I grew up most of my life in a troubled home, because I didn't have much confidence, because I wasn't living up to my potential. My brain was like, "You want to know why your life sucks? Well, I've got the answers for ya!"

These were the worst years of my life. But something seemingly miraculous happened the moment I asked a different question one night. I had just seen the latest in a series of physicians hoping that they would give me some good news... but it was the same bill of goods I'd already received: bedrest, back brace, drugs, potential surgery, and this is just something I'm going to have to live with. I shared with you the story of how I finally made the decision to get well while sitting on the side of my bed about to down my pain pills. But it was immediately after that decision that I asked myself a specific question for the first time in over two years. I asked, "What is it that *I* need to do to get better from this?"

It was as if a switch was flipped on in my mind and I started to think in terms of solutions rather than problems. I went to sleep with possible solutions and I woke up with possible solutions. And I had more empowering questions that drove me like, "Since they're telling me my spine is degenerating, what is my spine actually made of?" "What foods have the nutrients I need to regenerate these deficient tissues?" "Who really believes in me and believes that I can get better?" All of these questions drove my decisions on what I studied, what I ate, and who I chose to spend time with. Saying that questions are the answer is really an understatement. The questions that we ask are at the core of motivation in our lives. We have the science to prove how it entrains the brain, but the practical applications are intensely powerful.

For me, even when I was asking those seemingly disempowering questions, I was eventually able to find value in them. "Why won't anybody help me?" *Because you must learn to help yourself.* "Why did this have to happen to me?" *Because this was what you needed to be a better man. This is what you needed to unlock the dormant gifts and capacities that you didn't even know you had. This is what you needed to wake up.* "Why me?" *Because you are strong enough. Because you have the heart and courage to help other people with your experience. Because this is bigger than you.* These were the things I found in the questions I asked. Asking the right, empowering questions is the essential first step to transforming your results and cultivating a successful mindset. Asking the tough questions, with an optimistic view, is the step that helps us to find great gifts inside of our grief.

Here are some sample questions to practice asking yourself on a regular basis—especially when there's a challenge you're facing:

- What is this situation trying to teach me?
- What gift or talent do I have that can help create a solution?
- How can I make this awesome?
- How can I use this situation to help someone else?
- How good can this get?! (I love to ask this when things are going well.)
- Why do I have so much to be thankful for?
- How can I serve today? (I've been starting my day with this question for about a decade now and it's become a directive for how I live my life. It may be something small, it may be something big, but there's always an opportunity each day that we can make a positive difference.)

R: Reframe Your Challenges

Who do you feel is the GOAT? The greatest of all-time? LeBron? Jordan? Kobe? Someone else? At the end of the day, the debate will rage on, but one thing is for certain about all of them: They chose a path, fell many times along the way, got back up each time, and never gave up.

This recipe is true in sports, business, relationships, and anything else in life, including our diet. You don't give up because you had a tough day. Ten-year-old Kobe Bryant could've been rapping in Italian at the basketball court one day (ya know, Kobe things) when a much older, much more experienced player came onto the court and absolutely crushed young Kobe in a game of one-on-one. Young Kobe could've easily thought, nah, this basketball thing isn't for me. I'm just going to pick up Spanish and create a trilingual rap album and take over the music scene. Thankfully for Kobe (and our ears), he didn't quit when he had obstacles come up along the way. He *did* have more experienced players outperform him. He *did* have obstacles and injuries that tried to stand in his way. He *did* fail and fall down more than people will ever know. But he got up, brushed himself off, and got back in the game.

When you decide to take on a lifestyle change and improve your health and fitness, you will, without question, come up against obstacles along the way. As a matter of fact, you can bet on it! For whatever reason, most diet programs try to convince people that their plan will be the easiest thing in the world. All you have to do is just eat purple foods (a real diet), wear blue-tinted glasses while you eat to reduce your appetite (another real diet), or just eat jars of baby food (again, a real diet, plus having someone else feed you will get you extra crazy points). Conventional diets promote their ease of compliance, and if you just follow their simple advice, the path to your dreams is straight down easy street. Yet, the data shows that conventional diets fail *at least* 83 percent of the time. Even if the diet is backed by science and not by Barney the dinosaur's purple food menu, most diets fail. But, the failure often doesn't lie in the program or the efforts of the person, it resides in the omission of the fact that there's growth involved.

You can't bring the old you to the new results. And the challenges you face with any new diet and lifestyle change are some of the greatest gifts you can ever receive, although most people never open the gift. But this is about to change for you.

Eating smarter isn't just about the food that you eat, it's about the mindset you carry in relationship to food. Yes, our food choices can improve our metabolism, enhance our cognitive function, and increase our longevity. But, through our relationship with food, we can also become more resilient, more confident, and more resourceful. Our challenges in eating healthfully offer an opportunity to become better people and improve many other areas of our lives. We just have to learn to reframe our obstacles and use them to show what we're made of.

You will have easy days of making smart food decisions, and you will have some tough days. There will be days when you're relaxed and days when you're rushed. There will be days when you feel inspired and days when you feel demotivated. There will be days when things are going your way and days when it seems like life is giving you more than you can handle. You can call them good days and bad days, or good moments and bad moments, but it really depends on how you look at it.

Like young Kobe lacking experience, we all have this issue when we're taking on a new lifestyle change. We're new to it, so we should *expect* not to be perfect at it. If you have the perspective that you should have everything on point right out of the gate, you are leaving the gate open for quitting to follow you in. For many dieters, a couple of "bad" meals can mean that they're failing at the diet. They didn't perfectly execute the plan, so they might as well give up! This lack of experience can prevent you from getting the positive experience you need. And this calls for a reframing of your perspective.

First, we can look at the perspective of "bad" foods or "bad" meals. We create a big psychological booby trap when we give morality to foods and label them as inherently good or bad. We've already discussed earlier in the book how certain foods that are labeled "bad" can be lifesaving in the right context. True enough, it's absolutely clear that there are foods that have detrimental effects on human beings. But just because you eat something that's not considered healthy, doesn't mean that it's the end of the world. And if it *were* the end of the world, and there's no food around, a box of cream-filled croissants might just save our derrieres.

Have you ever considered what eating a "bad" food might mean to your beliefs about yourself? For many of us, bad things are linked together psychologically. Eating *bad* food is a *bad* behavior which could make you a *bad* person (at least in the context of dieting). When we give morality to food, never overlook the implications it could have on the morality we give ourselves. To move past mental pitfalls like these, we can choose to reframe how we see our food by changing how we label things. Instead of being so black and white and good and bad, we can see various foods on a spectrum from less ideal to more ideal. When you eat a meal that's less ideal, it doesn't make you a bad person or that you engaged in bad behavior. You can much more gracefully move to a more ideal choice next time instead of throwing yourself into a food prison for your crime and, of course, swallowing the key.

In our Kobe example, he did fail and fall down many times. But he got back up. Not because he was born with Mamba Mentality, but because he got better by persevering through each obstacle he faced. Say an obstacle like car problems, an unexpected dilemma with your family, or a stressful situation with work takes place and you are forced to miss a workout or pick up food that doesn't meet the quality of your program. We can easily see these situations as failures and getting knocked off our plan. But if we can reframe them, and see them as gifts dressed up in unattractive outfits, we can use them to strengthen our determination and take us even further.

If a random car problem or issue with your house takes place, it can throw off your whole day. I've seen people put their car in the shop and lose all of their drive. They can't make it to a few workouts, plus, time and financial constraints give them a permission slip to throw on the hazard lights and totally break down from their goals. If you're aware of your ability to reframe your perception of the situation, you'll not just overcome the obstacle, you'll be better equipped to handle similar mishaps in the future. Data cited in the journal *Behavior Modification* clearly demonstrates that reframing challenging experiences can lead us to better outcomes.

Instead of just being the victim of misfortune, you can take a moment and distance yourself from the situation. Instead of seeing this as a roadblock to your health goals, you can reframe it and see it as an opportunity. Hitting a U-turn and referencing back to our strategy of asking empowering questions, you can ask, "What's the gift in this situation?" or "What opportunity does this situation present for me?" You can reframe the situation to see that maybe this gives you the opportunity to take an Uber or cab to work tomorrow while you plan out your grocery list and meals for the week. You can see it as a chance to look up healthy food delivery options that you can now have on hand whenever you need them. You can see it as an opportunity to move past a history of making excuses (though they may be justified) that has stopped you from making the progress you want in the past. You can cultivate the attitude that everything is figureoutable and you can keep moving forward even when things don't go your way. As my oldest son always says when a tough obstacle comes up: "It's a minor setback for a major comeback."

You have the ability to *instantly* change your perspective on things and to start thinking in terms of solutions rather than problems. Don't get me wrong, it's not always easy to do when an apparently negative situation first presents itself. You are human! You are allowed to vent, to be upset, and to get caught up in your feelings. But, as soon as you can, bring yourself back to the awareness that there's an opportunity in the challenge somewhere. If you practice this over time, it will serve you in every area of your life. As the wise adage says, "We don't rise to the level of our expectations, we fall to the level of our training." To take another page out of the book of Mamba, practice daily, use the challenges as fuel to get better, and consistently work toward being the best version of yourself. Championships aren't won overnight. You're going to have some wins and losses. The most important thing is to learn from it all, stay in the game, and treat yourself with respect.

T: Treat Yourself with Respect

Respect is one of the most powerful words in the English language. It can be related to esteem, admiration, approval, appreciation, and even worship. But I like the association that respect has to *significance*. We all have an inherent human need to feel significant, to feel like we matter. However, today more than ever, we are turning to the external world to meet this need. In our hyper-connected society, we are no longer just seeking approval from the folks in our local neighborhood, tribe, or family circle, we are often seeking approval from virtual friends, acquaintances, and countless people who we will never even know. Keeping up with the Joneses has turned into *Keeping Up with the Kardashians* and our level of comparison is now pandemic.

What's more, the respect that we have for other people (even if we don't know them very well) typically towers over the respect that we have for ourselves (even though we've known ourselves our whole lives). How often do we see what other people are doing online and admire them while minimizing ourselves? Even if we have feelings of envy, jealousy, and "who do they think they are," it's still because we're giving them a power of significance that we often don't carry for ourselves.

Even in our day-to-day actions, the average person will treat other people with more respect than they'll extend to themselves. We'll speak kindly to other people, but speak to ourselves as if we don't matter. We'll respect other people's feelings, but will rarely respect our own. We'll respect other people's wishes, goals, and agendas, but will throw our own right out the window to avoid bothering anyone else. I can hear Aretha Franklin trying to get through to us right now... R-E-S-P-E-C-T.

Our tendency to compare, added to a deficiency of self-respect, is what many experts agree to be a melting pot for unhappiness and underachievement. Flipping the switch on this inner secret is a huge key to our long-term success. To do it is simple, but not necessarily easy. So, we'll tackle each component of that unhappiness melting pot so that you have the insights to break through it.

Theodore Roosevelt said, "Comparison is the thief of joy," and Teddy didn't even have social media. Today's level of comparison is so big it's at an *Ocean's Eleven* level of effectiveness. It's part of our primitive makeup to compare ourselves to others. It served us well in establishing where we fit in the structure of the tribe, in deciding who might be a threat and who's not, and in identifying who might throw the best cave party (every generation has their own P. Diddy). But seriously speaking, our brains are not yet wired to handle this level of comparison and to even discern what is real and what is not. Our minds are more vulnerable than we realize. Within a minute, you can swipe through your social feed and compare yourself and where you are to dozens of other people. At the surface, it's really just pixels on a handheld device controlling how you feel. At a deeper level, the images we see tell a story that, the vast majority of the time, just isn't true.

When we see the social media posts of both the people we know and of strangers, it's usually their life's highlight reel, and not their real reel. In talking with many of the people with millions upon millions of social media followers, many of them have shared with me that they struggle with problems in different areas of their lives. They struggle with health issues, financial issues, relationship issues, career issues, unhappiness, insecurities, and fears, just like most of us do. But, if all you see is their selfie from their trip to Dubai, you might just believe that their life is perfect, or at least better than yours, when it's often not even close to the truth.

And the thing about social media that we really need to get out into the open once and for all, is the mirage of it all. We can easily feel like the grass is greener on the other side where they are, but we don't even realize that sometimes it's fake grass! (There was a time that I didn't even know grass could be fake, then I went to Las Vegas and learned otherwise.) What we compare ourselves to today is often not even real. We see what others want us to see. And with filters, camera angles, special lighting, and a little editing, the final product can be drastically different from what the reality actually is. Sure, we all want to be seen in our best possible light, and there's nothing wrong with that. We just have to stand guard at the doors of our mind and remember that some stuff is trying to sneak in with a fake ID.

When you compare yourself, you negate yourself. In addition to reducing your haphazard comparison to others, I need you to truly work on understanding how valuable you really are. There is no more important work in the world to dedicate yourself to than this. Everything you think and everything you do is based on the beliefs that you carry about who you are. In the context of diet, we affirm our ideas we carry about ourselves through the food that we eat. In other words, we are driven to eat things that are congruent with who we believe ourselves to be. If you believe that you are a health-conscious eater who will go out of your way to eat organic, chances are you're not going to be at the Krispy Kreme every morning. If you believe that you don't digest dairy very well (which might well be true), chances are you're going to buy a dairy-free version of ice cream at the ice cream shop (or best of luck to the person who has to ride home in the car with you).

That's the thing: Our beliefs about ourselves can be based on factual experiences, or they can simply be made up based on the internal decisions we've made. There's no law that a health-conscious eater has to eat organic. But, if you decide that's a belief you'd like to take on, you can have it. You do have to give the belief "legs" to stand on. So, reading studies on the benefits of organic versus conventionally grown foods, learning about organic farming practices, and talking with farmers at your local farmers market are all ways to help affirm the belief you are taking in. In understanding the incredible value you carry, you have to affirm that belief, too. You can do this by proactively getting yourself around people who value and respect you, by journaling and writing out what you appreciate about yourself or one thing you respect about yourself each day, and by giving thanks to yourself for the things you've accomplished in your life—honoring where you are, where you've been, and where you'll be in the future. This comparison issue doesn't just stop with other people, it also involves comparing ourselves to ourselves. A before and after picture can be a massively valuable tool, but it can also be a hindrance if it's not viewed in the right way.

That before picture could be of a man who is a father, a son, a brother, and a friend. Someone who's always been there for everyone in his life. He's been a rock, someone you can count on, and if he had it to give, it's yours. He has a huge heart for others, but somewhere along the line he lost touch with his own health and well-being. He's realized that it's time for a change. He wants to be healthy so that he can continue to be there for the ones he loves. That before picture isn't someone to look down on—that's someone who deserves massive respect. He's a great human being with some of the best character you can ever ask for. And he's the one who made the decision to transform his health. Be thankful for that man. He's pretty freakin' awesome.

That before picture could be of a mother of some of the most amazing little kids in the world. They're her heart outside of her body. She never knew she could experience so much awe and joy by looking into someone's eyes. Her amazing body brought these little beings into the world and she deserves an endless amount of respect and admiration. Her skin is different, her metabolism doesn't work like it used to, and her "snap back" isn't what she's seen with others on social media. But, there's nothing wrong with her! She is beautiful, she is the greatest life-giving force on this planet, and she's also decided to take good care of herself now, too. Be thankful for that woman. She's everything and so much more.

Healthy self-comparison to honor the positive changes you're making is a good thing. But, looking at old pictures without respect, or wanting to "go back" to a time when your body was different, is not honoring what you've been through and who you are today. Today is where you start to move toward a brighter future. And doing that with a healthy sense of self-respect will make the process even better. You can't hate your body into submission and then expect to be happy *if* you get there. Long-lasting change is a collaborative effort that comes from growth, practice, self-respect, and the other inner insights we've been covering here in *Eat Smarter*. And, remember, there's also an *after* the after picture. The party doesn't stop because you hit a goal. You get to decide whether or not you keep moving forward each day. You've probably heard the statement that if you're not growing, you're dying. To continue to experience great health and to continue to move toward being the best version of yourself, you've got to be mindful to up-level that inner dialogue.

Our thoughts are powerful and they're also automatic. We have tens of thousands of thoughts each day, and the vast majority of them are the habitual thoughts we've been conditioned to think. These automatic thoughts stem from our beliefs about ourselves and the world around us. If you tend to carry more negative beliefs about yourself and the world, you will inherently produce more of what neuroscientist Dr. Daniel Amen calls *automatic negative thoughts* (or ANTs). He shared with me that he encourages people to exterminate those ANTs by doing three things:

1. Become aware of them—in the words of GI Joe, "Knowing is half the battle."
2. Challenge them—stand up to the ANTs and don't let them limit your life.
3. Replace them with a more positive affirmative thought (a PAT).

There is a metaphoric DJ booth in your mind that's spinning a pre-recorded playlist that you might not always like. You have the power to jump in the booth and play the music that *you* want. Being a good

DJ takes practice, but you'll make the entire party better for you and everyone else in your life.

One of the most powerful PATs that I implemented in my life many years ago was inspired by a quote that is attributed to Albert Einstein: "The most important decision we make is whether we believe we live in a friendly or hostile universe." When I was lost, when I was alone, when I was feeling like a victim, food was one of the major lifelines that helped me to truly take control of my life. But I eventually realized that food was just one piece of the diet I was feeding my mind. The mental food I was absorbing from the world around me was also giving me sustenance. And, most important, my beliefs about who I was and the world that I lived in were determining my thoughts and the actions I took, more than anything. I decided to take on the mantra that we live in a friendly universe, rather than a hostile one. It was not overnight, but I eventually became more comfortable in a world that I once felt disempowered in. And I became more committed to helping other people in this friendly world to experience the same things that I had. No matter how challenging things may seem on the surface, my wish for you is to take on the belief that things are not happening *to* you, they're happening *for* you. You are powerful beyond measure, and I hope that the tools and insights contained in this book serve you well on your journey moving forward.

Here's to your health and success,

Shawn Stevenson

Welcome to the Eat Smarter 30-Day Program!

This program enables you to personalize things to fit your unique goals and lifestyle. By utilizing the F.A.S.T. transformation tips that we covered on page 308, you can cater your eating windows to best fit *you*! Plus, I've got your back with sample eating/fasting schedules, a weekly meal plan, and delicious recipes.

You can follow the Smart Intermittent Fasting approach to take advantage of the incredible benefits you've discovered about intermittent fasting. Or follow a conventional breakfast, lunch, dinner approach (implementing smarter foods and nutrients). I just highly encourage you to have your meals within a 12-hour eating window to imbibe some of the benefits of Smart Intermittent Fasting whenever possible.

There is a delicious collection of recipes for you in the next section highlighting many of the amazing foods we've covered. But I've got even *more* recipes incorporating smarter foods and nutrients (as well as beautiful full color pictures of all the recipes!) for you in the Eat Smarter Bonus Resource Guide, so make sure to pop over there at eatsmarterbook.com/bonus and pick it up if you haven't done so already.

WHAT TO EAT DURING YOUR 30-DAY EAT SMARTER PROGRAM

We've covered a plethora of extraordinary foods and nutrients throughout this book. The following tables provide a compilation of Eat

Smarter–approved foods (including those that are highlighted in the book and many more). Your mission is to simply include a variety of these foods each day based on the servings and additional tips that follow.

Proteins

As we've discussed, this macronutrient is critical to fueling your brain, hormones, and overall metabolism. Just remember, your protein requirement is a unique part of your metabolic fingerprint. Review the protein calculating tips on page 100. Always keep in mind the subjective measurements (how you feel!) that we covered in Chapter Ten as well. If you're ever feeling unexpected hunger, not sleeping well, or not experiencing good levels of energy, dialing up your protein is usually the first place to go.

Beef, grass-fed	Lamb, grass-fed	Shellfish, wild-caught
Bison, grass-fed	Pork, pastured	Spirulina, Chlorella
Eggs, pastured	Poultry, pastured	(protein-dense algae)
Fish, wild-caught	Protein powder	Wild game
	(without artificial	
	ingredients)	

Note: Nuts, seeds, beans, dairy foods, and certain grains have a substantial ratio of protein. Although they are actually fat- or carbohydrate-dominant foods, as we've discussed, a variety of these foods can be added in to help you meet your protein requirements.

Fats

From cognitive function to the production of your sex hormones, we've learned how this macronutrient is a major key to performing at your best. Target at least four to five servings of healthy fats each day.

Almonds (and unsweetened almond butter)	Chia seeds	Pecans
Avocado	Coconut (meat, butter, and oil)	Peanuts (and unsweetened peanut butter)
Avocado oil	Dairy, grass-fed	Pine nuts
Barùkas	Eggs	Pistachios
Brazil nuts	Fatty fish	Pumpkin seeds
Butter, grass-fed	Flaxseeds	Salmon roe
Cacao nibs	Hazelnuts	Sesame seeds
Cashews	Macadamia nuts	Sunflower seeds
Caviar	MCT oil	Walnuts
Chestnuts	Olive oil	And others
	Olives	

Carbohydrates

Thanks to the clinical data we've delivered here in *Eat Smarter,* you are well aware that the category of carbohydrates is massively important to your health and fitness. The big reveal is that there are more styles of carbohydrates than Lady Gaga outfits. Putting a blanket (or a meat dress in the case of Lady Gaga) over the entire category of carbs and saying they're problematic is a huge mistake. Here is where you'll find a major source of the vital micronutrients that control everything from gene expression to energy production. To be clear, this category of macronutrients needs to be approached with intelligence.

The most underutilized carb-dominant foods are the non-starchy vegetables. Focus on green leafy vegetables like kale, collards, and spinach, as well as cruciferous vegetables like broccoli, bok choy, and cabbage. Target a minimum of five to seven servings a day from this camp. When you ensure that 50 to 60 percent of your plate is non-starchy vegetables, you can rest assured that you are crushing your nutritional performance.

Veggie-like fruits can be included in your non-starchy servings count too. As for the other carb-dominant foods, here are a couple rules of thumb. Hold your intake of sweet fruits to zero to two servings per day. Lower glycemic fruits like berries play nice at one to three servings per day, as do starchy vegetables. And if grains and beans work well with your system, then zero to one servings of grains and zero to two servings of beans per day is a smart place.

Non-starchy vegetables including:

Arugula	Cilantro	Spinach
Bok choy	Collard greens	Sprouts (like
Broccoli	Kale	broccoli sprouts,
Brussels sprouts	Mustard greens	clover, etc.)
Cabbage	Radicchio	Turnips
Cauliflower	Radishes	Watercress
Celery	Sea veggies (kelp,	And others
Chinese broccoli	dulse, nori, etc.)	

Starchy vegetables including:

Beets	Pumpkin	Winter squash
Parsnips	Sweet potatoes	And others
Potatoes	Turnips	

Veggie-like fruits including:

Cucumbers	Hot peppers	Zucchini
Bell peppers	Tomatoes	And others

Grains including:

Amaranth	Quinoa	Sprouted grains
Corn	Rice (brown,	And others
Oats	white, wild)	

Sweet fruits including:

Bananas	Oranges	Watermelon
Mangoes	Pineapple	And others

Lower glycemic fruits including:

Blackberries	Grapefruits	Raspberries
Blueberries	Lemons	And others
Cherries	Limes	

Beans and lentils including:

Black beans	Kidney beans	Pinto beans
Green lentils	Navy beans	And others

Beverages

What you drink has the potential to hit your cells faster than anything. Sipping on the right stuff can deliver some immediate and wide-ranging benefits as we've highlighted. Simply add one to four servings from any of these sources of liquid nutrition. Look for organic or wild-harvested whenever possible and feel free to mix-and-match to your heart's desire.

Black tea	Green juice (under 12 grams sugar)	Oolong tea
Bone broth		Rooibos tea
Chai	Gynostemma	White tea
Coffee	Herbal tea varieties	Yerba mate tea
Green tea	Matcha	And others
	Medicinal mushroom tea and coffee (like chaga, lion's mane, and others)	

Prebiotics and Probiotics

Hopefully our discussion on the microbiome–metabolism connection was enlightening and motivating. Hit ~two to three servings of prebiotic foods each day and ~four to five servings of probiotic foods and/or beverages each week. Here are some of the foods to look for in each category.

Prebiotics including:

Asparagus	Green banana	Onions
Cocoa/cacao	Jerusalem artichoke	Resistant starch
Garlic	Jicama	And others

Probiotics including:

Kefir (milk, coconut, or water-based)	Kombucha	Sauerkraut
	Miso	Yogurt, grass-fed, full-fat
Kimchi	Nondairy yogurt	
	Pickles	And others

Herbs and Spices

There is likely a fortune of nutritional assets in your spice cabinet right now. With the brain-boosting benefits of things like cinnamon and the metabolism-supportive effects of ginger, hopefully you're inspired to use them a lot more often now! Both fresh and dried versions of these spices can be utilized in generous amounts. They say that variety is the spice of life, but spice is also enlivened through variety! Be sure to add some herbs or spices to every meal you can.

Basil	Cinnamon	Ginger	Turmeric
Black pepper	Cloves	Mint	Salt
Cayenne	Cumin	Oregano	And others

SELECT YOUR FOUNDATIONAL EATING SCHEDULE

Standard Eat Smarter Format
(with 12-hour eating window)

Midnight	Sleeping and/or Fasting
4 a.m.	
8 a.m.	Eating
Noon	
4 p.m.	
8 p.m.	Sleeping and/or Fasting
Midnight	

Smart Intermittent Fasting Format I
(with 10-hour eating window)

Midnight	Sleeping and/or Fasting
4 a.m.	
10 a.m.	Eating
Noon	
4 p.m.	
8 p.m.	Sleeping and/or Fasting
Midnight	

Smart Intermittent Fasting Format II
(with 8-hour eating window)

Midnight	Sleeping and/or Fasting
4 a.m.	
10 a.m.	
Noon	Eating
4 p.m.	
8 p.m.	Sleeping and/or Fasting
Midnight	

Smart Intermittent Fasting Format + Fast Mimicking Nutrients
(with 8-hour eating window)

	Monday
Midnight	Sleeping and/or Fasting
4 a.m.	
6 a.m.	Tea/coffee fast: coffee, tea, MCT oil, and/or Superhero Coffee
Noon	Eating
4 p.m.	
8 p.m.	Sleeping and/or Fasting
Midnight	

Meal Plan Bonus Tips

- These eating/fasting schedules and recipes are designed to deliver you the remarkable benefits you've learned about in *Eat Smarter*. Simply have any of the recommended foods, meals, or beverages from this section within your chosen eating windows.

If you're feeling satisfied and energetic, you're always free to reduce the number of meals or snacks you have within your eating window. You can always choose to incrementally extend your fasting window, as well.

■ As a reminder, you can always slide these fasting windows around to fit your unique lifestyle. For example, if you tend to go to bed earlier due to your work schedule, you can opt to adjust Smart Intermittent Fasting Format I so fasting is from 6 p.m. to 8 a.m. Follow the format, but simply adjust the times to fit what works best for you!

■ Please note that the breakfast meal is always optional. You may opt to just have water, tea, and/or other recommended fast-mimicking nutrients (see page 316) until you want to break your fast later in the day. Keep in mind, the Superhero Coffee (page 389) provides fasting-mimicking nutrients that essentially extend your fast even later into the day when you're ready to have your first meal.

■ Breakfast doesn't have to be at a conventional time, nor does it have to be typical "breakfast foods." If the first meal you decide to break your fast with isn't the standard breakfast fare, you can simply call it a *first meal*. You might want to have one of our scrumptious burgers for your first meal, or a stir-fry, or maybe an omelet is calling your name. It doesn't matter what you call it, as long as you are fueling your body and brain with deep nutrition.

■ A great exercise program is an incredible complement to intermittent fasting. You can exercise any time you like. However, training during your fasting window can be especially effective at supporting fat loss. You can train in a fully fasted state in the morning (without anything except water, tea, and/or coffee). However, if you're not experienced with this, just be mindful of how your body feels and keep the intensity in check until your body is fully adapted. Alternatively, you can utilize fast-mimicking nutrients like MCT oil pre-workout, or even implement some BCAAs.

■ As we've talked about within the pages of this book, part of eating smarter is being fully aware that life will happen! Adhering to this sample meal plan perfectly is unlikely for most folks. So, plan for some days of ordering takeout or dining out, and simply choose program-equivalent meals. It's better to prepare and pro-actively take some days off to let someone else cook than to overstress yourself. This should be an experience that brings you more happiness and good health. Trying to be perfect all the time is unhealthy. Execute the plan, but give yourself permission to roll with the punches.

- Speaking of being prepared, having a day to complete a little meal prep is a great idea. My recommendation is to keep it short and simple. Maybe take a couple of hours on a weekend to pre-pare one or two different meals for lunch that week. I'm a huge fan of doubling and even tripling recipes to have extra for later. It's like meeting a meal you like and going on a second date.

- As you've learned, to really optimize the performance of your brain and metabolism, hydration is absolutely key. Be sure to drink at least 20 to 30 ounces of water within the first 30 min-utes of waking up. And ensure that you're staying hydrated dur-ing both your eating and fasting windows.

Standard Eat Smarter Format Example:

Any time between 8 and 10 a.m.:	Breakfast/first meal
Any time between noon and 2 p.m.:	Lunch
Any time between 3 and 5 p.m.:	Optional snack
Any time between 6 and 8 p.m.:	Dinner
8 p.m. to 8 a.m.:	Fasting window

Smart Intermittent Fasting Format I Example:

Any time between 6 and 10 a.m.:	Water only and/or fast-mimicking nutrients
Any time between 10 a.m. and 1 p.m.:	Breakfast/first meal
Any time between 1:30 and 4 p.m.:	Optional lunch/snack
Any time between 6 and 8 p.m.:	Dinner
8 p.m. to 10 a.m.:	Fasting window

EAT SMARTER SAMPLE MEAL PLAN

The next 30 days will provide you with some powerful nutrition for your mind and body. As always, it's encouraged to cater things for your lifestyle and unique goals. You can substitute any meal for one another from the recipe section, but the key is to ensure you're getting plenty of healthy fats, amino acids, and those priceless micronutrients. Utilize the following meal ideas (included in the Recipe Section!) for 15 days and then make a commitment to increase your fasting window (if you haven't done so already) and repeat to hit your target of 30 initial days of smarter eating.

Day 1

Breakfast: Southwest Chorizo Scramble + avocado OR Superhero Coffee/tea

Lunch/snack: Superfood Salad

Dinner: Honey Sriracha Salmon + steamed broccoli with grass-fed butter

Day 2

Breakfast: Triple-B Milkshake OR Superhero Coffee/tea

Lunch: Superfood Salad

Dinner: Bacon Bison Burger or Vegan Chipotle-Walnut Black Bean Burger + sweet potato fries and avocado

Day 3

Breakfast: Superhero Coffee/tea

Lunch: Leftover bison burger + side salad with Asante Sana Dressing (or dressing of choice)

Dinner: Slow-Cooker Chicken Curry + rice of choice and steamed broccoli with grass-fed butter

Day 4

Breakfast: Southwest Chorizo Scramble + avocado + sauerkraut OR Superhero Coffee/tea

Lunch: Leftover chicken curry + rice and vegetable of choice

Dinner: Beef and Broccoli Stir-Fry

Day 5

Breakfast: Triple-B Milkshake OR Superhero Coffee/tea

Lunch: Summery Chicken Salad

Dinner: Leftover beef and broccoli

Day 6

Breakfast: Post-Workout Easy Protein Pancakes + eggs OR Superhero Coffee/tea

Lunch: Summery Chicken Salad

Dinner: Honey Sriracha Salmon + steamed broccoli with grass-fed butter

Day 7

Breakfast: Smarter Green Smoothie OR Superhero Coffee/tea

Lunch: Leftover salmon + side salad

Dinner: Bacon-Ranch Buffalo-Chicken Casserole + rice or quinoa and veggie of choice

Day 8

Breakfast: Superhero Coffee/tea

Lunch: Leftover Buffalo chicken casserole + rice or quinoa

Dinner: Lean fish of choice + Garlic Brussels Sprouts and 1 Sweet Potato Muffin

Day 9

Breakfast: Classic Breakfast with Sautéed Curry Cabbage OR Superhero Coffee/tea

Lunch: Leftover fish + side salad

Dinner: Three-Ways Taco Bowl

Day 10

Breakfast: Triple-B Milkshake OR Superhero Coffee/tea

Lunch: Superfood Salad

Dinner: Bacon Bison Burger OR Vegan Chipotle-Walnut Black Bean Burger + Superfood Guacamole with organic tortilla chips or veggies for dipping

Day 11

Breakfast: Bacon Quiche + avocado OR Superhero Coffee/tea

Lunch: Large salad + protein of choice with Asante Sana Dressing

Dinner: Beef and Broccoli Stir-Fry + kimchi

Day 12

Breakfast: Smarter Green Smoothie OR Superhero Coffee/tea

Lunch: Leftover quiche + avocado

Dinner: Slow-Cooker Chicken Curry + rice of choice and steamed broccoli with grass-fed butter

Day 13

Breakfast: Superhero Coffee/tea

Lunch: Leftover chicken curry + rice of choice and steamed veggies

Dinner: Lean fish of choice + Garlic Brussels Sprouts + Chocolate Avocado Pudding

Day 14

Breakfast: Classic Breakfast with kimchi OR Superhero Coffee/tea

Lunch: Leftover fish + Garlic Brussels Sprouts

Dinner: Superfood Salad

Day 15

Breakfast: Smarter Green Smoothie OR Superhero Coffee/tea

Lunch: Summery Chicken Salad

Dinner: Three-Ways Taco Bowl

Increase your fasting window and repeat the meal plan for days 16 to 30!

SMART BREAKFAST MEALS (FOR ANYTIME!)

Southwest Chorizo Scramble

Breakfast scrambles are a great way to add a diversity of macro- and micro-nutrients to your diet. This Southwest-style scramble is super tasty, easy to make, and loaded with hormone-healthy ingredients.

MAKES 2 SERVINGS

Nutrition Facts

Calories 597

Protein 27g

Fat 50g

Carbs 12g

¼ pound ground chorizo

4 large organic eggs, whisked

¼ teaspoon turmeric

Sea salt and black pepper, to taste

¼ cup salsa of your choice

1 large avocado, peeled, pitted, and sliced

Heat a sauté pan over medium heat. Add the chorizo and cook until lightly browned. Add the eggs and turmeric and season lightly with salt and pepper. Cook, scrambling the eggs with a spatula, until the eggs are cooked to your preference. Transfer the eggs to plates and top with salsa and avocado slices. *Enjoy.*

Variations: *You can add anything you want to this scramble (that's what makes scrambles so awesome!). Mushrooms, sweet peppers, hot peppers, spinach, onions—the list goes on and on.*

Bacon Quiche

Contributed by Chalene Johnson

There isn't a word in the English language to describe how amazing Chalene Johnson is. She's a world record–breaking fitness instructor, business and marketing mogul, and bestselling author, and she will happily break off in a dance battle at any moment. She really hit the target with this quiche recipe. My family loves it so much that we'll often make it when we have guests for brunch. We took the liberty of adding spinach to the recipe, and if you wanted to make a vegetarian version of it, just nix the bacon and add an additional veggie with a little body to it, like black olives, bell peppers, and/ or cooked asparagus.

MAKES 6 SERVINGS

Nutrition Facts

Calories 473

Protein 17g

Fat 40g

Carbs 10g

CRUST

Coconut oil cooking spray

2 cups almond flour

1 large organic egg

2 tablespoons coconut oil, melted

1 teaspoon fine sea salt

FILLING

6 strips 100 percent grass-fed, pastured, nitrate-free bacon

1½ cups (12 ounces) canned full-fat coconut milk or heavy cream (see Tip)

4 large organic eggs

¾ cup chopped fresh spinach

¼ teaspoon fine sea salt

¼ teaspoon freshly ground black pepper

Preheat the oven to 350°F. Coat a 9-inch round pie plate with cooking spray.

To make the crust: Whisk together the almond flour, egg, coconut oil, and salt in a bowl until fully combined. Press the dough into the pie plate, pushing it evenly up the sides. Bake for 13 to 15 minutes, until the crust is lightly golden.

To make the filling: Fry the bacon strips in a large skillet over medium
  heat until crisp on both sides. Transfer to paper towels. When cool
  enough to handle, blot well, then crumble.
Whisk together the coconut milk, eggs, spinach, salt, and pepper in a
  bowl. Stir in three-fourths of the crumbled bacon. Pour the egg
  mixture into the baked crust and top with the remaining bacon.
Bake for 35 to 38 minutes, until the top is lightly golden, and the eggs
  are set. Cover the edges with aluminum foil if the crust begins to
  brown too much. Cool for 15 minutes before slicing.

*Tip: Use the heavy cream instead of coconut milk for a more neutral
  flavor.*

Classic Breakfast + Veggies

Adding some fresh veggies to the typical egg and protein breakfast can take
it from average to exceptional! Whether it's an omelet, a scramble, or simply
eggs over easy, this classic breakfast is revamped with a healthy dose of
micronutrients and fiber.

MAKES 1 SERVING

Nutrition Facts

Calories 413	Fat 28g
Protein 31g	Carbs 14g

2 large organic eggs	Sea salt and black pepper to
2 teaspoons coconut oil	taste
1 serving protein (bacon,	2 cups spinach
sausage, ham, etc.)	Garlic powder to taste

Cook your eggs any way you like (scrambled, over easy, etc.) using 1
  teaspoon of the coconut oil and salt and pepper to taste. Cook your
  protein of choice as well.
Heat the remaining 1 teaspoon coconut oil in a large skillet over
  medium heat. Add the spinach and garlic powder, plus salt and
  pepper to taste. Cook, tossing, until slightly wilted (do not overcook).
Arrange the eggs, spinach, and protein on a plate, grab a fork, and enjoy!

Variations: I recommend having fermented veggies like sauerkraut or kimchi as the veggie, or along with the spinach with this breakfast. Alternatively, instead of the spinach, you can have Sautéed Curry Cabbage, zucchini, or countless other veggies to add some color and nutrition to the classic breakfast.

Post-Workout Easy Protein Pancakes

These lower-carb easy-to-make protein-packed hotcakes are a great brunch item or treat after a workout.

MAKES 2 SERVINGS

Nutrition Facts

Calories 366	Fat 22g
Protein 34g	Carbs 26g

¾ cup pancake mix of choice (if you want to reduce the carbs, I recommend a lower carb mix that utilizes almond flour and/or coconut flour)

¾ cup unsweetened almond milk

2 scoops protein powder (vanilla whey works great here)

1 large organic egg

1 tablespoon extra virgin olive oil

Coconut oil cooking spray

Combine the pancake mix, almond milk, protein powder, egg, and olive oil in a bowl and mix thoroughly until there are no lumps. The batter should be pourable, but not too thin: Add more almond milk or mix as needed.

Heat a large skillet over medium-low heat. Off heat, spray with a bit of cooking spray. Return to the heat and spoon four portions of batter into the pan to make pancakes about 5 inches in diameter. Cook until bubbles start to form on top. Flip and cook until golden brown.

Variations: Top the pancakes with peanut butter, almond butter, grass-fed butter, chocolate coconut butter, berry preserves, or even a little maple syrup if you're feeling frisky.

Superfood Salad

What happens when your salad gets endowed with superpowers? You get this! The powerful combination of whole foods, superfoods, and flavor just might ignite your superhuman abilities too.

MAKES 1 SERVING

Nutrition Facts

Calories 370

Protein 42g

Fat 33g

Carbs 19g

Spinach, romaine, and/or other mixed salad greens

2 tablespoons Simple and Smart Vinaigrette (page 385)

1 teaspoon spirulina powder

½ ripe avocado, peeled, pitted, and chopped

1 grilled chicken breast (4 to 6 ounces), chopped or diced

1 small tomato, diced; or handful cherry tomatoes, halved

1 tablespoon shelled hemp seeds

2 tablespoons sprouted pumpkin seeds or sunflower seeds (optional, if you want a little extra crunch)

1 teaspoon honey

In a large salad bowl, combine the greens with the vinaigrette and spirulina and toss to coat. Add the avocado, chicken, tomato, hemp seeds, and pumpkin seeds (if using) and give it a light toss.

Drizzle the honey over top, grab a fork, and enjoy!

Variations: This salad is packed with plant-based proteins. You can easily omit the chicken and make it a satisfying vegan version. Also, I like to spice things up from time to time (literally), so I'll add a few dashes of cayenne pepper!

Garlic Brussels Sprouts

If there was a mascot for disliked vegetables, it would be the Brussels sprout. I get it. The problem is, this underappreciated vegetable is usually prepared in ways that don't complement its personality. I never thought I would like Brussels sprouts until my wife made these. Now, we absolutely love them and look forward to their performance on nutritional gamedays.

MAKES 4 SERVINGS

Nutrition Facts

Calories 116

Protein 4g

Fat 8g

Carbs 11g

1 pound Brussels sprouts, trimmed and halved (or quartered if large)

½ small lemon, sliced

2 tablespoons extra virgin olive oil

1 tablespoon garlic powder; or 2 cloves garlic, sliced

½ tablespoon dried thyme

½ teaspoon sea salt

¼ teaspoon black pepper

1 tablespoon finely shredded Parmesan cheese (optional)

Position two racks in the upper and lower third of oven and preheat oven to 425°F.

Toss together the Brussels sprouts, lemon slices, olive oil, garlic, thyme, salt, and pepper in a large bowl. Divide between two large rimmed baking sheets and spread in an even layer.

Roast on the two racks without stirring for 10 minutes. Switch the pans top to bottom and continue roasting, without stirring, until the sprouts are lightly browned and tender, 8 to 10 minutes longer. Transfer to a serving dish and sprinkle with the Parmesan.

Summery Chicken Salad

*Contributed by Natalie Jill

Natalie Jill is a fitness icon who graced her first magazine covers at around the age of 40! She's a true inspiration for me and has such a big heart. This colorful, nutrient-packed salad she created features tastes of summer that are delightful year-round.

MAKES 6 SERVINGS

Nutrition Facts

Calories 395
Protein 24g

Fat 29g
Carbs 10g

1 bunch asparagus
3 tablespoons extra virgin olive oil
Himalayan salt and freshly ground pepper to taste
2 tablespoons fresh lemon juice
1 tablespoon honey
2 tablespoons balsamic vinegar

2 cups fresh trimmed spinach leaves
2 cups fresh spring lettuce mix
2 cups fresh strawberries, sliced
2 cups shredded cooked chicken
2 tablespoons toasted walnuts, chopped

Preheat the oven to 350°F.

Prepare the asparagus by breaking off the tough ends, then cut into 2-inch pieces.

On a baking sheet, place the asparagus in a single layer and drizzle 1 tablespoon of the olive oil over top. Toss to coat and season with salt and pepper to taste. Roast for 15 to 20 minutes, until the asparagus is just crisp. Let cool.

In a small bowl, whisk together the remaining 2 tablespoons olive oil, the lemon juice, agave nectar, and vinegar. Season the dressing with salt and pepper to taste.

In a large salad bowl, combine the spinach and spring mix lettuce and toss. Add the asparagus, strawberries, and chicken, then the dressing. Toss again to thoroughly coat the vegetables with dressing. Divide among four bowls and sprinkle each serving with toasted nuts.

Variations: *If strawberries are out of season, raspberries or another berry will be equally delicious.*

Sautéed Curry Cabbage

This tasty cabbage recipe is easy to make and packed with metabolism-boosting nutrients.

MAKES 2 SERVINGS

Nutrition Facts

Calories 124	Fat 7g
Protein 3g	Carbs 15g

1 tablespoon coconut oil	1 teaspoon ground mustard
⅓ cup chopped onion	(optional, but good!)
½ head organic green	Couple pinches sea salt
cabbage, shredded	¼ cup water
1 tablespoon curry powder	

Heat the coconut oil in a large skillet over medium heat. Add the onion and cook until it begins to soften. Add the cabbage and cook for a few minutes, tossing lightly to be sure all sides are cooked. Add the curry powder, mustard (if using), and salt, mix thoroughly, then mix in the water.

Cover, reduce the heat to medium-low, and simmer, stirring occasionally, for 10 to 15 minutes, until soft (but not mushy!).

Variations: *For an added boost of micronutrients, you can sprinkle on some kelp granules or dulse flakes.*

Bacon-Ranch Buffalo-Chicken Casserole

Contributed by George Bryant

OK, since we're in a safe-space of sharing, I've got a confession to make. I'm in love with this recipe! Gifted from my friend, *New York Times*–bestselling author George Bryant, we've served this casserole up to just about all of our friends who stop by, and they leave hooked on it as well. I can't tell you how many friends have sent pictures of them making the casserole after we give them the recipe.

MAKES 4 SERVINGS

Nutrition Facts

Calories 394

Protein 43g

Fat 17g

Carbs 13g

1 large head cauliflower, cut into florets

3 tablespoons avocado oil

Sea salt and black pepper to taste

½ cup Frank's RedHot hot sauce

½ cup Primal Kitchen ranch dressing, plus more for drizzling

½ cup canned coconut milk

½ cup sliced green onions, plus more for garnish

4 slices bacon, cooked crispy and crumbled

3 cups shredded cooked chicken (see Note)

Preheat the oven to 450°F.

In a mixing bowl, toss the cauliflower florets with the avocado oil and season liberally with salt and pepper. Spread evenly on a parchment-lined baking sheet and bake until tender and lightly brown, 20 to 25 minutes. Reduce the oven temperature to 350°F.

In that same mixing bowl, stir together the hot sauce, ranch, coconut milk, green onions, and bacon until combined. Add the roasted cauliflower and shredded chicken and mix until incorporated.

Transfer the mixture to a large baking dish and bake for 20 minutes.

Let cool for 10 minutes, then drizzle with ranch and garnish with more green onions. Enjoy with a side of rice or quinoa and a side salad.

Note: For the chicken, we sometimes bake our own chicken thighs: Sprinkle 6 thighs with paprika, onion powder, garlic powder, black pepper, and salt to taste and bake at 425°F for 30 minutes. Other times we use a store-bought rotisserie chicken

Beef and Broccoli Stir-Fry

*Contributed by Drew Manning

Drew is a *New York Times*–bestselling author who rose to fame for his Fit-2Fat2Fit experiment where he, as a fit personal trainer, intentionally gained 70 pounds over the course of six months and then spent the following six months working to lose all the weight he gained. He revealed that this was a transformative experience of empathy and self-discovery, and his story has positively impacted the lives of countless people. Here Drew is sharing with you an upgraded take on the classic beef and broccoli stir-fry. Stir-frying is an excellent way to mix-and-match health-giving ingredients. For an additional infusion of nutrients, you can toss in some cashews for brain support in addition to topping your plate with sea veggies.

MAKES 1 SERVING

Nutrition Facts

Calories 635	Fat 50g
Protein 35g	Carbs 10g

2 tablespoons avocado oil

½ teaspoon sesame oil

Sea salt and black pepper

Ground ginger, to taste

½ cup broccoli florets

1 cup cauliflower rice

2 teaspoons coconut aminos

1 teaspoon minced garlic

1 teaspoon dulse flakes
 (optional)

6 ounces flat iron steak, sliced

Heat 1 tablespoon of the avocado oil and the sesame oil in a large skillet over medium heat. Add the steak and season with salt, pepper, and ginger to taste. Stir-fry until the steak reaches desired doneness, then remove from the pan and set aside.

Add the broccoli and remaining 1 tablespoon avocado oil to the pan and stir-fry until the broccoli is bright green and just tender, 4 to 5 minutes. Add the cauliflower rice, coconut aminos, garlic, and more ginger to taste. Stir-fry until the cauliflower just begins to color, about 3 minutes. Add the beef and thoroughly combine for 1 minute, then remove from the heat.

Plate the stir-fry and sprinkle on the dulse flakes or other sea veggies if desired. Enjoy immediately.

Vegan Chipotle-Walnut Black Bean Burgers

*Contributed by Kevin Curry

Kevin Curry is on a mission to make cooking fun and flavorful while making us fitter as a result. His epic brand, *Fit Men Cook*, has been inspiring millions of men and women all over the world the past few years. Here Kevin is sharing his plant-based burger that's high on the flavor chart while avoiding the highly processed stuff usually found in veggie burgers. You can top your burger with avocado for some additional brain-healthy fats.

MAKES 4 HEARTY PATTIES

Nutrition Facts

Calories 252

Fat 12g

Protein 11g

Carbs 29g

Olive oil spray

1 tablespoon minced garlic

½ cup minced onion (red or white)

½ cup raw walnuts

1¾ cups cooled drained pressure-cooked black beans

3 chipotle peppers with 1 tablespoon adobo sauce

⅓ cup chopped cilantro

2 tablespoons milled flaxseed mixed with 3 tablespoons water

½ cup raw oats

Sea salt and black pepper, to taste

Heat a nonstick skillet over medium heat. Off heat, spray with olive oil. Return to the heat and add the garlic and onion. Cook for 3 to 5 minutes, until the onion is golden brown and somewhat translucent, being careful not to burn the garlic.

Transfer the onions to a food processor and add the walnuts. Blend for about 1 minute, until minced. Add only half of the beans then the chipotle peppers and cilantro and blend for 1 to 2 minutes, until well combined.

In a large bowl, lightly mash the remaining black beans together with a fork (this creates some texture for the burger). Add the bean mixture from the processor, the flaxseed and water (flax egg) and oats. Mix everything together well, then season to taste with sea salt and pepper. Cover the bowl with plastic wrap and place in the fridge for 20 minutes.

Batter too wet? Add tablespoons of raw oats. Batter too "crumbly"? Add another flax egg (1 tablespoon milled flaxseed set in 1½ tablespoons water).

Form four equal patties with the batter and place on a baking sheet. Chill in the freezer for 20 minutes to set. (This will help the patties retain their form when cooking.)

Heat a large nonstick skillet over medium heat. Once hot, generously spray with olive oil. Add the patties and cook for 6 to 8 minutes on each side, until the outside edges turn brown and slightly crispy.

Enjoy the patties with a fresh salad or as a delicious post-workout hamburger.

Bacon Bison Burger

*Contributed by Drew Manning

Here's another one of Drew's most popular recipes. He takes his "animal style," wrapped in lettuce. If you're minding your unique carb tipping point, you might opt for a sourdough or gluten-free bun from time to time. Try this burger with some Superfood Guacamole (page 383) or chipotle mayo and thank me later. ;-)

MAKES 1 SERVING

Nutrition Facts

Calories 692	Fat 52g
Protein 49g	Carbs 6g

6 ounces ground bison	1 tablespoon Primal Kitchen
Garlic powder, to taste	chipotle lime mayo
Cumin, to taste	2 slices bacon, cooked
Paprika, to taste	1 large organic egg, fried
1 large leaf romaine	(optional)

Preheat a grill to medium heat and preheat the oven to 375°F.
Combine the bison and seasonings in a large bowl. Use your hands to form into a patty. Grill the burger, turning once, to desired doneness.
Place the burger on the lettuce leaf and top with chipotle mayo, bacon, and a fried egg (if you like). Enjoy with veggies of choice (and sweet potato fries if you're in the mood!).

Honey Sriracha Salmon

Salmon is the bona fide king of omega-3–rich fatty fish. And the great thing is, you don't have to swim upstream to find mouthwatering recipes to enjoy it. This spicy salmon recipe is one of my favorites.

MAKES 2 SERVING

Nutrition Facts

Calories 523   Fat 43g

Protein 40g   Carbs 5g

2 tablespoons avocado oil   ¼ teaspoon sea salt

2 tablespoons sriracha hot   2 skin-on salmon fillets, 6 to 8
  sauce, plus more for serving   ounces each

1 teaspoon raw honey   ½ small lemon

Combine 1 tablespoon of the avocado oil, the sriracha, honey, and salt in a small bowl.

Place the salmon in shallow bowl, add the hot sauce mixture, and turn to coat the fish. Let marinate for at least 20 minutes at room temperature.

Heat the remaining 1 tablespoon avocado oil in a medium skillet over medium. When hot, add the salmon fillets, skin side up, and cook until browned on the bottom. Flip to the skin side to cook for a couple additional minutes, or to desired doneness (I recommend medium). Add a small squeeze of fresh lemon to each.

Plate the salmon and top with a tiny amount of sriracha. Serve with desired veggies and enjoy.

Slow-Cooker Chicken Curry

My biggest food crush would have to be curry. I love the spice combinations, nutrient-dense ingredients, and saucy finished products. This slow-cooker chicken curry is a regular at our house.

MAKES 6 SERVINGS

Nutrition Facts

Calories 240

Protein 21g

Fat 10g

Carbs 14g

¾ cup coconut milk

1 (6-ounce) can tomato paste

3 garlic cloves, minced

4 to 6 tablespoons curry powder (I like lots so always use more than this)

Sea salt and black pepper, to taste

3 bell peppers (I use yellow and red), cored and chopped into 1-inch squares

1 yellow onion, thinly sliced

2 pounds boneless chicken (a mixture of skinless thighs and breasts), cut into 1- to 2-inch pieces

½ cup chicken broth

Grab your slow cooker, add the coconut milk, tomato paste, garlic, curry powder, salt, and pepper, and whisk together.

Add the peppers and onion, then the chicken. Pour the broth over chicken and mix everything together to completely cover the chicken in the curry mixture.

Cover and cook at low for 6 to 8 hours or high for 4 to 5 hours.

Serve with rice or quinoa and vegetables.

Three-Ways Taco Bowl

This is three ways because you can make the bowl using traditional proteins like chicken or beef, take it to the sea by utilizing white fish, or make it plant-based with spicy walnut taco "meat."

MAKES 1 SERVING

Nutrition Facts

Calories 670

Protein 39g

Fat 33g

Carbs 14g

½ cup cooked rice (optional — you can omit the rice or use cauliflower rice to go lower carb)

½ cup shredded grilled chicken or other protein of choice including beef, pork, white fish, or walnut "meat" (see Note)

Grilled fajita veggies

Shredded lettuce

2 tablespoons pico de gallo (or salsa of choice)

2 tablespoons Superfood Guacamole (page 383)

Spoon the rice into a bowl, then add the protein, veggies, and lettuce and top with pico de gallo and guacamole.

Note: For spicy walnut taco meat, soak 1½ cups walnuts in water for at least 1 hour and drain. In a food processor, Combine the walnuts with 1 tablespoon chili powder, 1 tablespoon ground cumin, ¼ cup stemmed cilantro, 1 small diced tomato, and 2 tablespoons coconut aminos and pulse until you achieve a ground meat texture.

Variations: Feel free to add black beans (ideally pressure cooked), sour cream, shredded cheese, and/or crumbled organic tortilla chips (if you'd like to add a little crunch).

Superfood Guacamole

There isn't another guac recipe that comes close to the simplicity and nutrient density of this Superfood Guacamole. It is one of my go-to snacks and toppings, and the secret ingredients in the recipe takes the green to another level!

MAKES 4 SERVINGS

Nutrition Facts

Calories 317	Fat 30g
Protein 3g	Carbs 15g

3 avocados, pitted and peeled
⅓ cup favorite salsa (we use the organic medium-heat salsa from Whole Foods)
1 teaspoon spirulina powder

¼ teaspoon cayenne pepper
2 teaspoons fresh squeezed lemon juice
½ teaspoon sea salt

In a bowl, mash up the avocados with a fork until smooth. Add the salsa, spirulina, cayenne pepper, lemon juice, and salt. Mix well and serve fresh, or chill in the refrigerator before serving.

Asante Sana Dressing

I used to think that salad dressing only came in a bottle. Then one day my beautiful mother-in-law made this dressing for me, and I was hooked! Being from Kenya, she taught me that *asante sana* means "thank you" in Swahili. I'm thankful for this recipe and thankful for her, too.

MAKES ABOUT 2 CUPS (4 TO 6 SERVINGS)

Nutrition Facts

Calories 117

Fat 10g

Protein 0.9g

Carbs 8g

¼ cup extra virgin olive oil

2 garlic cloves, peeled

2 tablespoons minced red onion

2 dates, pitted and soaked

1 tablespoon minced fresh ginger

1 cup raw almond butter

1 tablespoon raw honey

1 tablespoon noma shoyu or coconut aminos

Juice of 1 small/medium lemon

¼ teaspoon cayenne pepper

Combine all ingredients and ¼ cup water in a high-speed blender. Blend on high until smooth, adding more water as needed to reach your desired consistency. (We like it pretty thick, but still pourable!) The dressing will keep for up to 4 days in the refrigerator.

Variations: If you like it spicier, you can add some fresh jalapeño, or simply up the amount of cayenne.

Simple and Smart Vinaigrette

This quick and easy salad dressing features brain- and gut-friendly ingredients. Plus, its versatile flavor tastes great with just about any salad veggies you can imagine!

MAKES ABOUT 1½ CUPS (8 SERVINGS)

Nutrition Facts

Calories 121	Fat 13g
Protein 0.1g	Carbs 2g

½ cup extra virgin olive oil
½ cup apple cider vinegar
¼ cup coconut aminos

¼ cup fresh-squeezed lemon juice
2 garlic cloves, minced

Simply pour all ingredients into a bottle and shake it up before using. The dressing will keep 4 to 5 days in the refrigerator.

Sweet Potato Muffins

*Contributed by Michael Morelli

Sweet potato pie meets muffin, meets upgraded ingredients! Michael Morelli is one of the most popular fitness experts in the world right now. One of his biggest insights is the power of the sweet potato and all of the wonderful things you can do with this nutrient-dense food. My family absolutely loves his muffins. I highly recommend adding raisins or organic chocolate chips to the batter!

MAKES 12 MUFFINS

Nutrition Facts

Calories 114

Protein 2g

Fat 3g

Carbs 20g

- 1 cup mashed cooked sweet potato
- 1 apple, cored and shredded
- ½ cup maple syrup
- 2 large organic eggs
- 2 tablespoons butter, melted
- 1 teaspoon vanilla extract
- 1 cup flour (low carb and/or gluten-free if desired)
- 1½ teaspoons baking soda
- 1 teaspoon ground cinnamon
- ¼ teaspoon ground nutmeg
- ½ teaspoon sea salt

Preheat the oven to 375°F. Line the cups of a 12-cup muffin pan with liners.

In a large bowl, combine the sweet potato, apple, maple syrup, eggs, melted butter, and vanilla. In a separate bowl, combine the flour, baking soda, cinnamon, nutmeg, and salt. Fold the dry ingredients into the wet ingredients.

Spoon the batter into the lined cups, filling each two-thirds full. Bake for 15 minutes or until desired doneness.

Cashew Butter Planets

These little treats are out of this world. When you're orbiting your kitchen in search of a frozen treat, you'll find that Cashew Butter Planets will make your taste buds lift off while providing an array of micronutrients.

MAKES 10 PLANETS (5 SERVINGS)

Nutrition Facts

Calories 378

Protein 12g

Fat 30g

Carbs 21g

1 ripe banana, diced

2 cups cashew butter

2 tablespoons soaked flaxseeds (see Note)

2 tablespoons hulled hemp seeds

2 tablespoons pourable raw honey

¼ teaspoon sea salt

Combine all ingredients together in a large bowl and mix together. Grab enough of the mixture to make a golf ball–sized sphere and roll between your hands (it doesn't have to be a perfect ball at all!). Place in a freezer-safe container lined with parchment paper. Repeat to make about 10 balls, making sure that you don't place them too close together. (If your container isn't that big, place parchment paper on top of the first layer of cashew planets then add a second layer.)

Put a tight-fitting lid on the container and place in the freezer for at least 4 hours to become something special.

Take a Cashew Butter Planet out of the freezer for you or a loved one as needed and enjoy!

Variations: You can add lots of different things to this mixture, just like ice cream. Good options would be cacao nibs, coconut butter, and/or bee pollen.

Note: To soak flaxseeds, place a small amount (¼ cup is good) of whole flaxseeds in a bowl or cup. Add enough water to cover them, mix a bit, then let soak for at least an hour. This will create a nice flax "gel" that helps to make a nice consistency for the Cashew Butter Planets.

Chocolate Avocado Pudding

Contributed by Natalie Jill

If you're like me, you'll be surprised by how much chocolate and avocado can make beautiful music together. Healthy fats, micronutrients, and prebiotics hit nutritious notes, while your palate will want to hit the dance floor from the incredible flavors. Natalie Jill's Chocolate Avocado Pudding is a classic treat with an upgraded beat. Feel free to add fruit or other toppings of your choice.

MAKES 4 SERVINGS

Nutrition Facts

Calories 205	Fat 10g
Protein 3g	Carbs 31g

1 ripe avocado, pitted and peeled
1 cup unsweetened almond milk
¼ cup natural non-alkalized cacao powder or cocoa powder
6 pitted dates
½ teaspoon pure vanilla extract

Puree all ingredients in a high-powered blender on high until smooth and creamy, scraping down the sides if necessary.
Spoon into four bowls, chill before serving, or store in a covered container for up to 2 days.

Superhero Coffee

About ten years ago I came across a video from my friend Daniel Vitalis where he was making an "elixir," combining ingredients that blew my mind. He was using teas and herbs I was familiar with, like reishi and pau d'arco, but he said your tea can become a "meal" by adding high-quality fats to it. It should have been obvious, since folks have been adding milk and cream to tea and coffee for centuries, but it opened my eyes to adding things like grass-fed butter, coconut oil, coconut butter, and nut milks like cashew or almond milk. I typically don't just go for standard coffee, either. I love a coffee that is infused with other potent brain- and metabolism-boosting ingredients like medicinal mushrooms. As you've discovered in *Eat Smarter,* the quality of your coffee matters a lot! I list my favorite sources of coffees and teas for you in the Eat Smarter Bonus Resources Guide at eatsmarterbook .com/bonus.

MAKES 1 SERVING

Nutrition Facts

Calories 160	Fat 18g
Protein 0	Carbs 0

- 1 cup hot fresh brewed organic coffee of choice (ideally infused with medicinal mushrooms like chaga and lion's mane)
- 1 tablespoon MCT oil (emulsified if possible)
- 1 tablespoon grass-fed butter or ghee
- 5 to 10 drops flavored stevia (chocolate or English toffee are good choices), optional

Combine all ingredients in a coffee mug and mix with a hand mixer, or combine in a blender and blend for 5 to 10 seconds.

Variations

* Instead of coffee you can use a tea in this recipe. Yerba mate, black tea, and rooibos are all great options.

*If you want a boost of peptide support for your skin, bones, and joints, try adding a serving of collagen peptides.

*I regularly add cinnamon to my drinks for its brain-healthy attributes. Plus, it's pretty tasty!

*You can also add things like nut milk, cayenne, and/or cacao powder for additional benefits.

Triple-B Milkshake

The brain-boosting blueberry shake is one of my favorite things to have post-workout. It helps fuel my mind *and* my recovery so that I can bring my very best to the day.

MAKES 1 SERVING

Nutrition Facts

Calories 460

Protein 28g

Fat 20g

Carbs 40g

½ cup frozen blueberries

½ medium banana

1 scoop vanilla protein (at least 20g protein)

1 tablespoon soaked chia seeds

2 tablespoons full-fat yogurt

1 tablespoon emulsified MCT oil (I like vanilla or strawberry here)

¾ cup unsweetened almond milk

Handful of ice

Combine all ingredients in a blender and blend. Pour into a cup and enjoy!

Smarter Green Smoothie

Green smoothies are an excellent way to help you achieve your green veggie goals. This is my go-to recipe. It tastes great and is stacked with nutrition.

MAKES 1 SERVING

Nutrition Facts

Calories 374	Fat 15g
Protein 27g	Carbs 38g

½ medium banana
1 big handful spinach
½ cup frozen blueberries
1 scoop chocolate or vanilla protein (at least 20g protein)

1 tablespoon unsweetened peanut butter (salt added)
¾ cup unsweetened almond milk
Handful of ice

Combine all the ingredients in a blender and blend. Pour into a cup and enjoy!

Variations: There are so many cool variations for this recipe. I highly recommend adding one serving of a superfood "greens blend" for a major upgrade in micronutrients (my favorites are in the bonus resource guide at eatsmarterbook.com/bonus). I'd also recommend varying the leafy greens. Try kale, collard, or romaine lettuce (another one of my favorites). If you'd like to switch up your healthy fat, you could go for almond or walnut butter instead of peanut butter, or even use full-fat coconut milk in place of the almond milk. Again, lots of combinations to try!

Acknowledgments

A book like this requires the guiding hands and hearts of many people. I'd like to thank my family, first and foremost, for providing me with continued inspiration and a healthy space to create. I couldn't make this kind of impact without you!

I'd like to thank the incredible team at Little, Brown for helping to bring *Eat Smarter* to life. And my agents Scott Hoffman and Steve Troha, thank you for your dedication, wisdom, and support during this process. It's an adventure every time, and it's great having you in my corner!

What's more, a book like this doesn't just come from the time and energy that goes into writing it. It comes from the countless years of experiences in education (researching, experimenting, teaching, learning, etc.), but also the countless years building relationships (mentorships, friendships, fans, supporters, etc.). Thank you to the listeners and readers of my shows and books. Thank you for inspiring me to continuously grow, explore, and create. And to my incredible friends, mentors, and colleagues, thank you for inspiring me to always think bigger! We are all a patchwork quilt of our friends, families, and experiences. I'm so grateful for the warmth you've given me and the long-lasting difference you've made.

One-Click References

The transformational data in *Eat Smarter* is based on cutting-edge evidence from hundreds of peer-reviewed studies. If you'd like to access any of the studies from the book, you'll have easy, one-click access to them at eatsmarterbook.com/references.

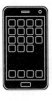 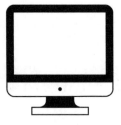

Index

Note: Page numbers followed by R indicate recipes

About the Author

Shawn Stevenson is a bestselling author and creator of *The Model Health Show*, frequently featured as the #1 health podcast in the U.S. with millions of listener downloads each year. A graduate of the University of Missouri–St. Louis, Shawn studied business, biology, and nutritional science, and went on to be the founder of Advanced Integrative Health Alliance, a company that provides wellness services for individuals and organizations worldwide. Shawn has been featured in *Entrepreneur* magazine, *Forbes, Muscle & Fitness,* ABC News, ESPN, and many other major media outlets. He is also a frequent keynote speaker for numerous organizations, universities, and conferences.